Sheila Young.

OXFORD MEDICAL PUBLICATIONS

CUNNINGHAM'S
MANUAL OF
PRACTICAL
ANATOMY

CUNNINGHAM'S MANUAL OF PRACTICAL ANATOMY

THIRTEENTH EDITION

REVISED BY

G. J. ROMANES
B.A., Ph.D., M.B., Ch.B., F.R.C.S.Ed., F.R.S.E.
Professor of Anatomy in the University of Edinburgh

VOLUME I

UPPER AND LOWER LIMBS

LONDON
OXFORD UNIVERSITY PRESS
NEW YORK   BOMBAY

Oxford University Press, Ely House, London W. 1

GLASGOW NEW YORK TORONTO MELBOURNE WELLINGTON
CAPE TOWN SALISBURY IBADAN NAIROBI LUSAKA ADDIS ABABA
BOMBAY CALCUTTA MADRAS KARACHI LAHORE DACCA
KUALA LUMPUR SINGAPORE HONG KONG TOKYO

Dissector's Guide, 1879
Manual of Practical Anatomy, 1889
Present Series
First Edition, 1893
Thirteenth Edition, 1966
Reprinted (with corrections) 1967 and 1969

Printed in Great Britain by R. & R. Clark, Ltd., Edinburgh

CONTENTS

PREFACE
TO THE THIRTEENTH EDITION

THE preparation of the 13th Edition of the Manual comes at a time when marked changes in the medical curriculum are being discussed throughout the world, and most courses in gross anatomy are being shortened to allow the inclusion of the great new developments in anatomy and in the allied sciences. In these circumstances the obvious solution might seem to be a drastic reduction in the content of the Manual; yet there is neither a consensus on the best method of giving a grounding in the structure of the human body which is sufficient to allow an intelligent approach to the examination of a patient, nor are the needs of the newly qualified doctor the same in every country, but vary greatly in relation to the degree of development of the medical services. In view of these varying requirements, and the different approaches to their solution which teaching departments are likely to follow, it is felt best to retain the greater part of the information which has been available in earlier editions, and to allow the individual schools to select and stress those elements which they feel are important, and to arrange the order of dissection to suit their particular requirements, as indeed they have always done.

One effect of shortening the course is to make it more difficult for the student to extend the scope of his reading, and it was felt necessary to make good some of the deficiencies in previous editions, which, by use and wont, have been filled by the larger textbooks, and which are yet essential to an understanding of gross anatomy. To this end there are included illustrations of bones with the major features labelled, a greater number of explanations of the functional significance of the structures, and the briefest references to development and microscopic anatomy which should be sufficient to give the student an entrée to further study in strictly limited fields.

One of the perennial problems for the student is the great number of unaccustomed names which he has to learn, and which form the basis of communication in medicine. In this edition of the Manual, the terms have been kept to the minimum by strict use of the New International Nomenclature without the corresponding older terms. It is appreciated that this may set a problem for teachers who are used to other terminologies, and that it will be some time yet before the new nomenclature is absorbed into clinical practice, but the new students, who will be the principal users of this book, are likely to benefit by the lack of duplication and confusion.

The greater part of the text has been rewritten with, it is hoped, an increase in clarity of those sections which have previously given difficulty, and, wherever possible, with the removal of those details which add little to the student's understanding of the arrangement of the various regions.

The illustrations have all been redrawn, and the number of descriptive captions reduced to a minimum so as to make the purpose of the illustration clearer and reduce the confusion of multiple leader lines where these are not strictly necessary. In addition to the new illustrations depicting bones, a considerable number of drawings have been added with the object of clarifying the dissections, and to illustrate the function of various structures. To the latter group belong the illustrations of bones in different positions during movement; many of these are prepared from radiographs which, though admirably suited to this kind of demonstration, are often difficult for the junior student to interpret without assistance. A number of radiographic illustrations have been omitted partly for this reason and because the great majority of departments have available a wide range of normal radiographs which are demonstrated and explained to the student in a manner which is difficult to achieve within the compass of this Manual.

The Editor is grateful to a number of the Staff of this Department for suggestions and help; and especially to Dr. H. S. Barrett for her careful correction of typescript and proofs, and a number of valuable suggestions.

It is a pleasure also to acknowledge the important contribution made by the artists, Mrs. C. Clarke and Mr. R. N. Lane, whose expert help in preparing illustrations of excellent quality has been invaluable.

Edinburgh
September, 1965   G. J. ROMANES

GENERAL INTRODUCTION

For descriptive purposes the HUMAN BODY is divided into Head, Neck, Trunk and Limbs. The trunk is subdivided into the Chest or Thorax and the Belly or Abdomen; the abdomen is further subdivided into the Abdomen Proper and the Pelvis; and the lower end of the trunk, where the pelvis comes to the surface between the buttocks and between the thighs, is called the Perineum.

Dissecting the body region by region, the student of Anatomy acquires first-hand knowledge of the situation and relations of the various structures that compose it— Regional or Topographical Anatomy. Before he begins, he should have an elementary knowledge of the kinds of structures he will encounter, and for accurate description he requires an anatomical vocabulary which must include terms that define relative position precisely. These things are usually explained in introductory courses of lectures; but it is well to summarize them in the Introduction to a Dissecting Guide.

TERMS OF POSITION

During dissection, the body, or any detached portion of it, usually lies horizontally on a table; but the dissector must remember that descriptive terms which refer to position are used as though the body were standing upright, with the upper limbs hanging by the sides but so rotated that the palms of the hands are directed forwards. This attitude is known conventionally as the 'anatomical position'.

Superior, cephalic or upper, therefore, does not refer to the position of a part that is nearer the dissector as he looks down on his dissection, but refers to the position of a part that is nearer the head of the supposedly erect body; **inferior** or **caudal** means nearer the feet.

Anterior means nearer the front of the body,

and **posterior** means nearer the back. In the trunk, **ventral** and **dorsal** may be used instead of anterior and posterior; these terms have the advantage of being applicable in any position of the body and are therefore used in Comparative Anatomy. (**Venter** = the belly; **dorsum** = the back.) In the hand, **dorsal** commonly replaces posterior, and **palmar** replaces anterior; in the foot, the corresponding surfaces are superior and inferior in the anatomical position, but those terms are usually replaced by **dorsal** (**dorsum** of foot) and **plantar**. (**Planta** = the sole.)

The **median plane** is an imaginary plane that divides the body into two apparently equal halves, right and left. The **anterior** and **posterior median lines** are the edges of that plane on the front and the back of the body. The term **median** usually refers to the position of a structure that is bisected by the median plane. **Medial** means nearer the median plane, and **lateral** means farther away from that plane. The ordinary English words, inner and outer, or their equivalents (derived from the Latin) internal and external, are to be used only in the sense of nearer the interior and farther away from the interior in any direction; in anatomical description they are not synonymous with medial and lateral, unless applied strictly at right angles to the median plane, and should not be used in place of these terms. External and internal (or outer and inner) are seldom used in the description of the structures in the limbs, for the words in common use are **superficial** for nearer the skin, and **deep** for farther away from it.

A plane through any portion of the body parallel to the median plane is called **sagittal,** and any vertical plane at right angles to these is called **coronal** (named from the position of two of the sutures of the skull).

In the different positions taken up by

1

mobile structures such as the limbs, it is not always apposite to use the terms superior and inferior; for this purpose **proximal** (nearer to) and **distal** (farther from) indicate the relative distances of structures from the root of the limb.

Middle, or its Latin equivalent *medius,* is the usual adjective denoting a position between superior and inferior or between anterior and posterior, but **intermediate** is commonly used instead of 'middle' for a position between lateral and medial.

TERMS OF MOVEMENT

All movements take place at joints and may occur in any plane, but are usually described in the sagittal and coronal planes. Movements in the sagittal plane are known as **flexion,** bending anteriorly, and **extension,** bending posteriorly. In the limbs, flexion is applied to the movement which carries the limb anteriorly and folds it, while extension is used for the reverse movement which straightens the limb and carries it posteriorly. Movements of the trunk in the coronal plane are known as lateral flexion, while in the limb they are called **abduction** (movement away from the median plane) and **adduction** (movement towards the median plane). The latter terms apply primarily to the proximal joints of the limbs, hip and shoulder, but are also used at the wrist where abduction refers to movement of the hand towards the thumb side (radial deviation) and adduction to movement towards the little finger side (ulnar deviation). In the fingers and toes, abduction and adduction are applied to the spreading and drawing together of these structures; in the hand this movement is away from or towards the middle finger, and in the foot is movement away from or towards the second toe. These movements occur in the plane of the finger and toe nails and in the case of the thumb are in an anteroposterior direction, the thumb being rotated relative to the fingers so that its dorsoventral axis is at right angles to that of the fingers. Thus abduction carries the thumb anteriorly and adduction carries it posteriorly. Circular

movements which pass through a number of planes are known as **circumduction.**

Rotation is the term applied to the movement in which a part of the body is turned around its own axis.

STRUCTURES MET WITH
IN A DISSECTION

The first step in a dissection is the removal of the skin. The skin consists of a superficial, avascular epithelium formed from layers of cells, the epidermis, and a deeper zone of vascular, dense fibrous tissue, the dermis, which sends minute peg-like protrusions into the epidermis. It is these which form the minute bleeding points which appear when a thin layer is cut from the surface of the skin and which help to bind the epidermis to the dermis. Between the skin and the underlying structures (muscles and bones) are two layers of fibrous tissue, the superficial and deep fasciae.

The Superficial Fascia

This is a fibrous network, the interstices of which are filled with fat. This fibrous mesh, which connects the dermis to the membranous layer of deep fascia sheathing the deeper structures, is particularly dense in the scalp, the back of the neck, the palms of the hands and the soles of the feet, thus holding the skin firmly to the underlying structures.

In all other parts it is loose enough to allow the skin to be freely moved, and its elasticity enables it to bring the skin back into place again. The thickness of the superficial fascia depends upon the quantity of fat in its meshes, and therefore varies greatly in different bodies and in different parts of the same body; fat is absent from the parts of it that underlie the skin of the eyelid, the nipple and areola of the breast, and some parts of the external genital organs.

The deeper parts of the glands of the skin and of the roots of the hairs penetrate into the superficial fascia, and the **mammary gland,** which is composed of modified and enlarged skin glands, is developed in it.

2

In some regions—for example, in the groin —the deeper part of the superficial fascia is in the form of a distinct membranous layer. In two regions, it contains muscle: (1) in the front and side of the face, neck, and the adjacent part of the chest, and (2) in the scrotum.

The superficial fascia is a warm garment underneath the skin, for fat is a bad conductor of heat. When moderately fatty, it fills up the hollows and rounds off the irregularities at the surface of the body. In a muscular man, however, it is seldom thick enough to obscure the outlines of the muscles that lie near the surface, whereas it is usually thick enough to do so in women. The rounded contours and smooth outlines of a woman's figure, due to the greater quantity of fat in the superficial fascia, are a secondary sex-character.

The superficial fascia contains also the cutaneous blood vessels, lymph vessels, and nerves on their way to and from the skin, and a few lymph nodes are embedded in it.

Vessels

Blood vessels are of three kinds—arteries, veins, and capillaries.

The **arteries** are the tubes that convey blood from the heart. Before the body is brought into the dissecting-room, it is embalmed by the injection of a preservative liquid into the arteries, and that is usually followed by the injection of coloured starch which distends the arteries and simulates the scarlet blood of arteries, making the smaller ones more apparent for dissection. The largest artery in the body is the elastic aorta, which springs from the heart. It is about 2·5 cm. in diameter. The largest artery of a limb is 6–8 mm. in diameter. Arteries branch and re-branch, and become successively narrower, less elastic, and more muscular, and those in the superficial fascia are so slender that the red injection seldom runs into them. The smallest arteries (<0·1 mm. in diameter), which open into the capillaries, are known as **arterioles.** In many parts of the body the smaller arteries join one another, forming tubular loops. The union of branches of arteries in this manner is called an **anastomosis.** Obvious anastomoses occur around the joints of a limb, and they may be of importance in maintaining the circulation if a main vessel has to be ligatured. In other places the anastomosis of arteries provides for an even distribution of blood to the parts supplied; notable examples are the 'arterial circle' on the base of the brain, and the series of arcades formed by the arteries of the intestines.

The **veins** are the tubes that carry the blood back to the heart. They are wider and more numerous than the arteries. They usually retain their blood after death, and are therefore bluish or purple in colour. The lesser veins unite, like the tributaries of a river, to form the larger veins, and veins anastomose even more freely than arteries, forming **venous plexuses** in some parts of the body, e.g., on the back of the hand. Every artery in a limb is accompanied by at least one vein. Most of the superficial arteries and all the larger deep arteries are accompanied by a single vein; the smaller deep arteries have two veins, one on each side, called **venae comitantes,** united by channels that cross the artery. But, in the superficial fascia, there are numerous veins that do not accompany arteries; they are fairly large, and can be easily seen, with their anastomoses, through the skin in the living forearm.

The **blood capillaries** are microscopic tubes that complete the circulatory system by forming a network in which the arterioles end and the smallest tributaries of veins begin. It is through the capillary walls that substances are exchanged between the blood and the tissues.

The pumping action of the heart sends the blood through the arteries and capillaries and onwards through the veins. The force of the heart beat is, however, becoming spent by the time it reaches the veins; the more sluggish flow of blood in them is aided by the movements of the muscles among which they lie and also by the movements of the thorax, for its enlargement with each inspiration draws venous blood into it as well as air. None the less, the flow in veins is liable to be

3

retarded by slight impediments; most veins, therefore, have valves to prevent or hamper any tendency to backward flow of the blood. The position of the valves of the superficial veins of one's own forearm can be seen if these veins are compressed at the elbow; the veins then become distended with blood, and the position of the valves is indicated by little, localized swellings or 'beads'.

It was the presence of these valves in the veins—first demonstrated publicly by Fabricius at Padua in 1579—that led William Harvey (1578–1657) to his great discovery of the circulation of the blood. The student should not omit to slit open veins in different parts of the body to observe the situation and structure of the valves.

In some parts of the body, e.g., in the pads of the fingers and toes and in the walls of some organs, there are direct connexions between small arteries and small veins without the intervention of capillaries. These **arterio-venous anastomoses** are under the control of the nervous system; relaxation of the arterioles concerned thus allows a greater blood flow through the organ without involving the capillary bed.

The **lymph nodes** are firm, gland-like structures that vary in size from a pin-head to a large bean; they are the main source of lymphocytes, a variety of white blood corpuscle. It is difficult to distinguish the smaller nodes from the pellets of fat amidst which they lie, but they are firmer in consistence, and though they vary in colour they are seldom yellow like fat. In the root of the lung they may be quite black owing to the presence of inhaled carbon particles which have been carried to them through the lymph vessels in scavenger cells (phagocytes) from the lung. In the limbs, they are largest and most numerous in the armpit and in the groin. Lymph nodes are found usually in groups of three or four; the groups are named after the places where they lie, and it often occurs that several groups are linked together by lymph vessels.

The **lymph vessels** are very fine tubes that contain a clear liquid called **lymph.** The lymph is exuded from the blood in the blood capillaries, and permeates all the tissues of the body to provide for chemical exchanges between tissues and blood. During activity of any organ or part of the body, the lymph vessels carry off any excess which cannot be dealt with by the blood capillaries and otherwise would accumulate in the tissues. The formation of lymph depends therefore on the activity of a part. There is a constant flow in the lymph vessels that drain the alimentary canal in the abdomen, some part of which is nearly always at work; but from parts that are sometimes at rest, e.g., the limbs, the flow is intermittent.

The lymph is collected from the tissues by a network of fine vessels, called **lymph capillaries,** which are wider than blood capillaries and are less regular in shape. They differ also in that they communicate with larger vessels in only one direction, whereas blood capillaries receive their contents from the arteries and pass them on to the veins. The smaller lymph vessels arise from the capillary network and carry the lymph to a lymph node, where they end. The lymph passes through the node and is collected by other lymph vessels that arise in the node. These vessels carry it onwards either to another node or to a larger lymph vessel. The vessels that carry lymph to a node are called **afferent** vessels; those that carry it from a node are **efferent.** (Ad = to; ex = from; fero = carry.) As the nodes are linked together the efferent vessels of one node are often the afferent vessels of another. The nodes that receive afferent vessels direct from a part of the body are known as the 'primary' nodes of that part. The larger lymph vessels unite together like the veins to form wider and wider vessels, but the resulting main lymph channels are no larger than small veins. The lymph is ultimately poured into the blood stream, for the largest lymph vessels (the longest and widest of which is called the **thoracic duct)** end by joining the great veins at the root of the neck.

There is no pumping force, like that of the heart, to drive the lymph onwards. Its flow through the lymph vessels depends merely upon the movements of the body aided by the

4

low pressure in the big veins in the root of the neck. Valves are provided for the maintenance of the flow in one direction, as in the veins; and they are so closely set that a distended, lymph vessel has a characteristic beaded appearance.

The lymph vessels that lie in the superficial fascia drain the lymph from the skin. For the most part they run along the superficial veins and ultimately converge upon the important groups of lymph nodes situated at the junction of the limbs and trunk. Only a few lymph nodes are found in the superficial fascia, and they lie in its deeper part, nearly all nodes are situated deeply, usually close to the deep veins, along which the deep lymph vessels also run.

The lymph vessels of the superficial fascia are like silken threads—so slender that often they are not detected during the dissection. Indeed, it should be mentioned that, with the exception of the main, terminal lymph vessels and some of the larger afferents of the principal groups of nodes, it is scarcely possible to display the lymph vessels unless special methods of injection have been employed. Nevertheless, because of their great importance in the spread of disease—either bacterial infection or cancerous tumours—the dissectors must make every endeavour to find the groups of lymph nodes as they dissect each part, and to learn which are the 'primary' nodes for any area or organ.

Nerves

The nerves are cords of a light grey colour or nearly white; they branch like arteries, and their branches often unite with one another. In a way, they resemble telegraph cables, because they are made of bundles of exceedingly fine filaments, called **nerve fibres**, bound together by fibrous tissue; and they carry messages, which are called **impulses**. The impulses are sent through them from the central nervous system (*i.e.*, brain and spinal medulla) to the various structures in the body, and from the structures to the central nervous system. The fibres that carry impulses from the central nervous system are called **efferent**, and those that carry impulses to it are **afferent.** The commonest outgoing impulses are those to muscles to make them shorten or contract to move some part of the body, and they are therefore called **motor.** The commonest incoming impulses are from the skin and other structures and convey information about sensations—touch, pain, heat, etc.—and are called **sensory.**

The largest nerve in the body is the **sciatic nerve,** which lies in the buttock and in the back of the thigh, and is about the width of the little finger and half its thickness. Most of the larger nerves in the limbs are much smaller, the finest branches being invisible to the unaided eye. In the superficial fascia, even the larger nerves are fairly slender. At first it may not be easy to distinguish a nerve from a small empty vein; but the vein is collapsed and can be easily stretched, while the nerve is cylindrical and firmer.

The nerves connected with the brain emerge from the skull or cranium, and are called **cranial nerves.** Those connected with the spinal medulla are called **spinal nerves;** they have to escape from the vertebral canal—*i.e.*, the tunnel in the backbone that lodges the spinal medulla. Nerves that supply a limb come from spinal nerves, and in the early stages of dissection reference has to be made to the names, numbers, and divisions of spinal nerves.

There are 31 pairs of **spinal nerves**—8 cervical, 12 thoracic, 5 lumbar, 5 sacral, and 1 coccygeal. They are named after the groups of vertebrae—*i.e.*, the segments of the backbone or vertebral column. But note that there are 8 cervical nerves and only 7 cervical vertebrae, and that there is only 1 coccygeal nerve though there are 4 segments in the coccyx.

Every spinal nerve is attached to the spinal medulla by **two roots**—an anterior or ventral and a posterior or dorsal [Fig. 1].

The **ventral root** consists of bundles of **motor fibres**.

The **dorsal root** consists of bundles of sensory fibres. It is distinguished by the fact that it has a swelling on it, called the **spinal**

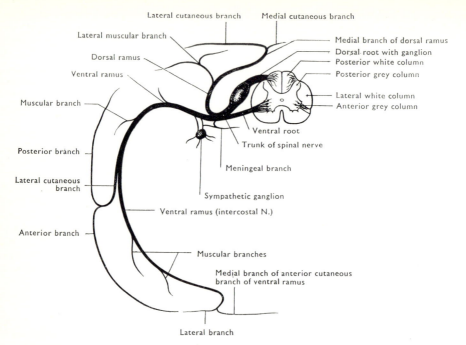

Lateral cutaneous branch   Medial cutaneous branch

Lateral muscular branch

Dorsal ramus

Ventral ramus

Muscular branch

Posterior branch

Lateral cutaneous
branch

Anterior branch

Medial branch of dorsal ramus
Dorsal root with ganglion
Posterior white column
Posterior grey column

Lateral white column
Anterior grey column

Ventral root
Trunk of spinal nerve

Meningeal branch

Sympathetic ganglion

Ventral ramus (intercostal N.)

Muscular branches

Medial branch of anterior cutaneous
branch of ventral ramus

Lateral branch

FIG. 1 Diagram of a typical spinal nerve. Note that the medial branch of the dorsal ramus is represented as distributed to skin, whilst the lateral branch terminates at a deeper level in muscle. Both branches, however, supply muscles; and in the lower half of the body it is the lateral branch that supplies skin.

ganglion, which is composed of **nerve cells** and their microscopic processes the nerve fibres.

The two roots unite, immediately beyond the ganglion, to form the **trunk** of the spinal nerve. The union takes place at the inter-vertebral foramen through which the nerve trunk leaves the vertebral canal.

The **nerve trunk** is very short. The union of the roots allows the mixture of motor and sensory fibres; and the nerve trunk, as it leaves the intervertebral foramen, splits into two divisions called the **ventral ramus** and the **dorsal ramus.** (*Ramus* = a branch.) Do not confuse the *roots* by which a spinal nerve arises with the *rami* into which it divides; nearly every ramus contains both motor and sensory fibres.

The **dorsal ramus** is the smaller. It passes backwards into the mass of muscle on the back of the body. There, it divides into a

lateral branch and a **medial branch.** Both of these branches supply muscles, and one of them sends a branch to the skin. These **cutaneous** branches of posterior rami form a row of nerves on both sides of the midline of the back [FIG. 21].

The **ventral ramus** runs in a lateral direction away from the vertebral column. The ventral rami of thoracic nerves run along the ribs; the upper eleven are **intercostal,** and the twelfth is **subcostal** (*costa* = a rib); they end as **anterior cutaneous** branches on the front of the trunk. Each gives off a **lateral cutaneous** branch, which divides into anterior and posterior branches. The ventral rami of the other spinal nerves are more or less pleated together to form what are called **nerve plexuses.** Those of the cervical nerves (with part of the first thoracic) form two plexuses called the **cervical plexus** and the **brachial**

6

plexus. Most of the nerves of the Upper Limb arise from the brachial plexus, and a few come from the cervical plexus. The brachial plexus lies in the neck and in the armpit; dissectors of the Upper Limb combine with the dissectors of the Neck in displaying it. Those of the lumbar, sacral, and coccygeal nerves form plexuses that have the same names. Nearly all the nerves of the Lower Limb come from the **lumbar** and **sacral plexuses.** These two plexuses lie near the backbone in the abdomen and pelvis; they will be exposed by the dissectors of the Abdomen.

The fibres of the ventral or motor root arise from nerve cells in the spinal medulla. They run out into the ventral root, and onwards through the nerve trunk and the rami into the various motor nerves. The fibres of the dorsal or sensory root arise in the nerve cells of the spinal ganglion. Each sensory fibre, while still in the ganglion, splits into two branches—a central branch and a peripheral branch. Central branches run to the spinal medulla, forming the dorsal root of the nerve, and end around nerve cells in the spinal medulla or in the brain. Peripheral branches run outwards through the rami. A sensory impulse starts at the end of a peripheral branch, runs in it to the ganglion, and onwards in a central branch into the spinal medulla.

Deep Fascia

Deep fascia is the name given to the bluish membrane that lies under cover of the superficial fascia. It is thin, but dense and strong, and the superficial fascia is loosely attached to it by fibrous strands. It clothes the muscles, investing them so closely that it forms a tight sheath around the limb and preserves the contours of the limb. From its deep surface it sends in wide sheets that form partitions or **septa** among the muscles. In that way the deep fascia provides fascial sheaths for many of the muscles, and for the vessels and nerves that lie among the muscles; parts of some muscles are attached both to the investing fascia and to the septa. Some of the septa are attached to the bones and to the

ligaments of joints that lie deeply among the muscles. The investing fascia is attached to the ligaments of joints and to the parts of bones that come to the surface between muscles. In certain places it is thickened to form strong, restraining bands, called **retinacula,** that hold tendons or sinews in position, and serve also as pulleys on which the sinews move—for example, at the wrist and ankle.

Muscles

The muscles are the red flesh of the body, and form nearly half the weight of the body. They are the active agents that produce movements, for they can be shortened or contracted at will to bring the parts to which they are attached closer together. The 'actions' of muscles, however, are by no means simple; and the student must learn the various capacities in which muscles act in combination in any movement of a limb or other part of the body.

Each muscle has at least two attachments—one at each end. When a muscle is activated it may either shorten, approximating its ends, or the tension in it may increase without shortening if the load against which it is acting is equal to the tension. In the latter case the muscle helps to fix a part of the body, but if the load is greater than the tension developed in the muscle, the muscle will lengthen while active, paying out gradually, as in preventing the uncontrolled activity of the muscles which produce the opposite movement, or in lowering a heavy weight to the floor. If the muscle shortens, either or both ends may move, but it is usual to consider one end, the origin, as fixed, while the other, the insertion, moves. Which end moves is determined by the other forces in action at the time and is not an intrinsic property of the individual muscle; it is best therefore, to use the term attachments, rather than origin and insertion, to avoid the spurious idea that a muscle invariably moves its 'insertion'. The limb muscles are attached mostly to bones and deep fascia, but some are attached also to cartilages and to the ligaments of joints.

The red, fleshy part of a muscle is called its **belly.** The belly is composed of bundles of red muscle fibres held together by white fibrous tissue. At the ends of a muscle the muscle fibres become continuous with white fibrous tissue, and through this they obtain their attachments. In many muscles, especially at the origin, those terminal, white parts are so short that the naked eye cannot see them; the muscle appears to be attached by red, fleshy fibres, and is, in fact, described as having a fleshy attachment. But many muscles terminate as long cords of white fibrous tissue by which they are attached. These cords have a greenish tinge, and are called **tendons** or sinews. Those on the back of the living hand are easily seen, for they raise the skin and fasciae into ridges when the fingers are bent back. In some cases, especially when the muscle is thin and wide, the tendon is not a slender cord but is a thin, wide sheet called an **aponeurosis.** (*Neuron* and *nervus* originally meant sinew.)

Tendons not only enable the power of a muscle to be transferred to a distance, as in the case of those that move the fingers, but they are related also to the structural form of muscles. The dorsal interossei of the hand [FIG. 80] and of the foot exhibit a simple **bipennate** type of structure, two heads converging on a tendon like the barbs of a feather. The deltoid and the subscapularis are typical **multipennate** muscles; tendinous sheets (intersections) between the parts of the muscles greatly increasing the area from which muscle fibres can arise.

In addition to a main vessel which enters many limb muscles with the nerve at a distinct **neurovascular hilum,** numerous small arteries enter most muscles at irregular points, and the blood is drained away by veins that accompany the arteries. Every muscle has at least one nerve of supply which conveys motor impulses to it to make it contract, and carries sensory impulses from it to inform the central nervous system about its state of contraction.

Individual muscles may be made to contract by appropriate electrical stimuli applied to the skin over or near the sites of entry of their nerves; a knowledge of these 'motor points', as they are called, is necessary for electrical diagnosis of the condition of a muscle.

When a muscle or a tendon passes over a bone or a ligament or another tendon, a bursa is placed between them to lessen friction and make movement easier. A **bursa** is a closed fibrous bag or sac, lined with a smooth membrane, called **synovial membrane,** which exudes a glutinous liquid called **synovia** to lubricate the surfaces. Normally the synovia is just enough to moisten the surfaces, but a bursa may be distended by excessive secretion caused by irritation, as in the case of 'housemaid's knee'. For the same purpose, many tendons are enclosed in **synovial sheaths** made of white fibrous tissue and lined with synovial membrane.

Ligaments are strong bands of inelastic white fibrous tissue that connect bony points. Most of them are found therefore at the articulations or joints.

Joints

A joint is where two bones come together whether there is movement between them or not. Joints without movement are those in which adjacent pieces of bone are separated by cartilage or fibrous tissue during development and subsequently fuse; examples are the developing long bones and the sutures of the skull [FIG. 2]. Joints with a small amount of movement are those where the bones are held together by a thick layer of fibrous tissue or fibrocartilage, *e.g.,* the discs between the bodies of the vertebrae. Joints with the maximum amount of movement are the **synovial joints.** Here the bearing surfaces of the bones are covered with hard, slippery, articular **cartilage** and ride on each other in a narrow space filled with synovia or lubricant fluid. They are enclosed in a tubular sheath of fibrous tissue (the **fibrous capsule**) which holds the bones together and is separated from the joint cavity, which it encloses, by synovial membrane. **Synovial membrane** lines all the structures bordering on the joint cavity except the articular surfaces. The

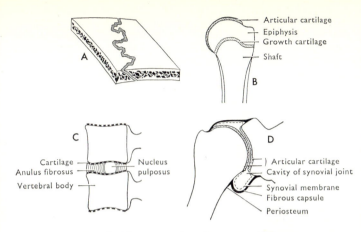

Articular cartilage
Epiphysis
Growth cartilage
Shaft

Cartilage — Nucleus
Anulus fibrosus — pulposus
Vertebral body —

) Articular cartilage
Cavity of synovial joint
Synovial membrane
Fibrous capsule
Periosteum

FIG. 2   Diagrams to show four types of joints.

A. A suture between two skull bones. In this the bones are firmly bound together by a thin layer of dense fibrous tissue which does not allow movement, but permits the addition of new bone to the adjacent surfaces, thus assisting in growth of the bones.

B. Section through the proximal end of the growing humerus; the two parts of the bone, epiphysis and shaft, are joined by a layer of firm, growing cartilage. No movement is possible, the joint is a temporary one concerned with the growth in length of the shaft, and is called a synchondrosis. When growth ceases this joint is replaced by bone, forming a synostosis, a fate which also overtakes sutures.

C. Section through an intervertebral disc joining two vertebral bodies. A thick, laminated, fibrous sheath (anulus fibrosus) of great strength encloses a pulpy central mass (nucleus pulposus). The flexibility of the disc allows limited movement between the vertebrae, the range increasing with the thickness of the disc.

D. Section through the shoulder joint to show the parts of a synovial joint. Such joints have a cavity which extends between the ends of the bones which are covered with slippery, hyaline cartilage, and the whole is enclosed in a fibrous sheath or capsule lined with synovial membrane. This type of joint allows the maximum freedom of movement which is limited only by the shape of the articular surfaces, and the length and strength of the fibrous capsule and ligaments.

amount of movement at any such joint is determined by the shape and extent of the bearing surfaces of the bones, and the length and strength of the fibrous capsule and any additional ligaments joining the bones. Such ligaments are usually named from their position, e.g., radial and ulnar collateral ligaments of the elbow.

The fibrous capsule is an inelastic sheath, but movement is permitted at synovial joints: (1) by increasing the length of those parts of the capsule which would otherwise become taut; (2) by the arrangement of the fibres in these regions, so that they run obliquely across the capsule and can be spread when

tension is applied. Powerful ligaments which maintain the stability of the joint are placed approximately as radii of the arc of movement and so tend to remain taut throughout. Thus the anterior and posterior parts of the fibrous capsule of the elbow joint are lax and are composed mainly of oblique fibres, the sides alone having the powerful radial and ulnar collateral ligaments. In joints where movement either can take place in many directions, or is of a range not easily achieved by the above methods, the strength of the joint is maintained by the surrounding muscles. These act as ligaments of variable length and tension, assuring stability in all positions even with a weak, loose fibrous capsule, e.g., the shoulder joint. In some cases tendons form part of the capsule of the joint, e.g., extensor tendons of the fingers, thus effectively increasing the available range of movement.

The stability and complexity of movement at a joint are sometimes increased by placing between the adjacent bones a disc of fibrous cartilage. This may have different curvatures on its two faces and turn a single joint into two, with different types of movement at each, e.g., the sternoclavicular joint.

Osteology

It is essential for the dissector to be fully conversant with the bones of the part being dissected as they form the essential basis of all topographical knowledge. He should be able to read the tell-tale marks which each shows: smooth areas, covered in life by articular cartilage, where a bone articulates at a synovial joint; roughened areas for the attachment of ligaments, aponeuroses, and tendons; smooth areas where bone is subcutaneous or gives rise to muscle fibres directly; grooves lodging vessels, and holes (foramina) where arteries enter and veins leave the substance of the bone, to supply it and the contained marrow which forms blood cells in many parts of the body (vertebral column, skull, ribs, sternum, hip bone, etc.). Many of the features of a bone are not readily seen but are easily felt on the dry bone; they are of importance because they give a clear indication of the functions of muscles and ligaments by pinpointing their exact attachments. The student should also determine the position of each bone in the living body and the parts which are readily visible or palpable, making use of radiographs to confirm his findings.

GENERAL DIRECTIONS
FOR DISSECTION

Instruments

The dissector should have at least one scalpel with a stout, sharp blade; two pairs of forceps, one with fine and the other with broad points; a strong blunt hook or seeker; and a hand lens. The blades of the forceps should not be so strong that they cannot be held compressed without fatigue, and the hand lens should be used frequently to bridge the gap between naked-eye and microscopic anatomy, to aid in the study of the minute arrangement of tissues which can throw much light on their function.

Beneath the skin, the body consists of a number of different organs embedded in a matrix of fibrous connective tissue, or fascia, which varies in density from a loose net to tough sheets or bundles of fibres. Dissection is the process of freeing the organs from this tissue and demonstrating the places where it is loose or dense. For this purpose blunt dissection with the points of the forceps or a

hook, stripping out the loose layers of fascia separating the organs, is the quickest and most satisfactory method, the knife being reserved for incising the skin and for dividing structures such as the dense layers of fascia which cover the organs and obscure them from view.

Care of Parts

Once the skin has been removed, drying of the underlying tissues occurs rapidly and must be avoided if dissection is not to become impossible. After each period of dissection the part should be moistened with preserving fluid, preferably containing some glycerin, and either enclosed in a plastic bag, or wrapped in cloths soaked in similar preservative.

Removal of the Skin

The flaps of skin to be removed are marked out by cuts made through it to the level of the superficial fascia. In bodies with plenty of fat in the superficial fascia it is easy to determine when the skin has been cut through, by the decrease in resistance when the knife enters the fascia, but in thin bodies it is best to check the depth of the incision by lifting the cut edge of the skin. Next lift up one corner of the flap and detach it from the superficial fascia, continuing to pull the skin away and separating the fascia from it with the edge of the knife directed towards the skin, so as to leave no fat attached to the skin and avoid injuring the superficial vessels and nerves which run in the superficial fascia. Now lift up one edge of the superficial fascia and strip it away from the membranous deep fascia using blunt dissection as far as possible. By this means the points at which the superficial nerves pierce the deep fascia to enter the superficial layer will be found, and they can then be traced towards their termination in the skin. Much time can be wasted trying to follow each tiny branch of the superficial nerves, and it is best to consult illustrations of the distribution of these nerves. The student should be aware that the arrangement of the cutaneous nerves is of great importance in the clinical testing for injuries to the peripheral or central nervous systems. Each small artery entering the superficial fascia is accompanied by one or more small veins; in addition larger veins may be found in the superficial fascia, and these pierce the deep fascia separately to end in the deep vein. These communications between the superficial and deep veins are usually guarded by valves which prevent the reflux of blood into the superficial veins.

Deeper Dissections

When you have removed all the superficial fascia from the area under dissection, and have studied the superficial structures, examine the characters and connexions of the deep fascia, and then remove it in order to expose the muscles and other deep structures. The deep fascia not only clothes the muscles but also gives attachment to, and passes deeply between many of them; the cleaning of a muscle—that is, the removal of the fascia from it—is therefore not always easy.

To Clean a Muscle. If necessary, put the muscle on the stretch by adjusting the limb. Define the margins of the muscle. Cut through the deep fascia until the red bundles of the muscle are exposed. Put slight traction upon the cut edge and divide the delicate strands which pass between the bundles of muscle fibres carrying the blade in the direction of these bundles.

The cleaning of the deeper muscles and of the deep surfaces of the more superficial muscles requires the removal of fat as well as of fascia. Take care throughout not to injure the nerves of supply. The nerves in the greatest danger are those that supply the more superficial muscles, for almost all of them enter the muscles through their deep surfaces.

It is more important to define the ends of a muscle and verify its attachments than to spend time in attempting to clean off every particle of fascia from its surface.

To clean the deeper vessels and nerves means merely the piecemeal removal of the fat and loose fibrous tissue in which they are embedded. Begin with the main trunks.

Clean them; trace their branches, and clean them also. This work is often very tedious, and dissectors often find that they are hampered (especially in the thigh) by the veins and by the branches of arteries that supply muscles. Keep the main venous trunks and most of the arteries; have no hesitation in removing the veins that accompany the smaller arteries, or in dividing the smaller arteries that supply muscles, if they are in the way. But be careful of nerves. They are much more constant in position and important than the arteries and veins, for the latter link up (anastomose) with adjacent vessels to give an alternative route of vascular supply, a feature which the nerves do not possess. Trace all of them to their destinations and leave them uninjured.

VARIATION

The human body, like all living things, is subject to variation. Apart from general features—stature, build, head-form, facial configuration—and fine details such as the well-known finger-prints, which together confer bodily individuality, all the systems and organs vary, more or less, from body to body. The student must not expect, therefore, to find everything exactly as described in a Dissecting Manual which, being primarily a guide, can deal only with the usual or average arrangement. The true bible of the student of Anatomy is the body itself; and he should welcome the opportunity that dissection provides of perusing it for himself as an original investigation. Thus he will cultivate that faculty of observation which will stand him in good stead in his later clinical work.

Some variations are of direct clinical importance, such as the arrangement of the superficial veins of the forearm and even the course of main arteries. Others, such as variations in the attachments of muscles (*e.g.*, an extra head of the biceps muscle of the arm), the absence of a usual muscle or the presence of an unusual one, may be chiefly of evolutionary significance. There is also the class of congenital malformations, not commonly seen in the dissecting room, which

11

may be of great functional importance. Position of organs, *e.g.*, in the abdomen, may vary too; and there are more subtle variations, such as the form of the living stomach, which can be demonstrated by appropriate X-ray methods. The systematic noting of variations as they are observed is a most useful exercise, notwithstanding that most of them will be found recorded in the larger textbooks and in special works which may be consulted as occasion serves.

ANATOMY OF THE LIVING BODY

It has sometimes been made a reproach to anatomical studies that they are concerned with dead, preserved material, and that the student thereby receives false impressions that he is in danger of transferring to the living body. But, apart from opportunities of attending autopsies of the recently dead or of observing living tissues at surgical operations, it is obvious that the student must have time to examine the structure of the body in detail, and that this implies embalming of the cadaver. It is true that embalming alters the texture and appearance of the tissues, and that hardening agents, such as formalin, produce an unnatural rigidity of muscles and organs. On the other hand, these agents, used in moderation, do preserve the form of organs at the time of death and thus maintain their relations to each other. No sensible student is likely to imagine that the healthy liver in the living body is incapable of moulding itself to other organs as the diaphragm rises and falls, or that the living lung is a static organ because he finds them so in the embalmed cadaver that he dissects.

These remarks are made, however, to emphasize the importance of cultivating an attitude of mind that looks to dissection as a means to an end, and that end is under-standing of the body as a living organism. The basis of that understanding is the topography of the body, of which real knowledge can be acquired only by personal contact. But it is not enough merely to supplement dissection by Surface Anatomy on the living model and by radiographic demonstration of the relations and changing form of organs in the living body. The student of Anatomy must always keep in mind the indissoluble relation between structure and function, as in the simple case of the valves in the veins or in the more complex arrangement of the heart, where gross structure is meaningless without reference to the circulation of the blood. So, in every system of the body, structure and function are but two aspects of the same study : the attachments of muscles must be related to the actions of which they are capable ; the form of joints and the arrangement of ligaments and muscles around them must be studied with reference to movements and stability ; and in tracing the nerves the student must constantly ask himself what functional groups of muscles they supply ; from what areas of skin they convey sensory information, and what would be the effect if this or that nerve were to be compressed by disease or severed by injury. These are simple examples of the relation between form and function which is manifest throughout the body and in the intimate details of the structure of organs—the most perfect example is the central nervous system, brain and spinal medulla. It is the attitude of mind that counts—the approach to Anatomy not as a dead subject but as the study of a living, functioning organism. Thus it is the indispensable foundation not only of Physiology and Pathology but also, with these subjects, of Clinical Studies, through appreciation of the anatomical basis of the signs and symptoms of disease.

THE UPPER LIMB

INTRODUCTION

The parts of the Upper Limb are the shoulder, the upper arm or brachium, the forearm or antebrachium, and the hand or manus.

The region of the **shoulder** includes more than the familiar prominence at the upper end of the arm. It includes also: (1) The **axilla** or armpit; (2) the **scapular region** or the parts around the shoulder blade; and (3) the **pectoral region** on the front of the chest. (*Pectus* = the breast.) The bones of the shoulder form the shoulder girdle. They are the **scapula** or shoulder blade and the **clavicle** or collar bone [FIGS. 18, 22, 33]. They articulate with each other at the top of the shoulder to form a joint called the **acromioclavicular joint,** and the clavicle articulates with the upper end of the sternum or breast bone to form the **sternoclavicular joint.**

The **upper arm** is the part between the shoulder and the elbow or cubitus. Its bone is called the **humerus,** which articulates with the scapula to form the **shoulder joint.**

The **forearm** extends from the elbow to the wrist. It has two bones—the **radius** and the **ulna.** They articulate with the humerus to form the **elbow joint,** and they articulate with each other, at both ends, to form the **proximal** and **distal radio-ulnar joints**. When the forearm is turned so that the palm of the hand looks forwards (supination), the two bones are parallel—the radius on the lateral side of the ulna. When the hand is turned so that the palm looks backwards (pronation), the distal end of the radius rotates around the ulna, and the radius lies obliquely across the front of the ulna.

The **hand** is subdivided into: (1) the wrist or carpus, (2) the hand proper or metacarpus, and (3) the digits (thumb and fingers).

The skeleton of the **wrist** is a group of eight little bones called **carpal bones,** arranged in two rows—a proximal and a distal [FIGS. 60, 84]. They articulate with one another to form **intercarpal joints,** and the proximal row articulates with the radius to form the **radiocarpal** or **wrist joint.** On the back of the wrist, they are near the surface, partially under cover of the tendons that pass over the lower ends of the radius and ulna; on the front, they are to a large extent obscured by the ball of the thumb (thenar eminence) and the ball of the little finger (hypothenar eminence).

The **hand proper** has a skeleton of five **metacarpal bones.** They correspond to the five digits and are numbered 1 to 5, beginning with the thumb. At their proximal ends or bases, they articulate with the distal row of carpal bones, forming **carpometacarpal joints;** and there are **intermetacarpal joints** between the bases of the medial four [FIG. 89].

The **digits** are named: thumb or pollex; forefinger or index; middle finger or digitus medius; ring finger or annularis; and little finger or minimus. The bones of the digits are called **phalanges.** The thumb has two phalanges; the other digits have three. The proximal phalanx articulates with the head of a metacarpal bone to form a **metacarpophalangeal joint.** The middle one articulates with the other two to form **interphalangeal joints.** On the front of some of the metacarpophalangeal joints there are, occasionally, little nodules of bone called **sesamoid bones** [FIG. 84].

THE PECTORAL REGION AND AXILLA

The dissection of the Upper Limb begins with the body supine, *i.e.*, lying on its back. Until the dissection of the axilla is completed, the dissectors of the Upper Limb and of the Head and Neck will find it advantageous to arrange to work at different hours. The

13

dissectors of the Head and Neck, at this stage, are engaged on the dissection of the posterior triangle of the neck, and that cannot be well done unless the limb is placed close to the side and the shoulder depressed. For the dissection of the axilla, the limb should be pulled away from the thorax, care being taken not to tear the muscles connecting it to the trunk.

<h2 style="text-align:center">SURFACE ANATOMY</h2>

The **clavicle** lies immediately deep to the deep fascia between the neck and the front of the chest, and can be both felt and seen. It extends from the top of the shoulder to the upper end of the **sternum.** Draw your finger along it from one end to the other. Note that, in its medial two-thirds, it is curved with its convexity forwards, to give room for the passage of vessels and nerves between the neck and the axilla. The medial end of the clavicle [FIG. 13] articulates with the superior surface of the sternum and projects above it, producing a prominence that is easily felt. The prominence is, however, slightly masked by a part of the **sternocleidomastoid muscle**— the muscle which extends from the sternum and the clavicle to the skull behind the ear and rises as a strong, blunt ridge on the living neck when the face is turned towards the other side.

Place the tip of the index finger in the **jugular notch,** i.e., the hollow at the upper end of the sternum between the clavicles, and draw it downwards along the median line. About 5 cm. below the upper end of the sternum, a blunt, transverse ridge is distinctly felt. That ridge marks the **sternal angle** at the union of the **manubrium** with the **body** of the sternum. It is the best landmark on the front of the chest, for it can be felt even in obese subjects, and it is often visible. The **cartilage of the second rib** joins the side of the sternum at the sternal angle. The second rib is therefore more easily identified than any other. To find one of the other ribs, find second and count downwards from it. The anterior part of the **first rib** is about 2·5 cm. above the second, and is masked by the

clavicle. Continue to draw the finger down over the sternum. At the lower end of the body of the sternum, the finger sinks into a shallow depression. That is the **epigastric fossa** or 'pit of the stomach'. The bony, but slightly yielding, structure felt on the floor of the fossa is the third or lowest piece of the sternum, the **xiphoid process.** The right and left boundaries of the epigastric fossa are the **cartilages of the seventh pair of ribs.** Verify all these points on the articulated skeleton.

The **nipple** is variable in position, even in the male, but usually it is opposite the space between the **fourth** and **fifth ribs,** and is a guide to their position; it is near their junction with their cartilages. Measure its distance from the median plane; it is usually about 10 cm. (The dissector's own hand is a rough measure. A man's hand is about 10 cm. across, and his thumb about 2·5 cm. wide.)

Below the junction of the lateral and intermediate thirds of the clavicle there is a depression called the **infraclavicular fossa.** The soft bulging at the medial side of the fossa is part of a large muscle, called **pectoralis major,** that lies on the front of the chest and axilla. The prominence on the lateral side is the anterior part of the **deltoid muscle,** which clasps the shoulder. In the infraclavicular fossa, 2·5 cm. below the clavicle, press your finger laterally under deltoid; the indistinct resistance is produced by the tip of the coracoid process of the scapula [FIGS. 12, 18].

The lateral end of the clavicle articulates with the medial margin of a subcutaneous flattened piece of bone about 2·5 cm. wide that lies in the top of the shoulder, the **acromion.** (Acron = summit; omos = shoulder.) The upper surfaces of acromion and clavicle lie in nearly the same plane; the **acromioclavicular joint** is therefore inconspicuous, but it can be detected easily if the limb is moved.

Abduct the arm. That is, draw it away from the trunk. The hollow of the **axilla** and the rounded folds that bound it in front and behind are brought into view. The **anterior fold** encloses part of the **pectoralis major** muscle and part of the **pectoralis minor,** which is behind the major. The **posterior fold** encloses two muscles, teres major and latissimus dorsi. The **teres major**—a stout, round muscle—extends from the lower angle of the scapula, which can be felt in the posterior axillary fold where it joins the trunk when the arm is raised above the head, to the upper part of the shaft of the humerus. The

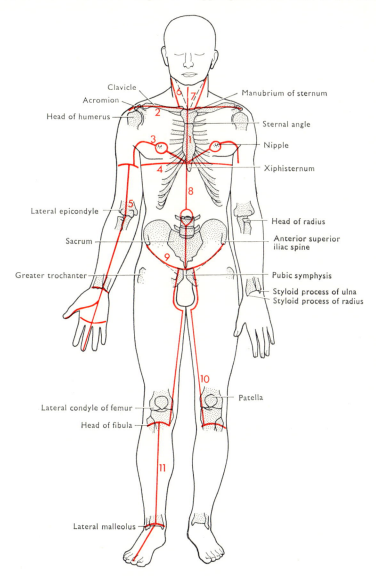

Clavicle
Acromion
Head of humerus
Manubrium of sternum
Sternal angle
Nipple
Xiphisternum
Lateral epicondyle
Head of radius
Sacrum
Anterior superior iliac spine
Greater trochanter
Pubic symphysis
Styloid process of ulna
Styloid process of radius
Patella
Lateral condyle of femur
Head of fibula
Lateral malleolus

FIG. 3 Landmarks and incisions. For the bony landmarks of the upper limb, see illustrations of individual bones.

latissimus dorsi—wide and thin—lies in the lower part of the back [FIG. 21], but narrows to form a flattened tendon, which, as it approaches the humerus, winds round the teres major [FIG. 12]. Draw the arm well from the side. The edge of the latissimus dorsi then raises up a distinct ridge of skin that runs downwards and backwards; the lowest rib that the ridge crosses is the **eleventh rib**. Grip the posterior fold between finger and thumb: the different consistence of the fleshy teres and the tendinous latissimus can be distinguished through the skin and fasciae. Note that the posterior fold reaches lower down than the anterior, and that therefore the structures in the lowest part of the axilla have no muscle in front of them.

Place the fingers in the **axilla** and examine its walls. The **anterior wall** is soft and fleshy. So is the **posterior wall**; but the lateral margin of the **scapula** can be felt in it. The **ribs** are felt in the **medial wall**—covered with a wide muscle called **serratus anterior**. The **lateral wall** is narrow. The softer parts felt in it are two muscles—the **biceps brachii** and the **coracobrachialis**; the hard part is the neck of the **humerus** and the upper part of its shaft. Some of the large nerves of the axilla can be rolled between the fingers and the bone; and in the living limb the **axillary artery** can be felt beating. Push the fingers well up into the axilla and rotate the arm: the globular **head of the humerus** can be felt indistinctly.

DISSECTION. Reflexion of Skin: Make skin incisions 1-4 shown in Figure 3. In making incision 2 avoid cutting into the superficial fascia and dividing the thin sheet of muscle, platysma, and the supra-clavicular nerves which lie deep to it [Fig. 4] both of which sweep down over the clavicle into the upper part of the chest wall.

Reflect the flaps of skin thus marked out (extend 4 to the posterior axillary fold), beginning in the median plane at one of the angles. Do not detach the flaps, but leave them hanging by their lateral ends, in order that they may be replaced when dissection for the day is finished. Leave the small patch around the nipple.

As the reflexion proceeds, note that the connexion between the superficial fascia and the skin is stronger in some places than in others. In the female, definite

fibrous strands will be found passing from the mammary gland to the skin; these extend through the gland to the deep fascia.

SUPERFICIAL FASCIA

In this region the fat of the superficial fascia is not usually very plentiful except in female bodies where it is abundant in the region of the mammary gland. Near the clavicle the vertical reddish striation of platysma is usually visible through the fat.

CUTANEOUS NERVES AND VESSELS

The nerves and vessels that pass through the superficial fascia to the skin must now be sought. They are:—

Supraclavicular nerves, from the cervical plexus.

Anterior cutaneous branches / from intercostal nerves, *i.e.*, from ventral / Lateral cutaneous branches / rami of thoracic nerves [FIG. 1].

Cutaneous arteries derived from deep arteries. Cutaneous veins.

DISSECTION. Cut through the superficial fascia along the margin of the sternum and strip it from the deep fascia by blunt dissection, finding the anterior cutaneous nerves as they pierce the deep fascia at the sternal ends of the intercostal spaces. They are very slender, but their greyish streaked appearance distinguishes them from surrounding tissues; and the accompanying arteries, if injected, are guides to them. Trace their branches medially and laterally as far as possible.

Next cut carefully through the superficial fascia and the platysma along the upper border of the clavicle, looking for the slender supraclavicular nerves as you reflect the fascia downwards. Trace the nerves as they stream downwards across the clavicle through the platysma into the superficial fascia of the shoulder and the front of the chest.

Thirdly, beginning at the arm, cut through the superficial fascia along the anterior fold of the axilla and continue the cut downwards and in a medial direction for 7-10 cm. Reflect the cut edges of the fascia, and look for the anterior branches of the lateral cutaneous nerves as they pierce the deep fascia at the lower border of the pectoralis major [Fig. 10]. Trace them medially through the superficial fascia.

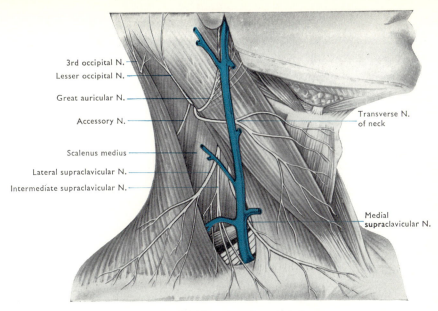

Labels on figure:
3rd occipital N.
Lesser occipital N.
Great auricular N.
Accessory N.
Scalenus medius
Lateral supraclavicular N.
Intermediate supraclavicular N.
Transverse N. of neck
Medial supraclavicular N.

Fig. 4 Superficial branches of cervical plexus.

The **supraclavicular nerves** arise in the neck from the third and fourth cervical nerves. They spread out as they descend, pierce the deep fascia of the neck, cross the clavicle under cover of the platysma, and run downwards to supply the skin that overlies the deltoid and pectoralis major muscles as far down as the level of a horizontal line drawn from the second costal cartilage. They are named, according to their positions [FIG. 4]: the **medial**—one or more—cross the medial part of the clavicle; the **intermediate**—two or three—pass over the middle of the clavicle; the **lateral**—one or more—cross the lateral third of the clavicle, and pass to the skin of the shoulder.

The **anterior cutaneous nerves** are the terminal branches of the intercostal nerves and are very slender. They emerge from the intercostal spaces, and pierce the pectoralis major muscle and the deep fascia close to the sternum. One will be found in each intercostal interval except the first and, occasionally, the second; they give slender twigs to the skin over the sternum, and larger branches which run laterally and may be traced as far as the anterior fold of the axilla.

The small arteries that accompany those nerves are the perforating branches of an artery—the **internal thoracic**—which descends in the thorax immediately behind the costal cartilages. The perforating arteries of the second, third, and fourth spaces are fairly large in the female (especially the third), for they send branches to the mammary gland.

The **lateral cutaneous nerves,** much larger than the anterior, also arise from the intercostal nerves, and appear on the side of the thorax a little behind the anterior fold of the axilla; they will be examined when the axilla is dissected.

If the subject is female, the mammary gland should now be dissected, but it is well to take note of its position and connexions before beginning. Dissectors of male subjects should take the first opportunity of studying a dissection of the gland in a female subject.

17

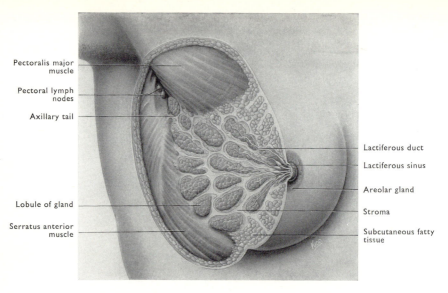

Pectoralis major
muscle

Pectoral lymph
nodes

Axillary tail

Lactiferous duct

Lactiferous sinus

Areolar gland

Lobule of gland

Stroma

Serratus anterior
muscle

Subcutaneous fatty
tissue

FIG. 5   Dissection of the right mammary gland.

THE BREAST

The mamma or breast is made up of:
(1) the mammary gland; (2) the superficial
fascia in which the gland is embedded; and
(3) the overlying skin, including the nipple
and the areola around the nipple.

In the male, the mammary gland is quite
rudimentary. The nipple is small and pointed,
and the areola is surrounded by sparse hairs,
which are never present in the female.

In the female, the **mammary gland** lies in the
superficial fascia, is composed largely of fat
in the non-lactating state, and is situated on
the front of the thorax and also, to some extent, on the side.

A little below its mid-point, and (unless it
is pendulous) at a level which usually corresponds to the fourth intercostal space, the
breast is surmounted by the **nipple,** which is
placed in the middle of a circular patch of
coloured skin known as the **areola** of the
breast. There is no fat under the areola or
in the nipple. A peculiar change of colour
occurs in this region during the second
month of a first pregnancy. At that time the

delicate pink colour of the skin of the nipple
and areola becomes converted to brown by
the deposition of pigment; and it never
again resumes its original appearance.

The base of the gland extends from the side
of the sternum almost to the mid-axillary line,
and from the second rib to the sixth costal
cartilage. About two-thirds of the gland is
placed on the pectoralis major muscle, whilst
the remaining part—its inferolateral third—
extends beyond the anterior fold of the axilla,
and lies on the serratus anterior muscle and
the external oblique muscle of the abdominal
wall. From the part related to the lower
border of the pectoralis major a prolongation
extends upwards into the axilla—the 'axillary
tail' of the breast—and reaches as high as the
third rib.

The mammary gland has no capsule, and
is not enclosed in a fascial sheath; in those
respects it differs from many other glands.
Its lobes and lobules are embedded in the
superficial fascia between strands of fibrous
tissue which pass through the superficial
fascia from the skin to the deep fascia. The
strands form the stroma or framework of the

18

gland, and the mammary blood vessels and some of its lymph vessels enter and leave the gland along these strands. They support and bind together the various parts of the true glandular tissue, which consists of branched tubes lined with cells, and they attach the gland both to the skin and to the deep fascia.

The main body of the gland is composed of gland tissue and stroma compactly arranged to form a wide-based conical mass. Many processes of stroma and gland substance project from the surface and borders of the central mass, and the fat deposited in the hollows between the projections gives the breast its smooth, rounded contour.

The gland tubes, which secrete the milk, are grouped together into distinct **lobes**—fifteen to twenty in number—each subdivided into **lobules,** and all separated from one another by the fibrous stroma. The **lactiferous ducts,** one from each lobe, converge upon the nipple. Under the areola, each duct expands to form a **lactiferous sinus,** and, narrowing again, opens independently on the summit of the nipple [FIG. 5].

In a well-injected body, twigs from the intercostal arteries and also from the perforating branches of the internal thoracic artery may be traced into the mammary gland. Mammary branches of the lateral thoracic artery may be seen winding round the edge of the pectoralis major, or piercing its lower fibres, to reach the gland.

Lymph Vessels of the Mammary Gland. The course of the lymph vessels of the mamma and the widespread situations of its primary lymph nodes are of the greatest importance in the spread of malignant growths and in determining the extent of tissue to be removed by the surgeon or the areas to be treated by the radiotherapist. The student should therefore study a textbook description of the lymph drainage of the mamma after they have dissected the axilla, where most of the nodes are situated [FIG. 11].

DISSECTION. Remove the fat from the surface of the gland, and define some of its lobes. Reflect the skin of the **areola** towards the nipple; if possible, pass a bristle into one of the ducts through its orifice on the nipple, and trace it to a lobe.

Next gradually detach the gland from the deep fascia. Begin at the upper border, and, as the gland is displaced, note the strands of the stroma which connect its deep surface with the deep fascia. Trace the process that extends from the lateral margin of the gland into the axilla.

Finally remove the gland by cutting the vessels at its margins, and then examine the deep fascia.

DEEP FASCIA

The **pectoral fascia** is a thin membrane which closely invests the pectoralis major It is attached above to the clavicle, and medially to the front of the sternum Below, it is continuous with the deep fascia that covers the abdominal muscles ; and, at the lower border of the pectoralis major muscle, it is continuous with the axillary fascia. Laterally, it is continuous with the fascia that covers the deltoid muscle. At the infraclavicular fossa, a process from its deep surface dips in between the deltoid and pectoralis major muscles to join the clavipectoral fascia, a membrane that lies behind the pectoralis major and forms part of the deeper layer of the anterior wall of the axilla [p. 23].

The **axillary fascia** is a dense, felted membrane which extends across the base of the axilla and is continuous with the fasciae of its walls. When the arm is raised, it is drawn up towards the hollow of the axilla due to the connexion of its deep surface with the fascial sheath of the pectoralis minor and the increased volume of the axilla.

DISSECTION. Cut through the deep fascia along the groove between the pectoralis major and the deltoid, and display the cephalic vein [Figs. 28, 30]. Follow it upwards to the infraclavicular fossa, where it disappears under cover of the pectoralis major. As you clean the vein, look for a small deltopectoral lymph node that sometimes lies alongside it.

Next clean the anterior part of the deltoid and the whole of the pectoralis major muscle.

Begin at the anterior border of the deltoid, and reflect the fascia until the base of the skin flap is reached. As the fascia is reflected, look for small cutaneous nerves : (1) lateral supraclavicular nerves over the upper part of the deltoid; (2) near the base of the skin flap, filaments of the upper lateral cutaneous

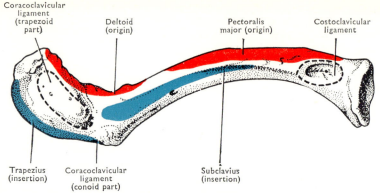

Fig. 6   Muscle attachments of inferior surface of right clavicle.

nerve of the arm; (3) other cutaneous twigs that pierce the anterior part of the deltoid [Figs. 28, 30].

To clean the pectoralis major: make the muscle tense by abducting the arm; begin at one or other border, and reflect the fascia upwards or downwards.

Deltopectoral Lymph Nodes. These nodes—one or two—lie in the groove between the deltoid and the pectoralis major [FIGS. 11, 26]. They are placed in the path of the superficial lymph vessels that run along the cephalic vein and convey lymph from the lateral side of the upper arm and shoulder, part of the forearm, and the upper part of the anterior thoracic wall and mammary gland, and transmit the lymph to the infraclavicular nodes, or direct to the apical nodes of the axilla [p. 27].

Pectoralis Major

The pectoralis major is a powerful muscle that extends from the front of the thorax to the humerus. It is divided by a deep fissure into clavicular and sternocostal portions. The **clavicular portion** arises from the medial half of the front of the clavicle. The **sternocostal portion** takes origin: (1) from the anterior surface of the sternum, (2) from the upper six costal cartilages, and (3) from the apo-neurosis of the external oblique muscle of the abdomen.

The muscle is inserted, by a flattened, bilaminar tendon, chiefly into the crest of the greater tubercle of the humerus.

The insertion is peculiar. The tendon of the sternocostal part is folded on itself to form a U, open superiorly and enclosing a bursa. The lowest fibres of the muscle pass into the upper part of the posterior layer, and the upper fibres into the upper part of the anterior layer; the rolled base of the U fills the edge of the anterior axillary fold. The

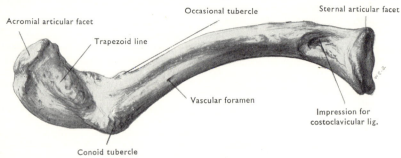

FIG. 7   Right clavicle (inferior surface).

20

clavicular part passes inferolaterally across the U-shaped tendon blending with its anterior layer and extending further inferiorly. Thus the whole muscle is V-shaped, the lowest sternocostal and the clavicular fibres lying at right angles to each other have separate, and even opposing, actions.

Nerve supply: the **lateral** and **medial pectoral nerves.** Action: as a whole it is an adductor and a medial rotator of the upper limb; when the limb is thrust backwards the pectoralis major assists in pulling it to the vertical position. The clavicular head, acting with the anterior fibres of the deltoid muscle [p. 56], is an active agent in flexion of the arm at the shoulder joint, a movement which can be reversed by the sternocostal head.

THE AXILLA

The axilla is the hollow between the upper part of the side of the thorax and the upper part of the arm. When the arm is abducted from the trunk, and the fatty tissue which occupies the axilla is removed, the space disclosed has the form of a truncated, three-sided pyramid. The apex is at the medial side of the coracoid process and is directed upwards towards the root of the neck; the base of the space looks downwards. The medial wall is the convex wall of the thorax, and the anterior and posterior walls converge on the blunt lateral edge formed by the humerus. The posterior wall is longer, from above downwards, than the anterior wall, and the posterior border of the base is therefore lower than the anterior.

Before beginning the dissection of the space, examine its boundaries and the manner in which the contents are disposed in relation to the boundaries.

BOUNDARIES AND CONTENTS OF THE AXILLA

The main walls of the axilla are anterior, posterior and medial.

The **anterior wall** consists of the two pectoral muscles, a small muscle below the clavicle called the subclavius, and the fascia which

encloses them. The pectoralis major forms the superficial stratum, and is spread out over the entire extent of the anterior wall. The pectoralis minor lies behind the middle third of the pectoralis major [Fig. 9]; and the fascia between it and the clavicle is the **clavipectoral fascia.** The lower border of the anterior wall is the **anterior fold** of the axilla and is formed by the pectoralis major.

The **posterior wall** of the axilla consists of: (1) the lateral part of the subscapularis muscle, (2) a portion of the latissimus dorsi and its tendon, and (3) the teres major muscle. The subscapularis covers the costal surface of the scapula. The latissimus dorsi winds from the back round the lower border of the teres major to gain its anterior surface; thus the lower border of the posterior wall—that is the **posterior fold** of the axilla—is formed in its medial part by the latissimus dorsi, and laterally by the teres major.

In the **medial wall** there is part of the serratus anterior muscle and, deep to it, parts of the upper five ribs with the intervening intercostal muscles.

The blunt lateral edge is formed by the humerus and the conjoined upper parts of the coracobrachialis muscle and the short head of the biceps muscle.

The **apex** of the space leads up into the narrow, triangular passage through which the axilla communicates with the neck. The passage is bounded anteriorly by the clavicle, medially by the outer border of the first rib, and posteriorly by the upper margin of the scapula; through it pass the axillary vessels and the big nerve cords of the brachial plexus on their way from the neck to the arm. Examine the boundaries of the passage from neck to axilla on the articulated skeleton.

The **base** or floor of the axilla is closed by the axillary fascia.

The most important **contents** are the axillary artery and vein, the large nerves of the upper limb, and the axillary lymph nodes. They are all embedded in soft fat. In the lower part of the axilla, the great vessels and nerves lie close to the lateral edge, and follow it in all the movements of the arm.

21

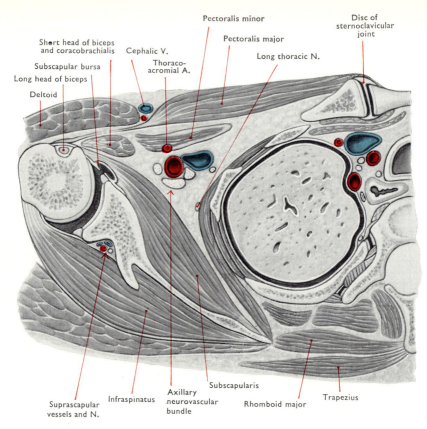

Short head of biceps and coracobrachialis
Subscapular bursa
Long head of biceps
Deltoid
Cephalic V.
Thoraco-acromial A.
Pectoralis minor
Pectoralis major
Long thoracic N.
Disc of sternoclavicular joint

Suprascapular vessels and N.
Infraspinatus
Axillary neurovascular bundle
Subscapularis
Rhomboid major
Trapezius

FIG. 8   Horizontal section at the level of shoulder joint (based on a section by Symington). The chief structures in the axilla and its walls are shown, and also the chief relations of the left sternoclavicular joint.

DISSECTION. Divide the clavicular head of pectoralis major below the clavicle, and turn it towards the insertion. As you do so, secure the branches of the lateral pectoral nerve as they pass into the muscle, and trace them back to the clavipectoral fascia. Follow the cephalic vein to the point where it pierces that fascia. Clean the small arteries in this region; they are branches of thoraco-acromial artery which also pierces the fascia. Clean the clavipectoral fascia and the fascia on the part of the pectoralis minor that has been exposed. Now cut vertically through the pectoralis major about 5 cm. from the sternum. Turn the medial part towards the median plane, and examine its attachments. Reflect the lateral part of the muscle towards the arm; while doing that, secure the medial pectoral nerve, which perforates the pectoralis minor and ends in the pectoralis

major. Clean the fascia that covers the remainder of the pectoralis minor. Reflect the pectoralis major fully, leaving a tag of muscle attached to the ends of its nerves; clean its tendon, and examine its insertion.

Complete reflexion of the pectoralis major exposes a thick, continuous sheet of fascia, which extends from the clavicle to the axillary fascia and from the wall of the thorax to the arm. It is because of the attachment of that fascial sheet to the clavicle above and to the axillary fascia below, that the floor of the axilla is raised as the arm is abducted and the clavicle is elevated. The pectoralis minor muscle, passing obliquely from its origin on the thoracic wall to its insertion into the coracoid process of the scapula, runs through the substance of the sheet and divides it into three parts: (1) The middle part encloses the muscle. (2) The lower part, as it extends downwards to blend with the axillary fascia, covers the lower parts of the axillary vessels and nerves. (3) The upper part is the clavipectoral fascia.

Clavipectoral Fascia

This fascia occupies the gap between the clavicle and the pectoralis minor, and extends from the first rib medially to the coracoid process laterally. Its upper part is split into two layers, an anterior and a posterior, which are attached to the clavicle, and enclose the **subclavius** between them. The strongest part of the membrane is that which extends along the lower border of the subclavius, from the first rib to the coracoid process. The membrane is continuous below with the fascial sheath of the pectoralis minor, and is connected posteriorly with the fascial sheath of the axillary vessels [Fig. 9]. It is perforated by the cephalic vein, the thoraco-acromial artery, and the lateral pectoral nerve. Note: (1) that the fibres of the membrane run horizontally; (2) that they are put on the stretch when the arm is abducted; and (3) that they are relaxed when the arm is by the side.

DISSECTION. Cut through the anterior layer of the upper part of the clavipectoral fascia, expose the subclavius muscle and examine the attachments of the fascia to the clavicle; then carefully remove the whole of the fascia.

Follow the cephalic vein to its junction with the axillary vein, and the thoraco-acromial artery and lateral pectoral nerve to their origins. Clean the proximal parts of the axillary artery and vein and the nerve cord from which the pectoral nerve springs. Find the small communicating nerve that connects the two pectoral nerves and crosses the axillary artery.

Clean the pectoralis minor muscle, without injuring the medial pectoral nerve, which pierces it.

Pectoralis Minor [Figs. 10, 12]

This is a triangular muscle which arises from the third, fourth and fifth ribs, close to their cartilages. Its fibres pass upwards and laterally, and its tendon of insertion is attached to the medial border and the upper surface of the coracoid process, near its tip.

Action: it draws the scapula downwards and forwards, and depresses the shoulder. In conjunction with other muscles it helps to fix the scapula and can assist in respiration by raising the ribs when the scapula is fixed. Nerve supply: **medial pectoral nerve.**

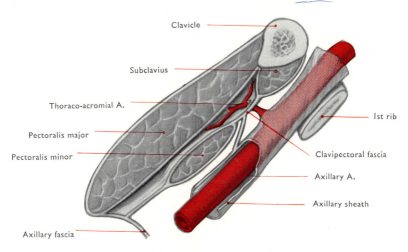

Clavicle

Subclavius

Thoraco-acromial A.

Pectoralis major

Pectoralis minor

Ist rib

Clavipectoral fascia

Axillary A.

Axillary sheath

Axillary fascia

Fig. 9   Diagram of clavipectoral fascia.

23

Lateral Cutaneous Branches of the Intercostal Nerves

These nerves emerge from the spaces between the ribs, divide into anterior and posterior branches under cover of the serratus anterior muscle and either pierce the muscle or appear between its digitations. The **anterior branches** appear, as a rule, about 2–3 cm. in front of the corresponding posterior branches,

and then pass forwards over the lower border of the pectoralis major muscle. From the lower members of this series some minute twigs are given to the external oblique muscle of the abdomen. The **posterior branches** run backwards over the latissimus dorsi muscle [FIG. 10].

The lateral cutaneous branch of the first intercostal nerve, though said to be constant, is seldom found. The lateral branch of the **second** nerve is the largest of the series, and differs from the others in not dividing into an anterior and a posterior branch. It is termed the **intercostobrachial nerve,** on account of its being distributed to the skin of the upper arm. To reach this destination it crosses the axilla and pierces the deep fascia of the arm a little below the posterior fold of the axilla. Before piercing the fascia it establishes communications with the medial cutaneous nerve of the arm and the lateral cutaneous branch of the third intercostal nerve. Branches from the plexus so formed supply the skin of the floor of the axilla.

The lateral cutaneous branch of the **third** intercostal nerve divides into an anterior and posterior part, which are distributed in the ordinary way, except that the posterior branch sends twigs to the skin of the floor of the axilla and of the upper part of the medial side of the arm.

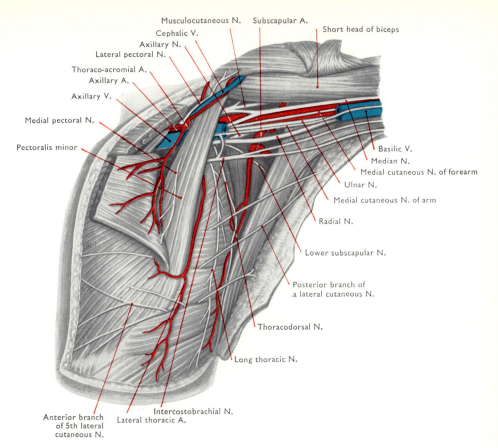

Musculocutaneous N.   Subscapular A.

Cephalic V.

Axillary N.   Short head of biceps

Lateral pectoral N.

Thoraco-acromial A.

Axillary A.

Axillary V.

Medial pectoral N.

Pectoralis minor

Basilic V.

Median N.

Medial cutaneous N. of forearm

Ulnar N.

Medial cutaneous N. of arm

Radial N.

Lower subscapular N.

Posterior branch of
a lateral cutaneous N.

Thoracodorsal N.

Long thoracic N.

Intercostobrachial N.

Anterior branch   Lateral thoracic A.
of 5th lateral
cutaneous N.

Fig. 10   Contents of axilla exposed by reflexion of pectoralis major and the fascia, and removal of fat and lymph nodes. Part of axillary vein has been removed to display the medial cutaneous nerve of forearm and ulnar nerve.

the axilla. Follow it next downwards and backwards, taking care not to injure the intercostobrachial nerve and the posterior branches of the 3rd, 4th and 5th lateral cutaneous nerves, as they cross in front of the artery. Near its lower end, secure the nerve (thoraco-dorsal) to latissimus dorsi, which crosses in front of the artery. Return to the angle between the subscapular artery and its circumflex branch; secure the lower subscapular nerve, and trace it into the teres major muscle.

Return to the radial nerve at the lower margin of the subscapularis muscle, and look for the branches that spring from the nerve near that point. They are the posterior cutaneous nerve of the arm and muscular branches to the long and medial heads of the triceps

muscle. They may arise separately or by a common stem. Trace them downwards.

The lateral thoracic and the subscapular branches of the axillary artery have now been found. Return to the axillary artery; find its other branches, and clean them.

After the lower part of the axilla has been thoroughly cleaned, divide the pectoralis minor midway between its origin and insertion, and turn the two parts aside. Secure the upper subscapular nerve as it enters the upper part of the subscapularis; and then clean the contents of the upper part of the axilla thoroughly.

When the dissection has been completed, the contents of the space must be studied in detail.

Axillary Lymph Nodes

These are spoken of, collectively, as the axillary nodes, but for convenience of description, they are divided into several subordinate groups each related to a particular drainage area. In the normal axilla, dissection seldom uncovers more than a few of the nodes, but representatives of three main groups are usually found: (1) A lateral or **brachial group** of six or more nodes which lie along the axillary vessels; they receive the lymph vessels from the greater part of the upper limb. (2) An anterior or **pectoral group** which lies in the angle between the anterior and medial walls of the axilla and is subdivided into upper and lower parts. Two or three upper pectoral nodes lie behind the pectoralis major in the region of the second and third intercostal spaces, and receive the main stream of lymph from the mammary gland through the sub-areolar and submammary lymph plexuses [FIG. 11]; the lower pectoral nodes lie along the lateral thoracic vessels, and receive

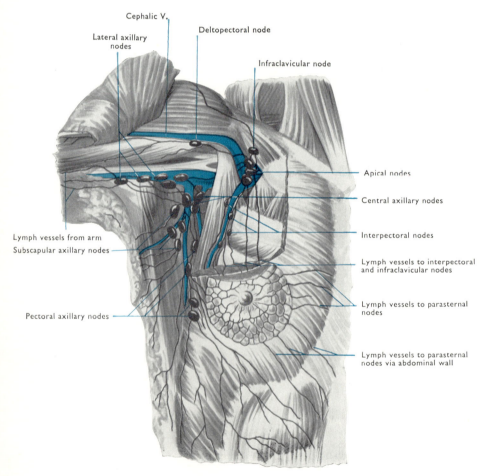

Cephalic V.

Lateral axillary nodes

Deltopectoral node

Infraclavicular node

Apical nodes

Central axillary nodes

Interpectoral nodes

Lymph vessels to interpectoral and infraclavicular nodes

Lymph vessels to parasternal nodes

Lymph vessels to parasternal nodes via abdominal wall

Lymph vessels from arm
Subscapular axillary nodes

Pectoral axillary nodes

FIG. 11   Lymph nodes and lymph vessels of axilla and mamma.

lymph from the side of the thorax. (3) A posterior or **subscapular group** which lies along the subscapular vessels on the posterior wall of the axilla, and receives lymph vessels mainly from the back.

The lymph nodes in the axilla drain a wide territory apart from the free upper limb—the pectoral region and the abdominal wall down to the level of the umbilicus, the side of the chest, the scapular region and the back down to the iliac crest. The regions above that territory are drained into the lymph nodes of the neck, and the regions below into the nodes of the groin—to which also there is a convergence of superficial lymph vessels from a wide area.

In addition to the lymph nodes which are usually seen in an ordinary dissection, there are three other groups of nodes: (1) The **central nodes,** which are very variable; they lie either on the surface of the axillary fascia, in a pocket of its substance, or deep to it in the fat of the middle part of the axilla; they have no afferents from any definite region, but connect the other groups together. (2) The *infraclavicular nodes,* which lie on the clavipectoral fascia in the infraclavicular fossa. One or two in number, they are associated with other nodes in two outlying situations— a few *interpectoral nodes* on the anterior surface of the pectoralis minor, which receive lymph from the deep part of the mammary gland by lymph vessels which pierce the pectoralis major, and the *deltopectoral nodes* [p. 20] and discharge into the next group. (3) The **apical nodes,** which lie in the apex of the axilla behind the clavipectoral fascia. They receive lymph from all the other groups, and their own efferents unite to form a vessel called the **subclavian lymph trunk,** which terminates usually in the subclavian vein.

Axillary Artery

The axillary artery is the chief artery of the upper limb. It begins, as a continuation of the subclavian artery, at the outer border of the first rib, enters the axilla through its apex, and runs along the lateral wall to the lower border of the teres major. There it leaves the axilla and becomes the brachial artery. The direction which the artery takes naturally varies with the position of the limb.

For convenience of description, the axillary artery is usually divided into parts—first, second and third; of these the second lies behind pectoralis minor. The three thick nerve cords that form the lower part of the brachial plexus are closely related to the first and second parts of the artery; and the large nerves that spring from the cords are grouped round the third part.

The **first part** of the axillary artery lies very deeply, behind the clavicular part of the pectoralis major, the clavipectoral fascia and the vessels and nerves superficial to it. Even when these are removed the vessel is not completely exposed, because it is enveloped, along with the axillary vein and brachial plexus, in a funnel-shaped sheath which is prolonged over them from the deep fascia of the neck [Fig. 15]. Posteriorly, it is separated from the first intercostal space and the first digitation of the serratus anterior by the nerve to that muscle and the medial cord of the brachial plexus. The axillary vein is on its medial side, and overlaps its anterior surface slightly; above and to its lateral side there are the lateral and posterior cords of the brachial plexus.

The **second part** is placed behind the two pectoral muscles, and has the three cords of the brachial plexus disposed around it. The axillary vein is still medial to it, but is separated by the medial cord.

The **third** is the longest part. It is superficial in its lower half, because the anterior wall of the axilla does not extend so far down as the posterior. The upper half is covered by the pectoralis major but its lower half by the skin and fasciae only. The medial root of the median nerve crosses in front of it at the lower border of the pectoralis minor. The axillary nerve and the radial nerve lie between it and the posterior wall of the axilla. The coracobrachialis muscle is on its lateral side, and also the median and musculocutaneous nerves, which lie between the muscle and the

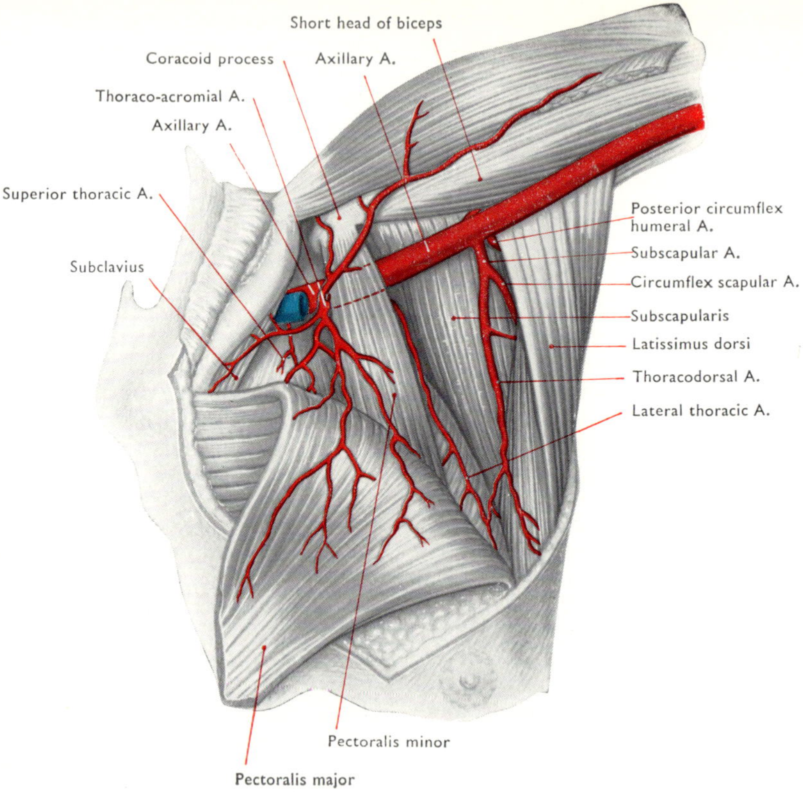
Short head of biceps
Coracoid process
Axillary A.
Thoraco-acromial A.
Axillary A.
Superior thoracic A.
Subclavius
Posterior circumflex humeral A.
Subscapular A.
Circumflex scapular A.
Subscapularis
Latissimus dorsi
Thoracodorsal A.
Lateral thoracic A.
Pectoralis minor
Pectoralis major

FIG. 12 Dissection of axillary artery and its branches.

artery. The axillary vein is on the medial side of the artery, with the medial cutaneous nerve of the forearm and the ulnar nerve between the artery and vein. More medially still, the medial cutaneous nerve of the arm lies along the medial side of the vein [FIG. 10].

Branches. The **superior thoracic artery** is a small branch that ramifies on the upper part of the medial wall of the axilla [FIG. 12].

The **thoraco-acromial artery** is a short, wide trunk which takes origin under cover of the pectoralis minor. It winds round the upper border of that muscle, pierces the clavipectoral fascia, and immediately divides into four small branches which diverge from one another and supply neighbouring structures; the largest of them runs downwards between the pectoral muscles. The **veins** that accompany those branches end in the cephalic vein.

The **lateral thoracic artery** skirts the lower border of the pectoralis minor on the side of the thorax. In the female, it is an important source of supply to the lateral part of the mammary gland.

The **subscapular artery** is the largest branch of the axillary. It runs downwards and backwards along the lower border of the subscapularis to the inferior angle of the scapula, giving off muscular branches. Note that it ends by entering the latissimus dorsi with the thoracodorsal nerve [FIG. 10]—a notable example of a neurovascular hilum [p. 8]. It gives off the **circumflex scapular** artery [FIG. 12], which takes a large share in the anastomosis around the scapula, and continues as the thoracodorsal artery.

The two circumflex humeral arteries arise at the same level—a short distance below the subscapular artery.

The **posterior circumflex humeral artery** is much the larger of the two. Only a small portion of it can be seen at the present stage. It springs from the back of the axillary artery, and at once passes backwards, with the axillary nerve, in the interval between the subscapularis and teres major muscles. It then curves round the surgical neck of the humerus, below the shoulder joint and under cover of the deltoid muscle [FIG. 32], supplying both.

The **anterior circumflex humeral artery** runs laterally, in front of the surgical neck of the humerus, under cover of the coracobrachialis and short head of the biceps brachii. Reaching the intertubercular sulcus, it divides into two branches, one of which runs up to the shoulder joint, while the other anastomoses with twigs of the posterior circumflex artery.

Axillary Vein

This vessel begins at the lower border of the teres major as the continuation of the basilic vein, and it becomes the subclavian vein at the outer margin of the first rib. It lies along the medial side of the axillary artery, overlapping it anteriorly ; and as the arm is abducted from the side the vein passes more and more in front of the artery.

At the lower margin of the subscapularis, it receives the two **venae comitantes** of the brachial artery ; and above the level of the pectoralis minor it is joined by the cephalic vein.

Subclavius

This small muscle lies immediately below the clavicle, enclosed between the two layers of the clavipectoral fascia. It takes origin, by a short, rounded tendon, from the upper surface of the first costal arch, at the junction of the bone with the cartilage ; and the fleshy belly is inserted into the floor of the shallow groove on the lower surface of the clavicle. Nerve supply is derived from the fifth and sixth cervical nerves and enters the posterior surface of the muscle. Action: it helps to steady the clavicle in movements of the shoulder girdle.

DISSECTION. When the subclavius has been examined divide it horizontally in order to find the costoclavicular ligament, which lies behind its medial end.

At this stage, examine the sternoclavicular joint with the aid of the dissectors of the Neck. Detach the clavicular head of the sternocleidomastoid from the clavicle, and pull the sternal head of the muscle towards the median plane in order to expose the upper and anterior surfaces of the joint.

Sternoclavicular Joint [FIG. 13]

This is a synovial joint at which the medial end of the clavicle fits into the shallow socket provided by the clavicular notch of the manubrium sterni and the upper surface of the first costal cartilage. It is the only point of articulation of the upper limb with the axial skeleton, and the clavicle, forming a strut to the shoulder, determines the range of its movements, and transmits to the trunk forces applied to the upper limb, *e.g.*, in falling on the outstretched hand. It is therefore a joint with a wide range of movement which carries heavy loadings and is consequently strengthened by powerful ligaments. The joint is enclosed in an articular capsule attached to the cartilage and the bones just beyond the margins of the articular surfaces. The anterior and posterior parts of the **fibrous capsule** are very strong and are called the **anterior** and **posterior sternoclavicular ligaments**. Associated with the joint there are an articular disc and two accessory ligaments— the interclavicular and the costoclavicular.

The **articular disc** is a nearly circular plate of fibrocartilage situated in the interior of the joint, which it divides into two separate **synovial cavities**. It is continuous with the anterior and posterior ligaments, but its main attachments are to the upper part of the medial end of the clavicle, and to the sternum and first costal cartilage at their junction ; it therefore acts as a ligament which prevents

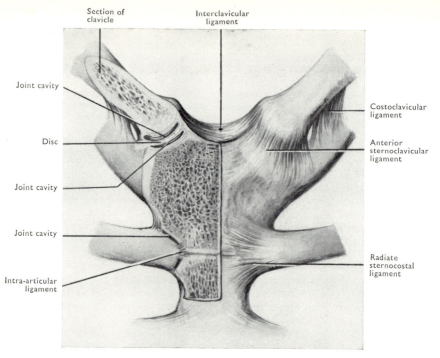

Section of clavicle

Interclavicular ligament

Joint cavity

Disc

Joint cavity

Joint cavity

Intra-articular ligament

Costoclavicular ligament

Anterior sternoclavicular ligament

Radiate sternocostal ligament

FIG. 13   Sternoclavicular and sternocostal joints.   A slice has been cut from the anterior surface of the sternum and clavicle, opening the sternoclavicular joint.

upward displacement of the sternal end of the clavicle.

The **interclavicular ligament** is fused with the upper part of the capsular ligament. It passes between the medial ends of the two clavicles, but dips down to be attached also to the upper border of the manubrium.

The **costoclavicular ligament** is a strong, thick, flattened band that lies behind the subclavius muscle. It is attached to the first rib and its cartilage at their junction, and extends upwards and laterally to a rough impression on the lower surface of the clavicle near its medial end.

Behind the joint there are two ribbon-like muscles of the neck—the **sternohyoid** and **sternothyroid**. They separate the right joint from a large artery called the **brachiocephalic trunk,** and the left joint from the **left brachio-cephalic vein** [FIG. 8].

DISSECTION. Cut through the anterior part of the capsule of the joint close to the sternum. Identify the sternohyoid and sternothyroid muscles in the root of the neck just above the joint, and a small vein, called the anterior jugular, that runs laterally in front of them. Push the vein out of the way, and detach the fibres of the sternohyoid that arise from the posterior ligament. Push the knife down behind the joint, cut the posterior ligament, and pull the clavicle laterally.

The articular disc is now exposed. Examine its attachments. Detach it from the costal cartilage; then carry the knife laterally below the clavicle and cut through the lower part of the capsule and the costoclavicular ligament. Displace the clavicle upwards and laterally to bring the whole of the brachial plexus into view.

THE BRACHIAL PLEXUS

This important plexus is formed by the ventral rami of the lower four cervical nerves and the greater part of the ventral ramus of the first thoracic nerve.   The plexus is rein-

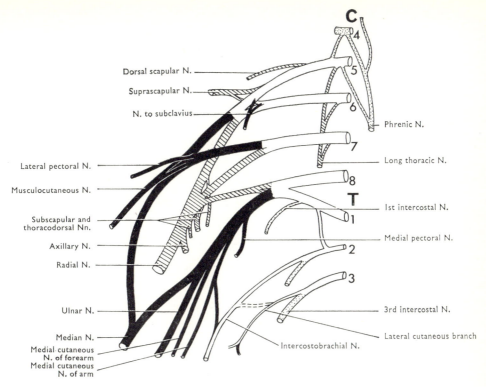

Fig. 14   Diagram of right brachial plexus.
Ventral offsets, black; dorsal offsets, cross hatched.   Cf. arrangement of the lumbosacral plexus, FIGS. 96,114.

forced, above, by a small twig of communication which passes from the fourth cervical nerve to the fifth, and, below, by a similar connecting twig that passes upwards, in front of the neck of the second rib, from the second thoracic nerve to the first.

The manner in which the nerves join to form the plexus is very constant. The **fifth** and **sixth cervical ventral rami** unite to form an **upper trunk**; the **seventh** remains single and proceeds laterally as a **middle trunk**; whilst the **eighth** and **first thoracic** join to form the **lower trunk**. A short distance above the clavicle each of the three trunks splits into an **anterior** and a **posterior division**. When the three anterior divisions are raised on the handle of a knife, it will be seen that the three

posterior divisions unite to form the **posterior cord** of the plexus and that the lowest or most medial of the posterior divisions is much smaller than the other two. Of the three anterior divisions, the upper two unite to form the **lateral cord** of the plexus, and the lower passes distally by itself as the **medial cord.** The three cords give off most of the branches that supply the upper limb [FIGS. 10, 14].

The plexus may be divided, therefore, into four stages:

First Stage .   Five separate ventral rami (viz., lower four cervical and first thoracic).

Second Stage .   Three trunks (viz., upper, middle and lower).

31

Third Stage . Three anterior divisions and three posterior divisions.

Fourth Stage . Three cords (viz., lateral, medial and posterior).

The plexus begins at the lateral border of the **scalenus anterior** muscle in the neck, behind the lower third of the posterior border of the sternocleidomastoid. It passes through the lower part of the posterior triangle of the neck, and through the cervico-axillary canal [FIG. 15] behind the middle third of the clavicle, into the upper part of the axilla. It ends behind the lower border of the pectoralis minor near the coracoid process, where it breaks up into the large nerves of the upper limb. Its termination is therefore at the junction of the second and third parts of the axillary artery. Consequently, the first and second parts of the artery are related to the cords of the plexus, and the third part is related to the large nerves that spring from them.

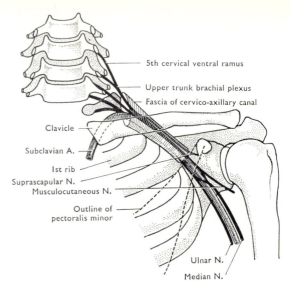

5th cervical ventral ramus
Upper trunk brachial plexus
Fascia of cervico-axillary canal
Clavicle
Subclavian A.
1st rib
Suprascapular N.
Musculocutaneous N.
Outline of pectoralis minor
Ulnar N.
Median N.

FIG. 15 A diagram to show the route of entry of the nerves and subclavian artery into the upper limb. The fascial sheath which binds these structures into a narrow bundle as they pass through the cervico-axillary canal is continuous medially with the prevertebral fascia and laterally with the axillary fascia. Compare with FIG. 98, and note how this single compact bundle is arranged to allow free movement of the upper limb without traction on its contents.

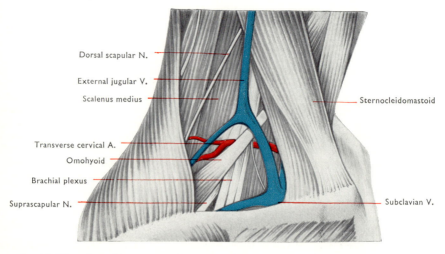

Dorsal scapular N.
External jugular V.
Scalenus medius
Transverse cervical A.
Omohyoid
Brachial plexus
Suprascapular N.
Sternocleidomastoid
Subclavian V.

FIG. 16 Dissection of lower part of posterior triangle of neck showing the supraclavicular part of brachial plexus. For the superficial branches of the cervical plexus, see FIG. 4.

As a rough guide to their position, it may be stated that the first two stages are in the neck, the third stage is behind the clavicle, and the last stage is in the axilla [FIGS. 15, 16]. The study of the plexus should therefore be undertaken jointly by the dissectors of the Upper Limb and of the Head and Neck.

The limb plexuses are so arranged that the branches which arise from the roots (in the neck) and cords (in the axilla) are composed of nerve fibres from more than one spinal or segmental nerve. A glance at FIGURE 14 shows that the segmental value of each cord is limited; the lateral cord to cervical (C.) 5–7, the medial cord to C. 8 and thoracic (T.) 1 (and 2), and the posterior cord to C. 5–8 (and T. 1). Thus the branches arising from each of these cords can only contain fibres from the same limited range of spinal nerves. A knowledge of these values is of importance in the diagnosis of injuries to the spinal nerves and the spinal medulla from which they arise. The lateral and medial cords, formed from ventral divisions, supply the ventral or flexor parts of the limb, while the dorsal divisions in the posterior cord supply the dorsal or extensor parts of the limb, there being some overlap in the case of the cutaneous nerves.

Branches of the Brachial Plexus

The following four branches *arise in the neck and are distributed in the upper limb.*

The **dorsal scapular nerve** (C. 5) runs downwards and laterally a little above the brachial plexus, disappears among muscles, and will be encountered again when the back is dissected.

The **suprascapular nerve** (C. 5, 6) runs laterally and downwards immediately above the plexus, disappears under the trapezius muscle, and will be further dissected in the scapular region.

The **nerve to subclavius** (C. 5, 6) descends in front of the plexus to enter the back of the subclavius muscle.

The **long thoracic nerve** (C. 5, 6, 7) runs most of its course in the axilla. It arises by three separate roots, which descend behind

the cervical part of the brachial plexus, and are therefore concealed by it. The upper two roots unite to form one stem which enters the axilla by crossing the first digitation of the serratus anterior behind the first part of the axillary artery, and gives twigs to the upper part of the muscle. The lower root descends close by that stem and joins it in the axilla. The nerve then runs downwards over the surface of the serratus anterior, about the junction of the anterior and middle thirds of the medial wall of the axilla, giving off twigs to each of its digitations.

Pectoral Nerves. These two nerves, which pass forwards on the lateral and medial sides of the first part of the axillary artery, communicate in front of it, and supply the pectoral muscles.

The **lateral pectoral nerve** (C. 5, 6, 7) springs from the lateral cord, pierces the clavipectoral fascia, and breaks up into branches which enter the deep surface of the pectoralis major.

The **medial pectoral nerve** (C. 8, T. 1) is smaller than the lateral. It springs from the medial cord, gives twigs of supply to the pectoralis minor, then pierces that muscle and ends in the pectoralis major.

The pectoralis major is thus supplied by both pectoral nerves, the pectoralis minor by the medial nerve alone.

Subscapular Nerves. The subscapular nerves (C. 5, 6) are two in number—the upper and the lower. They spring from the posterior cord of the plexus. After a very short course the upper nerve sinks into and supplies the upper and posterior part of the subscapularis. The lower subscapular nerve passes downwards and laterally, gives branches to the lower part of the subscapularis, and ends in the teres major, which it supplies.

Thoracodorsal Nerve. This nerve (C. 6, 7, 8) springs from the posterior cord between the two subscapular nerves, passes obliquely downwards and laterally through the axilla, and crosses in front of the subscapular artery to enter the deep surface of the latissimus dorsi at the inferior angle of the scapula. It is

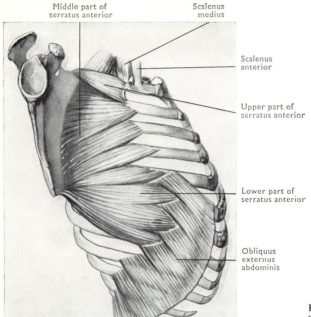

Middle part of
serratus anterior

Scalenus
medius

Scalenus
anterior

Upper part of
serratus anterior

Lower part of
serratus anterior

Obliquus
externus
abdominis

FIG. 17   Serratus anterior and origin of external oblique.   The
scapula is drawn away from the
side of the chest.

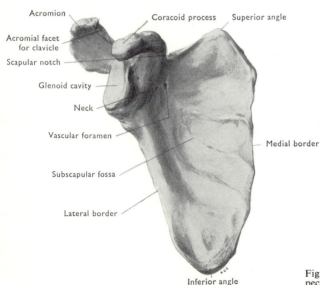

Acromion

Coracoid process   Superior angle

Acromial facet
for clavicle

Scapular notch

Glenoid cavity

Neck

Vascular foramen

Medial border

Subscapular fossa

Lateral border

Inferior angle

Fig. 18   Right scapula (costal aspect).   See also FIGURE 33.

accompanied into the muscle by the terminal branch of the subscapular artery [p. 28].

The other branches which spring from the cords will be described later.

THE SERRATUS ANTERIOR

This large and powerful muscle arises by fleshy digitations from the upper eight ribs about midway between their angles and cartilages. The slips are arranged on the chest wall so as to present a gentle curve convex forwards. The lower three interdigitate with the external oblique muscle of the abdomen. The serratus anterior sweeps posteriorly round the thorax and is inserted

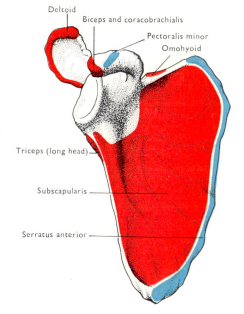

Deltoid
Biceps and coracobrachialis
Pectoralis minor
Omohyoid
Triceps (long head)
Subscapularis
Serratus anterior

FIG. 19 Muscle attachments to costal surface of right scapula. See also FIGURE 34.

into the entire length of the medial margin of the scapula [FIG. 19], and it falls naturally into three parts [FIG. 17]. The scapular attachments will be more fully examined when the subscapularis muscle is dissected [p. 59].

(1) The **upper part** is composed of the first digitation, which is the largest of the series. It arises from the first and second ribs and from a tendinous arch between them; its fibres converge to be inserted into a triangular area on the costal surface of the upper angle of the scapula. (2) The **middle part** consists of the two digitations from the second and third ribs, and its fibres spread out to be inserted into the anterior lip of the medial margin of the scapula. (3) The **lower part** is composed of the remaining digitations of the muscle. They converge to form a thick mass which is inserted into a rough area on the costal surface of the inferior angle of the scapula.

The deep surface of the serratus anterior is in contact with the chest wall.

Action: it is the most powerful protractor of the whole upper limb and holds the scapula against the chest wall, so that when paralysed the scapula stands out like a wing on pressing forwards with the outstretched arm. It assists in the upward rotation of the scapula that accompanies the raising of the arm above the head [FIG. 51]. Its usual action may be reversed so that, acting from the scapula, it raises the ribs in forced inspiration. Nerve supply: the long thoracic nerve from the ventral rami C. 5, 6, and 7 [p. 33].

CARE OF THE DISSECTION. After the dissectors have examined the serratus anterior and carefully revised the contents of the axilla, they must replace the clavicle, pack the axilla with tow or rags soaked in preservative fluid, and fix the skin flaps to the wall of the thorax with a few stitches.

THE DISSECTION OF THE BACK

Turn the body face downwards, and examine the structures which connect the limb with the back of the trunk.

This dissection should be completed before the dissectors of the Head and Neck continue the deeper dissection of the back.

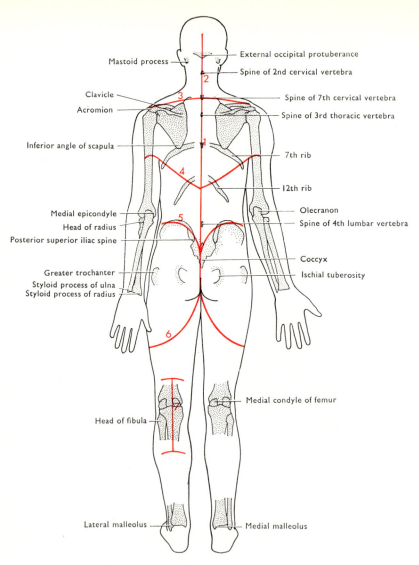

Mastoid process

External occipital protuberance

Spine of 2nd cervical vertebra

Clavicle

Acromion

Spine of 7th cervical vertebra

Spine of 3rd thoracic vertebra

Inferior angle of scapula

7th rib

12th rib

Medial epicondyle

Head of radius

Posterior superior iliac spine

Olecranon

Spine of 4th lumbar vertebra

Coccyx

Ischial tuberosity

Greater trochanter

Styloid process of ulna

Styloid process of radius

Medial condyle of femur

Head of fibula

Lateral malleolus

Medial malleolus

FIG. 20   Landmarks and incisions.   For the bony landmarks of the upper limb, see illustrations of individual bones.

SURFACE ANATOMY

The **scapula** is obliquely placed at a tangent to the posterolateral part of the upper thorax, covering parts of the second to the seventh ribs; and, though it is thickly covered with muscles, a great part of its outline can be made out.   Find the **acromion** at the top of the shoulder.   Draw your finger along the bony ridge (**crest of the spine** of the scapula) that runs in a medial direction and slightly downwards from the acromion to the **medial** border of the scapula. Palpate the medial border through the muscles that cover it, and trace it to the **upper** and **lower angles** of the scapula. The scapula is very movable. When the arms are folded across the chest, the scapulae are drawn apart, and their medial borders are 10–12 cm. from the median line. When the arm hangs by the side, the medial border is 3–5 cm. from the median line. The upper angle overlies the **second rib;** the lower angle—much more easily felt than the upper—usually overlies the **seventh rib.**

The rib felt inferior to the scapula is therefore usually the **eighth rib;** and the lower ribs can be counted from it. If the **twelfth** is long enough to reach beyond the lateral edge of the erector spinae (*i.e.*, the mass of muscle in the small of the back), its tip is about 3 cm. above the iliac crest.

The **iliac crest** is the bony ridge felt below the waist. Trace it backwards. Its posterior end is called the **posterior superior iliac spine,** and is the bone felt in the shallow dimple in the skin above the buttock about 5 cm. from the median line. The uneven bone felt between the right and left dimples is the back of the **sacrum.** Usually it has three spines that can be felt in the median line. The **coccyx** is the bone felt deeply between the buttocks.

The **median furrow** of the back varies in depth with the muscularity of the body. It is deepest in the upper part of the loin; it fades away inferiorly and is succeeded by the cleft between the buttocks. The **spines** of the vertebrae are felt in the furrow: pass the finger over them. Note that their tips do not all lie in the median line: some are deflected to one side or the other. The spines are the only parts of the vertebral column that are felt easily, but it is very seldom possible to identify individual spines directly. Some of them, however, can be identified because they are at the same level as recognizable landmarks; and the positions of the others can be gauged from them. The **second sacral** spine is at the level of the posterior superior iliac spine; the **fourth lumbar** is at the level of the highest part of the iliac crest; the

seventh thoracic is at the level of the lower angle of the scapula; and the **third thoracic** is at the level of the point where the crest and medial border of the scapula meet. The **seventh cervical** spine can be identified directly: it is the uppermost of the knobs in the median line at the root of the back of the neck; hence it is called the **vertebra prominens.** Pass your finger upwards in the nuchal groove over the other cervical spines. The uppermost one felt is the spine of the **second cervical** or **axis** vertebra (the first, or atlas, has no spine); it is about 5 cm. below the **external occipital protuberance** on the lower part of the back of the head at the top of the nuchal groove. Run your finger from the protuberance in a lateral direction and feel the curved ridge on the back of the skull called the **superior nuchal line.** Between the muscles of the two sides of the back of the neck there is a fibrous partition called the **ligamentum nuchae**; its posterior edge stretches from the occipital protuberance to the seventh cervical spine. The upper part of the first muscle encountered in the dissection of the back—the **trapezius**—arises from the superior nuchal line, the external occipital protuberance and the ligamentum nuchae.

DISSECTION. Reflexion of the Skin: Make incisions 1, 3, 4 and 5 [Fig. 20]. The two large flaps which are now mapped out on the back must be carefully reflected laterally together with the superficial fascia which may be infiltrated with fluid if the body has lain long on the back. As far as possible separate the superficial fascia from the deep by blunt dissection to expose the cutaneous nerves as they pierce the latter; this is difficult because of the greater density of the connexions between the two fasciae on the dorsal surface, particularly in the lumbosacral region. Trace the cutaneous nerves through the superficial fascia laterally [Fig. 21].

CUTANEOUS NERVES

The cutaneous nerves of the back are derived from the dorsal rami of the spinal nerves. As the dorsal rami pass backwards, they divide into medial and lateral branches (FIG. 1, p. 6). Both branches supply twigs to the muscles amongst which they lie; but the

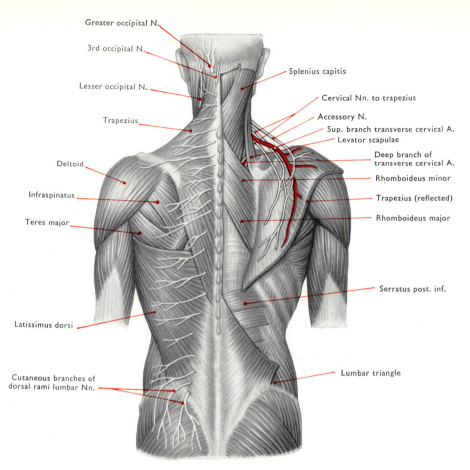

Greater occipital N.

3rd occipital N.

Lesser occipital N.

Trapezius

Deltoid

Infraspinatus

Teres major

Latissimus dorsi

Cutaneous branches of
dorsal rami lumbar Nn.

Splenius capitis

Cervical Nn. to trapezius

Accessory N.

Sup. branch transverse cervical A.

Levator scapulae

Deep branch of
transverse cervical A.

Rhomboideus minor

Trapezius (reflected)

Rhomboideus major

Serratus post. inf.

Lumbar triangle

FIG. 21   Dissection of superficial muscles and nerves of the back.

upper six or **seven thoracic** cutaneous nerves are the terminations of the medial branches and therefore lie near the median plane, though one or more may pierce the trapezius 3–5 cm. lateral to the line of the others. The second thoracic branch is the largest of the series, and may be traced, across the spine of the scapula, as far as the shoulder. The **lower five** or **six** come from the lateral branches of the dorsal rami of the thoracic nerves, and lie at some distance from the median line. The upper nerves of this group pierce the latissimus dorsi muscle on the line of the angles of the ribs. The lower nerves appear at the lateral margin of the erector spinae muscle by piercing the **thoracolumbar fascia,** which is the very thick deep fascia of the small of the back.

Each of these cutaneous branches divides into a small medial branch and a larger lateral branch, which runs laterally and downwards for a varying distance in the superficial fascia. Thus the area of skin supplied by each of these cutaneous nerves is placed at a lower level than the origin of the dorsal ramus from which it arises.

In the **lumbar region,** three cutaneous nerves reach the surface after piercing the lumbar part of the thoracolumbar fascia at the lateral margin of the erector spinae muscle, a short distance above the iliac crest. They are the terminal twigs of the lateral branches of the dorsal rami of the upper three lumbar nerves, and they differ from the nerves above them in that they turn downwards over the iliac crest to supply the skin of the gluteal region [FIG. 21].

The **cutaneous arteries** which accompany the cutaneous nerves of the back are derived from the posterior branches of the intercostal and lumbar arteries.

DORSAL MUSCLES THAT ATTACH THE UPPER LIMB TO THE TRUNK

There are five muscles in this group, arranged in two strata. The trapezius and the latissimus dorsi form the **superficial stratum.** Both are broad, and they cover the greater part of the back of the trunk from the occiput to the iliac crest. The trapezius lies in the back of the neck and the thorax ; the latissimus dorsi lies in the thorax and in the loin. The **deeper stratum** of muscles, composed of the levator scapulae and the two rhomboid muscles, is under cover of the trapezius.

DISSECTION. Clean away the deep fascia from the trapezius, taking care of the cutaneous nerves. That muscle belongs only in part to the dissectors of the Upper Limb. The portion of it which lies above the spine of the seventh cervical vertebra is the property of the dissectors of the Head and Neck, and should be dissected by them. The dissectors of the two parts should work in conjunction; and when the whole of the trapezius is exposed they should give one another an opportunity of studying it in its entirety.

During this dissection keep the trapezius on the stretch by placing the arm close to the trunk and depressing the scapula.

As the deep fascia is removed from the trapezius— and indeed throughout the whole dissection of the back—the cutaneous nerves must be carefully preserved, in order that the dissectors of the Head and Neck may have an opportunity of establishing their continuity with the dorsal rami from which they arise.

Trapezius

The trapezius is a triangular muscle which lies, in its entire extent, immediately subjacent to the deep fascia. It has a very long origin which extends, along the median plane, from the occiput to the spine of the last thoracic vertebra. It arises from : (1) the medial third of the superior nuchal line and from the external occipital protuberance ; (2) the ligamentum nuchae and the spine of the seventh cervical vertebra ; (3) the tips of the spines of all the thoracic vertebrae, as well as the supraspinous ligaments which bridge across the intervals between them [FIG. 21].

In the lower cervical and upper thoracic regions the tendinous fibres by which the two muscles arise lengthen out to form a flat tendon which is oval or diamond-shaped in outline, thus increasing the effective area of origin for a bulky portion of the muscle ; in the living body this is indicated by a depression of corresponding shape when the muscles are contracted.

As the fibres of the trapezius pass laterally they converge upon their insertions into the two bones of the shoulder girdle. The **occipital** and **upper cervical fibres** incline downwards, and then turn forwards over the shoulder to be inserted into the lateral third of the clavicle [FIG. 23]. The **lower cervical** and **upper thoracic fibres** pass more or less transversely to gain an insertion into the medial aspect of the acromion and the superior margin of the crest of the spine of the scapula. The **lower thoracic fibres** are directed upwards, and, at the medial border of the scapula, end in a flat, triangular tendon which plays over the smooth surface at the medial end of the scapular spine and is inserted into a rough tubercle on the crest immediately lateral to that surface [FIG. 34, p. 60]. To facilitate the movement of the tendon upon the bone, a small synovial bursa is interposed between them.

Nerve supply: page 41. Action: from its extensive origin this muscle acts on the scapula in a variety of ways, controlling its position in movements of the upper limb as a whole, and of the arm at the shoulder joint. Its upper

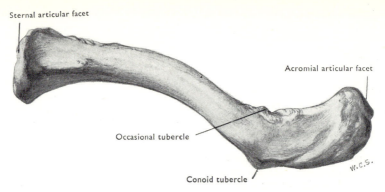

Sternal articular facet

Acromial articular facet

Occasional tubercle

Conoid tubercle

W.C.S.

FIG. 22 Right clavicle (superior surface).

fibres elevate the shoulder, its lower fibres depress the medial part of the scapula. Acting together, these two parts rotate the scapula when the arm is raised above the head, and its middle fibres retract the scapula as the shoulders are braced backwards.

DISSECTION. The latissimus dorsi is now to be dissected. It is a difficult muscle to clean, not only on account of the varying direction of its fibres, but also because its upper part is generally very thin, and its upper border ill-defined.

Define the attachment of the muscle to the thoraco-lumbar fascia [Fig. 21], and clean that fascia. Next

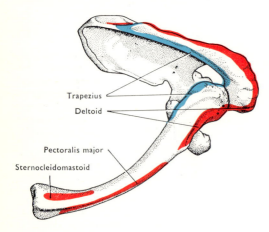

Trapezius

Deltoid

Pectoralis major

Sternocleidomastoid

FIG. 23 Shoulder girdle from above showing muscle attachments

40

define the attachment of the muscle to the iliac crest; and, when the lower part of the lateral border of the latissimus is reached, note the costal slips attached to the lowest three or four ribs, and also the slips of the external oblique muscle of the abdomen which interdigitate with them.

Evert the upper margin of the muscle as it crosses the inferior angle of the scapula, and display the slip which springs from that angle. This scapular slip is liable to be mistaken for a piece of the teres major muscle, upon which it lies.

Latissimus Dorsi

The latissimus dorsi is a wide, thin muscle which covers the back from the level of the sixth thoracic vertebra down to the iliac crest [FIG. 21]. The greater part of it is immediately beneath the deep fascia, but its upper part, near the spines, is under cover of the trapezius. It arises: (1) from the tips of the lower six thoracic spines and the corresponding supraspinous ligaments; (2) from the thoracolumbar fascia [FIG. 24]; (3) from the outer lip of the iliac crest, in front of the fascia [FIG. 21]; (4) from the lower three or four ribs; and (5) by a fleshy slip from the back of the inferior angle of the scapula [FIG. 34].

Its fibres converge rapidly towards the lower part of the scapula, and it sweeps over the inferior angle in the form of a thick, fleshy band which winds round the flat margin of the teres major and terminates in a thin, flat tendon, which is inserted chiefly

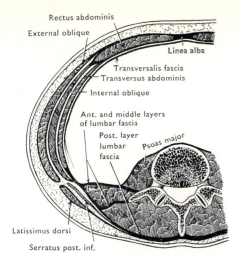

Rectus abdominis
External oblique
Linea alba
Transversalis fascia
Transversus abdominis
Internal oblique
Ant. and middle layers
of lumbar fascia
Post. layer
lumbar
fascia
Psoas major
Latissimus dorsi
Serratus post. inf.

Fig. 24   Diagram of thoracolumbar fascia in a section through the trunk at level of second lumbar vertebra.

into the floor of the intertubercular groove of the humerus [Fig. 40]. The insertion cannot be studied at present, but will be seen later [p. 61].

With the teres major muscle, the latissimus dorsi forms the posterior fold of the axilla. At first it is placed behind the teres major, then it is folded round its lower border, and finally it is inserted in front of it. To the peculiar relationship of the two muscles is due the full, rounded appearance of the posterior axillary fold.

Nerve supply: the **thoracodorsal nerve** (C. 6, 7, 8) from the posterior cord of the brachial plexus. Action: it is an adductor, retractor, and medial rotator of the upper limb, but its most powerful action is in drawing the arm down from above the head, as in climbing.

Intermuscular Space

A triangular space bounded by the trapezius, the latissimus dorsi, and the scapula [Fig. 21] exposes a small portion of the rhomboideus major muscle, and also a varying amount of the wall of the thorax—the borders of the sixth and seventh ribs and the space between

them. This is the only part of the back of the thorax which is not covered with muscles; and has been called the **triangle of auscultation** because, with the stethoscope, breath sounds are supposed to be heard better there than anywhere else on the back.

DISSECTION. Reflect the trapezius, working, if possible, with the dissectors of the Head and Neck. Divide the muscle about 5 cm. from the median plane, and turn it towards its insertion. The trapezius is very thin at its origin ; take great care, therefore, not to injure the subjacent rhomboid muscles. Clean and preserve the vessels and nerves on the deep surface of the muscle; and look for the bursa that lies between its tendon and the medial end of the spine of the scapula.

Nerves and Vessels of Trapezius. The trapezius gets its nerve supply from two sources, a motor supply from the **accessory nerve** (11th cranial) and sensory branches from the **third** and **fourth cervical nerves** as they cross the posterior triangle of the neck. On the deep surface of the trapezius they form a plexus from which twigs proceed into the muscle. The accessory nerve can be traced nearly to the lower end of the trapezius, and it is accompanied by the **superficial branch of the transverse cervical artery** [Fig. 21]. Twigs from the **deep branch** of the same artery appear close to the medial border of the scapula.

DISSECTION. Divide the trapezius into upper and lower parts by a transverse cut equidistant between the clavicle and the spine of the scapula, and examine the insertion of the muscle. Next, clean away the fat in the area exposed, and display the inferior belly of the omohyoid muscle, the suprascapular vessels and nerve, and the fascia over the supraspinatus. The supraspinatus covers the scapula between the spine and the upper border of the bone. The inferior belly of the omohyoid is attached to the lateral part of the upper border. The superior transverse scapular artery crosses the suprascapular ligament immediately lateral to the omohyoid, and the nerve is below the ligament; clean the parts of them seen now.

The next step is to define the muscles that connect the medial margin of the scapula to the vertebral column. From above downwards, they are (1) the **levator scapulae**, (2) the **rhomboideus minor**, (3) the **rhomboideus major**. Put them on the stretch and clean their surfaces.

Omohyoid, Levator Scapulae and Rhomboid Muscles

The **omohyoid** muscle stretches from the scapula to the hyoid bone in the neck, and has two slender bellies united by an intervening tendon. The **inferior belly** arises from the superior transverse scapular ligament and the upper border of the scapula, and passes upwards and forwards into the neck to join the tendon.

The **levator scapulae** is a thick, elongated muscle that arises by slips from the posterior tubercles of the transverse processes of the upper four cervical vertebrae and passes downwards and backwards to be inserted into the medial margin of the scapula from the upper angle to the spine. Nerve supply: the **dorsal scapular nerve** and by branches from the **third** and **fourth cervical nerves**.

The two rhomboid muscles extend as parallel bands obliquely downwards and laterally from the spines of the vertebrae to the scapula. The **rhomboideus minor** runs from the ligamentum nuchae and the seventh cervical spine to the medial margin of the scapula opposite its spine [Fig. 34].

The **rhomboideus major**, about twice the width of the minor, extends from the upper thoracic spines and supraspinous ligaments to the medial margin of the scapula from the spine to the inferior angle [Fig. 34].

Nerve supply: the **dorsal scapular nerve** from the fifth cervical ventral ramus. Action: they pull the scapula upwards, draw it towards the midline and, acting with latissimus dorsi, rotate the glenoid downwards.

DISSECTION. Complete the cleaning of the levator scapulae, taking care not to injure its nerves. With the dissectors of the Head and Neck, study its attachments and nerve supply; then divide the muscle across its middle and turn the lower half towards its insertion. Secure the dorsal scapular nerve and the deep branch of the transverse cervical artery, which lie deep to the muscle, and follow them to the rhomboideus minor.

Next cut through the rhomboids midway between the scapula and the spines of the vertebrae; remember that they are very thin, and take care not to injure the thin muscle, serratus posterior superior, which is immediately subjacent to them. Turn the medial part of each muscle towards the vertebral spines and examine its attachment. Turn the lateral parts towards the scapula, and follow the dorsal scapular nerve and the deep branch of the transverse cervical artery to their terminations.

The **dorsal scapular nerve** (C. 5) is a long, slender nerve and usually arises in common with the upper root of the long thoracic nerve. It passes downwards and laterally and, accompanied by the **deep branch of the transverse cervical artery**, descends under cover of the levator scapulae and the two rhomboids, near the scapula. It supplies one or two twigs to the levator scapulae and ends in the rhomboids.

DISSECTION. Divide the latissimus dorsi from the inferior angle of the scapula to a point below the origin of the muscle from the last rib. Remember that the muscle is thin, and do not injure the parts subjacent to it. Turn the medial portion towards the vertebral spines—avoiding injury to the thin muscle, serratus posterior inferior, which runs from the thoracolumbar fascia horizontally to the lower four ribs—and examine the origin of the latissimus [p. 40]. Throw the lateral part of the muscle forwards and, at the inferior angle of the scapula, find its nerve supply.

The upper limb should not be removed from the trunk unless it is essential to allow access to the thorax, in which case the limb is removed as follows:

1. Divide the suprascapular artery and nerve and the inferior belly of the omohyoid at the upper border of the scapula.

2. Divide the dorsal scapular nerve and the deep branch of the transverse cervical artery near the upper angle of the scapula.

3. Pull the scapula away from the ribs, and cut through the posterior part of the serratus anterior about 2 cm. from its medial margin.

4. Pull the scapula still further away from the thorax and divide the axillary vessels and the brachial plexus at the outer border of the first rib; also the intercostobrachial nerve.

5. Detach the anterior skin flap previously stitched to the anterior wall of the thorax, and take the limb to another table.

6. In preparation for further dissection, separate the axillary vessels and the cords of the brachial plexus from one another; tie them to a short piece of wood in their proper relative positions, and fix it to the coracoid process.

THE FREE UPPER LIMB

SURFACE ANATOMY

Place the fingers on the lateral side of the arm just below the acromion, and move the arm in any direction. The upper end of the humerus is felt moving under cover of the deltoid muscle; the part of it felt is the **greater tubercle** [FIG. 39]; the **lesser tubercle** is felt on the front. Follow the shaft downwards until, about half-way down on the lateral side, the **deltoid tuberosity** can be felt rather indistinctly. Immediately below and behind the tuberosity the **radial nerve** can usually be felt against the bone, though the nerve is covered with muscle. As the elbow is approached the humerus widens from side to side, and acquires fairly sharp margins— the **lateral** and **medial supracondylar ridges**; the lateral ridge is the more outstanding and the more easily felt. The projecting ends of the ridges are the epicondyles of the humerus. The **lateral epicondyle** is not prominent, but is easily felt in the upper part of a shallow depression on the back of the limb. The **medial epicondyle** is prominent. It can be seen as well as felt. Grip it between finger and thumb, and note that it inclines slightly backwards. The **ulnar nerve** passes behind the medial epicondyle and can be rolled between the finger and the bone. When the arm hangs loosely by the side, the medial epicondyle fits into the curve of the waist and the humerus is then so placed that the lateral epicondyle is well round to the front. It is only when the arm is held with the palm looking forwards that the epicondyles occupy the relative positions indicated by their names. It should be noted that in this position, owing to the obliquity of the plane of the elbow joint, the forearm is not in line with the upper arm but is directed outwards at the so-called 'carrying angle'.

The fleshy, bulging mass on the front of the upper arm is composed chiefly of the **biceps brachii**. Place your fingers on the medial margin of the biceps near the elbow, push the biceps away, press the fingers backwards and move them from side to side. The cord felt is the **median nerve** and, in the living limb, the pulsations of the **brachial artery** are felt. On each side of the biceps there is a faint, shallow groove. The vein seen through the skin on the surface of the biceps, in front of the lateral groove, is the **cephalic vein**. The vein seen in the medial groove is the **basilic vein**. At the upper part of the medial groove there is a narrow ridge produced by the **coracobrachialis muscle**; the lower part of the **axillary artery** and the upper part of the **brachial artery** lie close behind and medial to the ridge, and can be seen beating in the living limb. The **tendon of insertion of the biceps** is readily felt in the middle of the front of the elbow when the elbow is bent, and on the medial side of it the edge of the **bicipital aponeurosis** can be felt also.

The **coronoid process** of the ulna is hidden under muscles, but the tubercle on its medial margin can be felt about 2·5 cm. below the medial epicondyle. The **olecranon** of the ulna is the bony prominence at the back of the elbow; the skin moves freely over the back of it, because a bursa is placed between them. Note the relative positions of the olecranon and the epicondyles during the movements of the elbow. It is with reference to their normal relative positions that the surgeon can distinguish among the different forms of fracture and dislocation that occur so often at the elbow. When the elbow is straightened out to its full extent, the three prominences lie in the same horizontal plane; when it is bent to a right angle, they are at the angles of a triangle that is nearly equilateral.

The **posterior border of the ulna** is subcutaneous from end to end, and can be felt as a sharp edge that runs downwards from the olecranon. It ends at the styloid process of the ulna [FIGS. 76, 84, 88]. The **styloid process** makes a blunt ridge on the medial side where the forearm joins the wrist. When the palm faces forwards or upwards, the process is seen and felt at the medial margin of the back of the forearm; when the palm faces backwards or downwards, the process is on the medial surface of the forearm, and, in its place on the back, there appears a smooth, rounded prominence which is the **head of the ulna.** The distal third of the medial surface of the shaft of the ulna also is subcutaneous and easily felt.

The **head of the radius** lies below the lateral epicondyle in the lower part of the depression on the back of the limb. Place your finger tip in the depression and feel the transverse groove between the humerus and the head of the radius. Rotate the hand backwards and forwards: the head of the radius can be felt rotating, though it is covered by a strong ligament called the **anular ligament.** The **shaft of the radius** is buried among muscles, but can be felt through them. The **distal end of the radius** is a block of bone that can be felt at the distal end of the forearm, on both back and front and also on the lateral side. Feel for its **dorsal tubercle** on the back towards the lateral side. When the living thumb is stretched out from the palm a hollow appears between the tendons on the lateral side of the back of the wrist. This hollow is popularly known as the 'anatomical snuff-box', and the **styloid process of the radius** is the bone felt in the upper part of its floor.

Now, examine the palm of your own hand. The **hypothenar eminence** or ball of the little finger is the smooth, soft elevation along the medial side of the hollow of the palm. It overlies the fifth metacarpal bone, and is composed of the short muscles of the little finger. Feel the **pisiform bone** at the upper end of the eminence; the tendon which is felt above it is the **flexor carpi ulnaris.** Grip the pisiform bone between finger and thumb, and note that it can be moved slightly on the **triquetrum,** which is the bone concealed behind the pisiform. The **hook of the hamate bone** also may be felt obscurely a little below and lateral to the pisiform (FIG. 60).

The **thenar eminence** or ball of the thumb is the ovoid, fleshy elevation that overlies the first metacarpal bone, and is composed of three of the small muscles of the thumb. The tendons of two muscles, called the **flexor carpi radialis** and the **palmaris longus,** are seen descending side by side in the middle of the forearm towards the wrist. The flexor carpi radialis is the more lateral of the two, and it disappears at the upper medial part of the thenar eminence. Place your finger in the angle between the eminence and the tendon; the bone felt there is the tubercle of the scaphoid. Immediately distal to this tubercle of the trapezium is felt indistinctly in the thenar eminence immediately distal to the scaphoid. The skin crease that runs across the front of the limb at the level of the uppermost parts of the pisiform and the tubercle of the scaphoid marks the junction of the forearm and the wrist, and marks also the position of the upper border of a very strong ligament called the **flexor retinaculum.**

The Palm. Note that the skin of the palm is relatively immobile as compared with that over the rest of the limb. When the fingers are forcibly straightened it becomes taut and fixed and retains its concavity. This is due to its firm adherence to a thickened layer of deep fascia, the palmar aponeurosis, which extends distally on to the fingers and is attached proximally to the flexor retinaculum and the tendon of the palmaris longus muscle. The skin over the palmar surfaces of the fingers is similarly bound down and firmly packed with fat, especially at the tips, and this immobility of the skin allows of a firm grip. The several creases in the palmar skin are of no service as landmarks, but act as joints for this immobile skin.

The distal boundary of the hollow of the palm is a low, uneven elevation that overlies the **metacarpo-phalangeal joints** of the four fingers. The creases at the root of a finger are about 2 cm. distal to the metacarpo-phalangeal joint. The proximal of the two (or more) creases at the middle of a finger is opposite the first (proximal) **interphalangeal joint,** but at the second (distal) joint the creases are proximal to the joint.

On the lateral surface of the wrist, the **scaphoid** and the **trapezium** lie in the floor of the 'snuff-box', between the styloid process of the radius and the first metacarpal, and can be felt if the hand is bent towards the medial side. On the medial surface, the **triquetrum** is easily felt behind the pisiform; The **dorsal branch of the ulnar nerve** can be rolled between the finger and the triquetrum. The triquetrum overlaps the hamate bone so that the hamate bone can scarcely be felt on the medial side.

On the back of the hand, the **carpal bones** are hidden by the extensor tendons as they pass off the radius and ulna. These tendons ridge the skin when the fingers are extended, and they are best identified after they have been dissected. The **metacarpal bones** can all be felt through the tendons. The muscles between them are the **dorsal interossei,** of which the first is the largest and the only one visible in the living hand; it can be seen and felt contracting if you bend the forefinger or abduct it from the others. The **bases** or proximal ends of the metacarpal bones form small uneven prominences about 2·5 cm. below the radius and ulna. Their distal ends or **heads** are the first row of **knuckles.** The **metacarpo-phalangeal joints** are distal to the knuckles. The **heads** of the **phalanges** are the second and third rows of knuckles, and the **interphalangeal joints** are immediately distal to them.

SUPERFICIAL STRUCTURES

The whole of the skin should now be removed from the limb while the subcutaneous tissues are still in good condition, and in order that a general view of the superficial veins and the cutaneous nerves may be obtained. The main superficial veins carry blood to the axillary vein; the cutaneous nerves are either direct branches of the brachial plexus or they spring from the main terminal branches of the plexus.

DISSECTION. Make an incision on the anterior surface of the limb, and incise the skin along the middle of the index, ring, and little fingers [Fig. 3(5)].

Next, remove the flaps, taking great care not to injure the cutaneous vessels and nerves. Reflect the flaps to the margins of the limb and the margins of the digits, and then dissect them from the back of the limb, including the digits.

When the skin is completely removed the limb must be kept moist and enclosed in an impervious bag when the dissection is not proceeding.

Superficial Fascia

The superficial fascia presents no peculiarities in the upper arm, the forearm and the back of the hand. The amount of fat in it varies considerably in different subjects; and the dissector will have found that the skin is readily separated from it, except over the epicondyles and the olecranon. In the palm and on the front of the digits, the superficial fascia is dense and binds the skin to the deep fascia by fibrous septa which pass through, dividing it into small loculi occupied by separate lobules of fat. Over the hypothenar eminence some transverse muscle fibres will be brought into view; they connect the skin on the ulnar border of the hand with the deep fascia of the palm, and constitute the **palmaris brevis muscle.** It can be brought into action, with obvious puckering of the skin, by abducting the little finger against resistance. A loose, slender band of fibres, called the **superficial transverse metacarpal ligament** [FIG. 62], lies in the superficial fascia across the roots of the fingers and in the webs between them. When the hand is put into the position in which it grasps a spherical object, this ligament is put on the stretch and the palmaris brevis contracts, deepening the 'cup' of the palm.

Superficial Veins

The subcutaneous veins should be dissected first, because they are, except here and there, the most superficial structures [FIGS. 28, 29]; but be careful to preserve any nerves met with as the veins are being cleaned.

DISSECTION. Follow the cephalic vein downwards from the groove between the pectoralis major and the deltoid, and preserve its tributaries. At the bend of the elbow, secure and clean a large communicating branch called the median cubital vein, which runs obliquely upwards to join the basilic vein. Secure also a vein which pierces the deep fascia and connects the median cubital vein with the deep veins of the forearm.

Follow the cephalic vein down the forearm and round its radial margin to its origin from the dorsal venous arch. Trace the dorsal venous arch across the back of the hand to the ulnar side, where the basilic vein arises from it. Follow the basilic vein proximally through the forearm, in front of the medial epicondyle, and to the middle of the upper arm where it pierces the deep fascia. As you clean it, look for the superficial cubital lymph nodes, which lie in the superficial fascia a little above the medial epicondyle. Note any variations of the superficial veins that may be present.

Return to the dorsal venous arch and clean its tributaries.

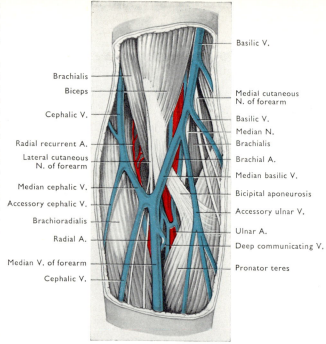

FIG. 25 Superficial veins at bend of elbow in a specimen in which the median vein was large.

The superficial veins must now be studied.

Dorsal Venous Arch. This arch usually lies across the distal part of the back of the hand, but it is inconstant in position and shape, as the dissectors may see if they compare their own hands. It gives origin to the basilic and cephalic veins, and it receives numerous tributaries including the three **dorsal metacarpal veins**, which lie in the spaces between the metacarpal bones of the fingers and are formed by **dorsal digital veins** which lie along the margins of the back of each digit, and are connected by venous arches. Communicating veins that pass through the intermetacarpal spaces connect the veins of the back of the hand with the veins of the palm.

Cephalic Vein. The cephalic vein begins at the radial end of the dorsal venous arch. It receives the two dorsal digital veins from the thumb, and then turns round the radial border of the distal part of the forearm and ascends to the front of the elbow. There, the greater part of its blood is transmitted to the basilic vein by the median cubital vein. It then ascends along the lateral surface of the biceps to the lower border of the pectoralis major, pierces the deep fascia [FIG. 28], and proceeds upwards in the groove between the pectoralis major and the deltoid to the infraclavicular fossa. It then pierces the clavipectoral fascia [p. 23] to join the axillary vein [p. 29].

Basilic Vein. The basilic vein begins at the medial end of the dorsal venous arch. It receives the dorsal digital vein from the medial side of the little finger, and then ascends along the medial surface of the forearm—often as two channels which unite before they reach the elbow. Near the elbow it inclines forwards to ascend in front of the medial epicondyle. Two to three centimetres or more above the medial epicondyle it is joined by the median cubital vein, and runs

46

along the medial margin of the biceps to the middle of the upper arm, where it pierces the deep fascia. After it has pierced the deep fascia, it runs along the medial side of the brachial artery to the lower border of the teres major, where it becomes the axillary vein. Only the termination of this, upper, part of the vein can be seen at present; the remainder will be displayed in a later dissection.

Median Cubital Vein. This is a large communicating vein which springs from the cephalic vein about 2·5 cm. below the bend of the elbow, and runs obliquely up to join the basilic vein about 2·5 cm. above the medial epicondyle. As it crosses from the cephalic to the basilic vein, it receives tributaries from the front of the forearm, is connected with the deep veins, and is separated from the distal part of the brachial artery by a portion of deep fascia thickened by an expansion from the biceps tendon called the **bicipital aponeurosis** [FIG. 25].

Variations of Superficial Veins. A **median vein of the forearm** may be larger than the cephalic vein in that region, in which case it divides in front of the elbow into a **median basilic** (which replaces the median cubital) and a **median cephalic** which joins the cephalic [FIG. 25]. The median cubital (or median basilic) is the usual vein for venesection or intravenous injections as in blood transfusion.

LYMPH VESSELS AND LYMPH NODES OF UPPER LIMB

In an ordinary dissecting room part, it is impossible to display the lymph vessels of the limb in a satisfactory manner. The dissectors will have seen some of the axillary nodes, and may have found a superficial cubital and possibly a deltopectoral node. But they will not have been able to trace the lymph vessels except for short distances near those nodes.

At this stage it is, however, worth their while to review the general arrangement of lymph vessels and lymph nodes in the limb, since it has a certain general relation to the pattern of the main superficial veins.

As in other parts of the body, both the vessels and the nodes are arranged in two main groups—superficial and deep.

Superficial Lymph Nodes. These are: (1) the infraclavicular [p. 27] and deltopectoral nodes [p. 20], and (2) the superficial cubital nodes, which are two small nodes that lie a little above the medial epicondyle near the medial side of the basilic vein, and are liable to become inflamed and painful when wounds of the ulnar border of the hand fester.

Deep Lymph Nodes. These lie along the course of the main blood vessels. The chief groups are in the axilla, but there are a few along the medial side of the brachial artery and at its bifurcation (deep cubital). Occasionally, small nodes are found in relation to the arteries of the forearm.

Deep Lymph Vessels receive the lymph from all the structures that are deep to the deep fascia, but they are much less numerous than the superficial vessels. They accompany the main blood vessels and end in the axillary nodes—some of them being interrupted in the nodes related to the brachial artery.

Superficial Lymph Vessels. These collect the lymph from the skin and the subcutaneous tissues, and they also ultimately reach the nodes in the **axilla.** As they traverse the limb they anastomose with one another to some extent, but each retains a definite individuality throughout its course. FIGURES 26 and 27 show the general arrangement of the lymphatic vessels of the upper limb. The points to be noted are: (1) The dense plexus on the palm and fingers drains mainly to the dorsal surface of the hand through vessels passing round its margins and between the fingers. Only a few vessels from the palmar plexus join those of the forearm directly. (2) The vessels from the dorsum of the hand join those of the forearm which sweep round its radial and ulnar borders to reach the ventral aspect and run up the arm in the general direction of the axilla, converging on it with vessels which turn round the medial and lateral aspects of the arm from its dorsal surface. (3) Some of the vessels on the medial aspect of the forearm enter the cubital nodes and from them drain through the deep fascia

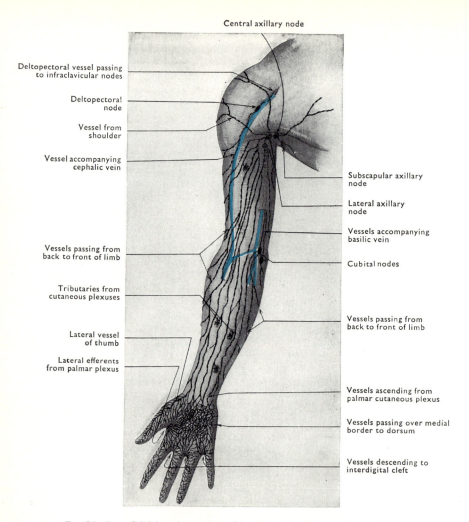

Central axillary node

Deltopectoral vessel passing to infraclavicular nodes

Deltopectoral node

Vessel from shoulder

Vessel accompanying cephalic vein

Vessels passing from back to front of limb

Tributaries from cutaneous plexuses

Lateral vessel of thumb

Lateral efferents from palmar plexus

Subscapular axillary node

Lateral axillary node

Vessels accompanying basilic vein

Cubital nodes

Vessels passing from back to front of limb

Vessels ascending from palmar cutaneous plexus

Vessels passing over medial border to dorsum

Vessels descending to interdigital cleft

FIG. 26   Superficial lymph vessels and lymph nodes of front of upper limb.

with the basilic vein, the majority remaining in the superficial fascia till they reach the floor of the axilla. (4) A few of the vessels from the lateral side of the forearm and arm join the cephalic vein and run with it to enter the deltopectoral or infraclavicular nodes. Apart from these, all the superficial vessels end in nodes around the axillary blood vessels, including those from the shoulder which

cross the anterior and posterior axillary folds to reach the axilla and pierce the deep fascia.

The student should compare the arrangement of the superficial lymph vessels of the Upper and Lower Limbs [cf. FIGS. 26, 27, and FIGS. 136, 137]. They begin in a similar manner in the hand and in the foot; and in each limb two streams are formed—a chief and a subsidiary—each associated with a vein.

48

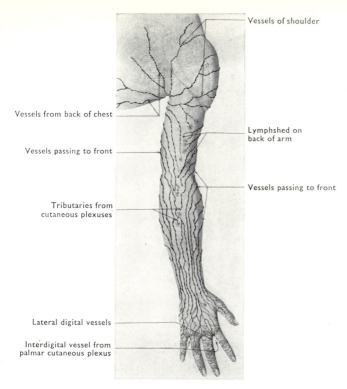

Vessels of shoulder

Vessels from back of chest

Vessels passing to front

Tributaries from cutaneous plexuses

Lymphshed on back of arm

Vessels passing to front

Lateral digital vessels

Interdigital vessel from palmar cutaneous plexus

FIG. 27   Superficial lymph vessels of back of upper limb.

CUTANEOUS NERVES OF UPPER ARM AND FOREARM

When the superficial veins and their connexions have been studied, the cutaneous nerves of the upper arm and the forearm must be identified and cleaned [FIGS. 28, 29]. It should be appreciated that cutaneous nerves supplying adjacent areas of skin share a considerable area by the overlapping of their fine terminal branches which cannot be followed by dissection.

DISSECTION. Find the intercostobrachial nerve and trace this nerve downwards through the medial side of the upper arm.

Next identify the two cutaneous branches of the medial cord of the brachial plexus. Pull gently on the medial cutaneous nerve of the arm. Note that it does not pierce the deep fascia till it is near the middle of the

upper arm. From that point, trace it downwards as far as the elbow.

The medial cutaneous nerve of the forearm is the thicker of the two. It does not pierce the deep fascia till it reaches the middle of the upper arm. Look for small branches that pierce the deep fascia above that level. Secure the nerve where it pierces the deep fascia, and follow it downwards. Near the elbow it divides into two branches. Trace them downwards through the fat on the medial side of the forearm to their terminations at the wrist.

Look for the remains of the lateral supraclavicular nerves [Fig. 4], and trace them through the fat over the upper half of the deltoid.

Identify the posterior cutaneous nerve of the arm, which springs from the radial nerve in the axilla. Trace it downwards through the fat of the back of the upper arm.

Next examine the back of the scapular region and find the posterior border of the deltoid muscle. Make an incision through the fascia along the lower half of that border, and secure the upper lateral cutaneous nerve of the arm (a branch of the axillary); trace its branches through the fascia over the lower half of the deltoid [Figs. 28, 29].

Now look for the lower lateral cutaneous nerve of the arm. It is often difficult to find. It pierces the deep fascia about 2–3 cm. below the insertion of the deltoid. Trace it downwards through the lateral part of the front of the upper arm. The posterior cutaneous nerve of the forearm pierces the deep fascia 2–3 cm. lower. Follow it downwards behind the lateral epicondyle, and along the back of the forearm. The origins of these two branches of the radial nerve will be displayed when the back of the upper arm is dissected [Fig. 44].

Turn to the front of the limb again, and find the lateral cutaneous nerve of the forearm. It appears at the lateral border of the biceps, under cover of the cephalic vein about 2–3 cm. above the bend of the elbow, and soon divides into two branches; trace them along the lateral side of the forearm to the hand.

49

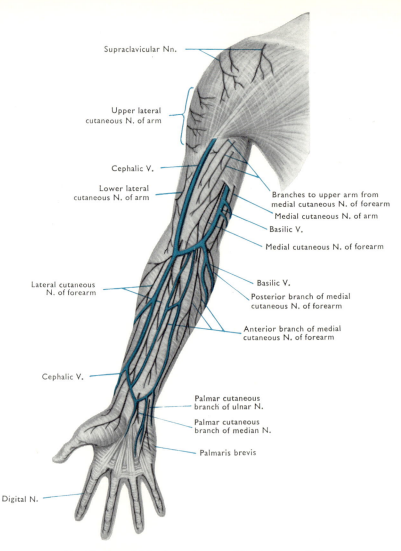

Supraclavicular Nn.

Upper lateral cutaneous N. of arm

Cephalic V.

Lower lateral cutaneous N. of arm

Branches to upper arm from medial cutaneous N. of forearm

Medial cutaneous N. of arm

Basilic V.

Medial cutaneous N. of forearm

Lateral cutaneous N. of forearm

Basilic V.

Posterior branch of medial cutaneous N. of forearm

Anterior branch of medial cutaneous N. of forearm

Cephalic V.

Palmar cutaneous branch of ulnar N.

Palmar cutaneous branch of median N.

Palmaris brevis

Digital N.

FIG. 28   Superficial veins and nerves of front of upper limb.

The **lateral supraclavicular nerves** (C. 4) cross the lateral third of the clavicle, and diverge from one another to supply the skin over the upper half of the deltoid.

The **upper lateral cutaneous nerve of the arm** (C. 5, 6) springs from the axillary nerve under

cover of the posterior border of the deltoid muscle, curves round that border at the junction of its lower and middle thirds, runs forwards, divides, and supplies the skin over the lower half of the deltoid.

The **medial cutaneous nerve of the arm** (T. 1,

2) springs from the medial cord of the brachial plexus, and supplies the skin on the medial side of the lower half of the upper arm (behind the basilic vein) and the adjoining part of the back of the arm.

The **intercostobrachial nerve** (T. 2) emerges from the second intercostal space, crosses the axilla, pierces the deep fascia of the upper arm about 2·5 cm. below the posterior fold of the axilla, and descends almost to the olecranon. Its branches supply the skin of the floor of the axilla, the skin on the proximal part of the upper arm behind the brachial artery, and a variable area of skin on the back of the upper arm. It communicates with the preceding nerve.

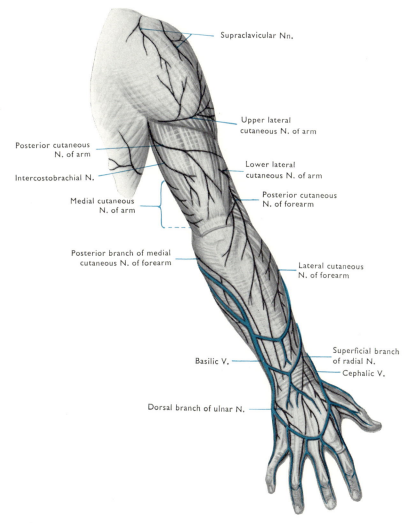

Supraclavicular Nn.

Upper lateral cutaneous N. of arm

Posterior cutaneous N. of arm

Intercostobrachial N.

Lower lateral cutaneous N. of arm

Posterior cutaneous N. of forearm

Medial cutaneous N. of arm

Posterior branch of medial cutaneous N. of forearm

Lateral cutaneous N. of forearm

Superficial branch of radial N.

Basilic V.

Cephalic V.

Dorsal branch of ulnar N.

FIG. 29   Superficial veins and nerves of back of upper limb.

The **posterior cutaneous nerve of the arm** (C. 5) arises in the axilla from the radial nerve. It pierces the deep fascia a little below the posterior fold of the axilla, and runs towards the olecranon. It supplies a wide area of skin on the back of the upper arm from the level of the deltoid tuberosity to the elbow.

The **lower lateral cutaneous nerve of the arm** (C. 5, 6) takes origin from the radial nerve before it leaves the radial groove of the humerus, pierces the deep fascia 2–3 cm. below the deltoid tuberosity, and supplies the skin of the front of the upper arm, lateral to the cephalic vein, from the deltoid tuberosity to the elbow.

The **posterior cutaneous nerve of the forearm** (C. 6, 7, 8) arises with the preceding nerve and pierces the deep fascia 2·5 cm. or less lower down. It passes downwards behind the lateral epicondyle and descends on the back of the forearm to the wrist. It gives a few branches to the skin of the lateral part of the upper arm, and supplies the skin of the middle of the back of the forearm from the elbow to the wrist.

The **lateral cutaneous nerve of the forearm** (C. 5, 6) is the continuation of the musculo-cutaneous nerve. It pierces the deep fascia at the lateral side of the biceps, about 2 cm. above the bend of the elbow, behind the cephalic vein. It soon divides into two branches—**anterior** and **posterior**—which run to the lateral side of the wrist. They supply the skin of the lateral side of the forearm both on the front and on the back, and the anterior branch supplies the skin of the proximal part of the ball of the thumb.

The **medial cutaneous nerve of the forearm** (C. 8, T. 1) arises from the medial cord of the brachial plexus. It pierces the deep fascia about the middle of the upper arm, in close relation to the basilic vein [FIG. 28]. At a varying point above the elbow it divides into **anterior** and **posterior** branches which descend along the medial side of the forearm to the wrist. The anterior branch as it enters the forearm is usually behind but may pass in front of the median cubital vein. Small branches supply the skin of the front of the

upper arm between the basilic and cephalic veins. The terminal branches supply the skin of the medial half of the forearm.

CUTANEOUS NERVES OF THE HAND
[FIGS. 28, 29, 68].

DISSECTION. Find the palmar cutaneous branches of the median and ulnar nerves.

The palmar cutaneous branch of the median nerve pierces the deep fascia between the tendons of the flexor carpi radialis and palmaris longus [p. 44], or near them; trace it to the middle of the palm. The palmar cutaneous branch of the ulnar nerve pierces the deep fascia near the lateral margin of the tendon of the flexor carpi ulnaris [p. 44]; trace it also into the palm.

Define the superficial transverse metacarpal ligament [p. 45], and then remove the superficial fascia from the area between the ball of the thumb and the roots of the fingers in order to expose a thick sheet of deep fascia called the palmar aponeurosis.

Opposite the distal ends of the metacarpal bones, the palmar aponeurosis divides into slips—one for each finger. Look for the three palmar digital nerves between those slips. Divide the superficial transverse ligament in order to expose them more fully, and trace their branches along the sides of the fingers, cleaning also the digital arteries which accompany them. Find another digital nerve on the hypothenar eminence and trace it to the medial side of the little finger. Pass to the other border of the palm and find the digital branch for the radial side of the forefinger at the lateral margin of the slip of the aponeurosis for that finger, and trace the nerve onwards. Distal to the thenar eminence, look for the two digital nerves of the thumb and follow them along the sides of the thumb. Careful dissection will show that some of the finer branches of the digital nerves end in minute, ovoid bodies called lamellated corpuscles.

Turn now to the back of the hand. Scrape away the fat on the medial side of the wrist below the styloid process of the ulna, and find the dorsal branch of the ulnar nerve; trace its branches to the little finger and the ring finger. Next, pass to the lateral surface of the lower end of the radius; find the terminal part of the superficial branch of the radial nerve, and trace its branches to the back of the thumb, the forefinger, the middle finger, and the ring finger.

The upper part of the skin of the ball of the thumb is supplied by the terminal twigs of the anterior branch of the lateral cutaneous nerve of the forearm ; the palmar digital nerves of the thumb supply the lower part. The rest of the skin of the palm is supplied by the palmar cutaneous branches of the median and ulnar nerves. At present, the dissectors can see only the lower parts of these two nerves [FIG. 28]; their upper parts will be seen when the deeper parts of the front of the forearm are dissected.

The **palmar cutaneous branch of the median nerve** (C. 6, 7, 8) arises about 2 cm. above the wrist and descends, branching, to supply the skin of the hollow of the palm.

The **palmar cutaneous branch of the ulnar nerve** (C. 7, 8) is a very slender nerve that arises at a variable point below the middle of the forearm, pierces the deep fascia near the wrist, and supplies the skin of the medial third of the palm.

The **dorsal branch of the ulnar nerve** (C. 7, 8) is larger. It also arises at a varying point below the middle of the forearm, and its origin will be examined later. It descends with the ulnar nerve, under cover of the flexor carpi ulnaris, almost to the pisiform bone. Then, inclining backwards, it descends obliquely across the medial surface of the carpus. It divides into two **dorsal digital nerves** which supply the skin of the medial third of the back of the hand, and the skin of the back of the little finger and medial half of the ring finger as far as the end of the second phalanx. The nerve can often be felt through the skin as it crosses the medial surface of the carpus.

The **terminal part of the superficial branch of the radial nerve** (C. 6, 7, 8) pierces the deep fascia about 5 cm. above the styloid process of the radius. It descends towards the 'anatomical snuff-box', crossing the tendons that overlie the lateral surface of the distal end of the radius, and divides into five **dorsal digital nerves**—two for the thumb and three for the fingers. They supply the skin of the lateral two thirds of the back of the hand, and the skin of the back of the thumb, forefinger, middle finger, and lateral half of the ring finger as far as the end of the proximal phalanx. The superficial branch of the radial nerve and some of its branches can often be felt through the skin as they cross the distal end of the radius and the extensor tendons of the thumb.

The dorsal branch of the ulnar nerve often contains fibres of the seventh cervical nerve received by communication with the median nerve in the axilla. When that is the case it gives off a branch that either replaces or assists the radial nerve in the supply of the contiguous halves of the ring and middle fingers.

The terminal parts of the backs of the digits are supplied by twigs that curve backwards from the palmar digital nerves. But the extent to which the dorsal and the palmar digital nerves supply the backs of the digits is variable, and the dorsal nerves of the thumb and little finger may reach the root of the nail.

Palmar Digital Nerves

There are seven palmar digital nerves. Two of them spring from the ulnar nerve and are distributed to the little finger and the medial half of the ring finger. The others arise from the median nerve and are distributed ot the other three and a half digits [FIGS. 62, 64]. They are visible only on the digits at present; their origin and course in the palm will be seen when the hand is dissected. They are accompanied by the palmar digital vessels, which are in front of them in the palm and behind them on the sides of the digits. They supply the joints and the soft parts on the sides and the front and, to a variable extent, on the distal part of the back of the digits. Each terminates at the end of the digit by dividing into two branches, one of which ramifies in the pulp of the digit and the other in the bed of the nail.

The **palmar digital branches of the ulnar nerve** (C. 7, 8) arise from the superficial terminal branch of that nerve. They begin on the hypothenar eminence about 2 cm. distal to the pisiform bone under cover of the palmaris brevis. The medial branch runs to the medial side of the little finger. The lateral branch divides near the cleft between the little finger and the ring finger into two branches which run along the contiguous sides of those fingers.

The **palmar digital branches of the median nerve** (C. 6, 7, 8) spring from the two terminal divisions of the median nerve in the upper part of the hollow of the palm. The medial two run towards the webs between the fore, middle, and ring fingers and divide to run along the contiguous sides of those fingers. The third runs to the radial side of the forefinger. The lateral two branches curve laterally round the distal margin of the thenar eminence, and run along the two sides of the thumb. The most medial of the digital branches of the median nerve sends a communicating twig to the adjoining branch of the ulnar nerve.

Lamellated corpuscles are minute ovoid bodies that lie amidst the fat on the digits, and are attached to the ends of the terminal branches of digital nerves. They are end-organs associated with the sense of pressure.

Dermatomes. Most cutaneous nerves contain nerve fibres from more than one spinal nerve, yet if the cutaneous pattern of distribution of the spinal nerves is mapped out on the limb, it is found to follow a definite plan, each spinal nerve innervating a particular area of skin called a dermatome. Adjacent dermatomes overlap as do the individual cutaneous nerves, but the pattern of their distribution is very different from that of the cutaneous nerves, and this is of importance in differentiating between spinal and peripheral nerve injuries.

DISSECTION. Remove the remains of the superficial fascia from all parts of the limb, and examine the deep fascia. On the back of the hand it is very thin, so be careful not to remove it with the superficial fascia.

DEEP FASCIA

The deep fascia of the upper limb consists chiefly of transverse fibres which are bound together by oblique and longitudinal fibres. The oblique and longitudinal fibres become specially developed in certain situations which will be noted later.

Turn first to the **scapular region,** and identify the deltoid, teres major and minor, and the infraspinatus. The first two have been examined already. The infraspinatus almost fills the infraspinous fossa. The teres minor is a narrow muscle that lies on the dorsum of the scapula along its lateral margin so closely applied to the infraspinatus that it may appear to be part of it. The deep fascia on the anterior and lateral surfaces of the deltoid is fairly strong. On the posterior surface of the deltoid and on the other three muscles, it is very strong and dense, especially over the infraspinatus. From its deep surface, it sends in a strong septum between the infraspinatus and the teres minor to be attached to the dorsum of the scapula, and another between the two teres muscles to be attached to the lateral margin of the scapula. As this fascia extends over the two teres muscles towards the deltoid, it splits into two layers which enclose the deltoid.

In the **upper arm,** the deep fascia consists largely of transverse fibres. On the front, where it covers the biceps, it is thin, but it is much stronger at the back, over the triceps. From its deep surface, it sends in septa between muscles, including two strong sheets, called the **lateral** and **medial intermuscular septa,** which bind it to the lateral and medial supracondylar ridges of the humerus. Those septa will be examined when the upper arm is dissected.

At the **elbow** it is thickened and strengthened by tendinous fibres which pass to it from the biceps and triceps muscles; and it is closely attached to the lateral and medial epicondyles of the humerus and to the olecranon. A special thickening, the **bicipital aponeurosis,** is found at the front of the elbow [FIG. 25]. It springs from the medial border of the tendon of the biceps muscle and is part of its insertion. It blends with the deep fascia on the medial side of the upper part of the forearm and separates the median cubital vein, which lies superficial to it, from the brachial artery, which is deep to it.

In the **forearm,** the deep fascia is dense except in the lower part anteriorly. It is especially strong near the elbow, where it gives partial origin to the muscles which arise from the epicondyles. It sends in strong septa between the fleshy bellies of those muscles; the positions of the septa are indicated on the surface by white lines. At the back it is firmly bound to the posterior border of the ulna in its whole length, and thus separates the muscles on the medial surface of the ulna from those on the back.

At the wrist the transverse fibres of the deep fascia become very obvious. On the back they form a well-marked band called the extensor retinaculum; on the front they are incorporated in a shorter but much thicker band called the flexor retinaculum [FIGS. 66 and 69].

Both bands are attached to the adjacent bones; they act as straps which bind down tendons, and prevent them from springing away from the bones when the hand is bent forwards or backwards.

The flexor retinaculum [FIGS. 55, 64] is a thick, strong band, about 2·5 cm. square, continuous above and below with the deep fascia of the forearm and palm. It lies immediately distal to the best marked crease at the lower end of the front of the forearm, and it bridges across the carpal groove, converting it into a tunnel for the long flexor tendons to pass through. It is attached to the bones that form the sides of the carpal tunnel—the pisiform and the hook of the hamate on the medial side, the tubercle of the scaphoid and the front of the trapezium on the lateral side. The retinaculum is hidden to a large extent at present by the structures that cross it and by the muscles of the thenar and hypothenar eminences that arise from it. Its connexions and relations will be examined fully when the hand is dissected.

Turn now to the back of the limb and identify the extensor retinaculum [FIG. 71]—

a thickened part of the deep fascia, nearly 2·5 cm. wide, that lies obliquely across the back of the limb where the forearm joins the wrist. Its deep surface sends off septa that divide the space under its cover into six compartments which transmit the extensor tendons and are lined with their synovial sheaths.

Before you leave the back of the limb, note again how thin the deep fascia is on the back of the hand; as it passes on to the backs of the digits it may become indistinguishable by adhering to the extensor tendons.

Turn again to the front and examine the deep fascia of the palm. The portions that cover the thenar and hypothenar eminences are thin; the intermediate, triangular portion is dense and strong, and is called the palmar aponeurosis.

The palmar aponeurosis conceals and protects the main vessels, nerves and the tendons, as they pass towards the fingers. Its apex blends with the distal border of the flexor retinaculum, and, more superficially, receives the tendon of the palmaris longus. From its distal border processes pass to the fingers where they blend with the fibrous sheaths of the flexor tendons.

The deep fascia on the palmar surfaces of the digits is thick and strong. It forms dense, curved plates or shields, called the fibrous flexor sheaths. These plates are attached by their edges to the margins of the phalanges, with which they thus form a tunnel in which the flexor tendons of the digit lie protected. The tunnel is lined with the synovial sheath of the tendons. The arrangement and connexions of the palmar aponeurosis and the flexor sheaths will be studied in more detail when the hand is dissected.

THE SHOULDER (SCAPULAR REGION)

Before proceeding with this dissection review the attachments of pectoralis minor to the coracoid process; trapezius to the clavicle, acromion and spine of scapula; inferior belly of omohyoid from the upper border of the scapula; levator scapulae and

the rhomboids to the medial border; and serratus anterior to the costal aspect of that border and to the upper and lower angles.

DISSECTION. Place a small block in the axilla, and bend the arm over the block to make the fibres of

55

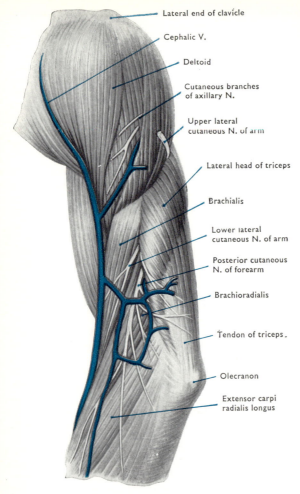

Lateral end of clavicle

Cephalic V.

Deltoid

Cutaneous branches
of axillary N.

Upper lateral
cutaneous N. of arm

Lateral head of triceps

Brachialis

Lower lateral
cutaneous N. of arm

Posterior cutaneous
N. of forearm

Brachioradialis

Tendon of triceps

Olecranon

Extensor carpi
radialis longus

FIG. 30   Deltoid muscle and lateral aspect of arm.

separated by tendinous intersections; and, as its name implies, it is triangular in outline. It arises, by its upper end or base, from the external margins of : (1) the lateral third of the clavicle ; (2) the acromion ; and (3) the crest of the spine of the scapula. Its origin corresponds closely with the insertion of the trapezius. Its bundles or fasciculi converge rapidly as they pass to a pointed, tendinous insertion into the **deltoid tuberosity** of the humerus [FIGS. 39, 40]. Nerve supply: branches of the <u>axillary nerve</u> which enter its deep surface.

Action: the form of the deltoid and the manner in which it clasps the shoulder determine its actions. Its anterior and posterior portions are opposed to each other : the anterior fibres act with the pectoralis major (clavicular head) in flexing the arm at the shoulder joint [p. 21], and in medial rotation ; the posterior fibres, acting with other muscles, reverse these movements. The acromial part of the deltoid is the chief agent in abduction at the shoulder joint; it can raise the arm to the horizontal position but not further, though this movement at the shoulder joint is invariably associated with rotation of the scapula [FIG. 51].

DISSECTION. Place the limb on its back and clean the angle between the humerus and the scapula. Follow the axillary nerve and the posterior circumflex humeral artery backwards to a cleft between the subscapularis and the teres major. Separate those muscles and note that a thick strap of muscle, the long head of the triceps, crosses the triangular interval between them and divides it into a lateral part called the quadrangular space and a medial part called the triangular space [Fig. 31]. The axillary nerve and the posterior humeral circumflex artery pass backwards through the quadrangular space. Now reverse the limb, push the posterior border of the deltoid forwards and find them as they emerge from the quadrangular space to curve forwards round the surgical neck of the humerus.

the deltoid muscle tense. Detach the upper lateral cutaneous nerve of the arm from the deep fascia and, turn it backwards to the posterior border of the deltoid; then clean the deltoid. On the left side begin at its posterior border and reflect the deep fascia forwards. On the right side begin in front and reflect the fascia backwards.

Deltoid Muscle

The deltoid is a typical multipennate muscle, being composed of short, coarse fasciculi,

56

At this stage cut the deltoid from its origin and turn it towards its insertion, taking care not to injure the circumflex artery and axillary nerve, and then clean the vessel and nerve.

Clean the axillary nerve with caution. Secure a small articular twig that springs from it in the quadrangular space and passes up to the capsule of the shoulder joint. Note that the nerve splits into two branches after this twig is given off. Secure the nerve to teres minor, which springs from the posterior branch before it turns round the posterior border of the deltoid. Trace the branches of the anterior division into the deltoid.

Clean the teres major and minor muscles from end to end, preserving their nerves of supply. Clean also the long head of the triceps—upwards to its origin and downwards to its junction with the other heads of the triceps—and preserve its nerve supply, which is found arising from the radial nerve in the axilla

and entering the front of the head.

Then examine the subacromial bursa. It lies below the acromion. Thrust a blowpipe into it. If its wall is uninjured it can be distended with air. Open it, gauge its extent with the finger, and note whether it is single or subdivided.

Turn the limb on to its back once more. Pull the coracobrachialis and short head of the biceps medially, and expose the tendon of the long head of biceps in the intertubercular groove. Then, pull them laterally to expose a thick tendon—the tendon of the subscapularis. Clean that tendon to its insertion. Clean also the anterior humeral circumflex artery, which runs laterally deep to the short head of biceps and the coracobrachialis.

Now, re-examine the structures that lie under cover of the deltoid, and note their relative positions.

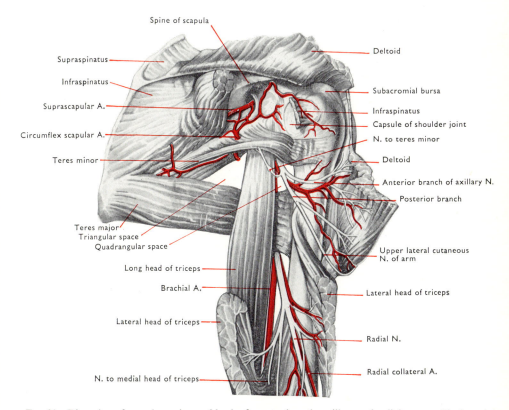

FIG. 31   Dissection of scapular region and back of arm to show the axillary and radial nerves. The lateral head of triceps has been divided and turned aside to expose the spiral groove on the humerus for the radial nerve.

STRUCTURES UNDER COVER OF THE DELTOID

The deltoid covers the upper part of the humerus, and envelops the region of the shoulder joint behind, laterally and in front; its anterior border covers the coracoid process and the muscles and ligaments attached to it. It is separated from the shoulder joint by the muscles attached to the upper end of the humerus and by the subacromial bursa; it covers also the long head of the biceps in the intertubercular groove and the greater part of the axillary nerve and circumflex vessels.

The full, rounded appearance of the shoulder is due to the deltoid passing over the upper end of the humerus. When the head of the humerus is dislocated, the muscle passes vertically from its origin to its insertion, and the dislocation is recognized by the squareness or flatness of the shoulder.

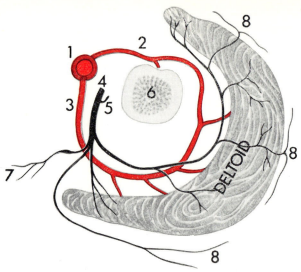

FIG. 32   Diagram of circumflex arteries and axillary nerve.

1. Axillary A.
2. Anterior circumflex humeral A.
3. Posterior circumflex humeral A.
4. Axillary N.
5. Articular branch
6. Transverse section of humerus immediatley below the tubercles
7. Branch to teres minor
8. Cutaneous branches

Subacromial Bursa

This is a large bursal sac that separates the acromion and the upper part of the deltoid from the muscles that lie on the upper surface of the capsule of the shoulder joint. It varies in size in different bodies, but, when distended, may be as large as a hen's egg; it may be a single sac or divided by fibrous partitions, and it may communicate with a smaller **subdeltoid bursa** between the muscle and the greater tubercle of the humerus. These bursae facilitate the play of the upper end of the humerus and the attached muscles on the under surface of the coraco-acromial arch and deltoid.

Intermuscular Spaces

The **quadrangular space** has no real existence until its boundaries are artificially separated from one another. These boundaries, as seen from the front, are the subscapularis above, the teres major below, the long head of the

triceps medially, and the surgical neck of the humerus laterally. At the back, the teres minor replaces the subscapularis as the upper boundary. Between the subscapularis and the teres muscles, *a loose fold of the capsule of the shoulder joint appears in the upper boundary of the space* [FIG. 45]. The axillary nerve and the posterior humeral circumflex vessels pass backwards through the space, directly below the capsule.

The **triangular space** [FIG. 31] is of less importance.

Circumflex Humeral Arteries

The **posterior circumflex humeral artery** was seen in the axilla [p. 29], springing from the axillary artery a short distance below the subscapular branch. It at once passes backwards through the quadrangular space, and, winding round the surgical neck of the humerus, it is distributed in numerous branches to the deep surface of the deltoid muscle. Several twigs are given also to other muscles, to the shoulder joint, and to the skin. It anastomoses with neighbouring arteries, the most important anastomosis being effected by a branch which it sends down to the profunda branch of the brachial artery.

The **anterior circumflex humeral artery** is described on page 29. It is much smaller than the posterior circumflex artery. By the anastomosis of their branches, an arterial circle is formed around the surgical neck of the humerus.

Axillary Nerve (C. 5, 6)

This nerve supplies : (1) an articular twig to the capsule of the shoulder joint ; (2) muscular branches to the deltoid and teres minor ; and (3) cutaneous branches to the skin over the lower half of the deltoid.

It springs from the posterior cord of the brachial plexus, turns round the lower border of the subscapularis, and passes backwards, with the posterior circumflex humeral vessels, through the quadrangular space to the back of the limb. There, it divides into an anterior and a posterior branch.

The **articular twig** takes origin from the trunk of the nerve in the quadrangular space, and enters the joint from below.

The **posterior branch** gives off the nerve to the teres minor, and, after furnishing a few twigs to the posterior part of the deltoid, curves round its posterior border as the **upper lateral cutaneous nerve of the arm,** which runs forwards branching to supply the skin over the lower half of the deltoid [FIGS. 29–32].

The **anterior branch** proceeds round the humerus with the posterior circumflex artery, and ends near the anterior border of the deltoid. It is distributed to the deltoid by numerous branches which enter the muscle through its deep surface and send a few fine filaments through it to the skin.

DISSECTION. Clean the coraco-acromial ligament, which extends from the coracoid process to the acromion. First examine the pectoralis minor and see whether or not its tendon sends a slip through the ligament to the capsule of the shoulder joint.

Coraco-acromial Ligament and Arch

The coraco-acromial ligament is a strong, flat band of a triangular shape. Its base is attached to the lateral border of the coracoid process ; its apex is attached to the extremity of the acromion [FIGS. 47, 48, 50]. Its upper surface is covered by the deltoid. Its lower surface is related to the sub-acromial bursa, which separates it from the supraspinatus muscle.

The **coraco-acromial arch** should be examined at the present stage, in order that its relationship to the subacromial bursa and the supraspinatus may be appreciated. It is the arch which overhangs and protects the shoulder joint. It is formed by the coracoid process, the acromion, and the coraco-acromial ligament. It is separated from the shoulder joint by the subacromial bursa, the tendon of the supraspinatus, and the upper parts of the tendons of the infraspinatus and sub-scapularis.

The coraco-acromial arch plays a very important part in the mechanism of the shoulder ; for, with the subacromial bursa, it might almost be said to form a secondary synovial socket for the humerus.

DISSECTION. Clear away the subacromial bursa and clean the supraspinatus, following it laterally to the humerus and medially below the coraco-acromial arch and trapezius. Then, clean the fascia from the surface of the subscapularis, noting its multipennate arrangement, and examine the attachments of the serratus anterior [Fig. 19]. Now, turn the limb and remove the fascia from the infraspinatus; and define the origin of the teres major.

SCAPULAR MUSCLES

Supraspinatus

The supraspinatus muscle arises from the medial two-thirds of the floor of the supra-spinous fossa. From this origin the fibres pass laterally under the acromion and end in a short, stout tendon which is inserted into the top of the greater tubercle of the humerus [FIG. 40, p. 69].

The supraspinatus is covered by the trapezius, the coraco-acromial arch, and the deltoid. Its tendon is closely adherent to the capsule of the shoulder joint, a feature common to the scapular muscles which prevents the capsule being folded into the joint when they contract.

Nerve supply: the **suprascapular nerve**. Action: it is an abductor of the arm and shares with the other scapular muscles the important function of maintaining the head of the humerus in the glenoid cavity during movements of the shoulder joint.

Infraspinatus

This muscle arises from the floor of the infraspinous fossa. Its tendon is closely adherent to the capsule of the shoulder joint, and is inserted into the greater tubercle behind the supraspinatus [FIG. 43]. Its lateral part is covered by the deltoid. Occasionally there is a small bursa between its tendon and the capsule of the shoulder joint, and, if present, it may communicate with the joint cavity. Nerve supply: the **suprascapular nerve**. Action: it is a lateral rotator of the arm, and it helps to steady the head of the humerus during abduction by the deltoid and supraspinatus.

Teres Minor

This small muscle lies along the lower border of the infraspinatus. It arises from an elongated flat impression on the dorsum of the scapula along the lateral border [FIG. 34]. It is inserted by tendon into the back of the greater tubercle of the humerus, and also, by fleshy fibres, into the shaft for 1 cm. below the tubercle [FIG. 43]. As it approaches its insertion it is separated from the teres major by the long head of the triceps brachii, and it is adherent to the capsule of the shoulder joint. Nerve supply: a branch from

60

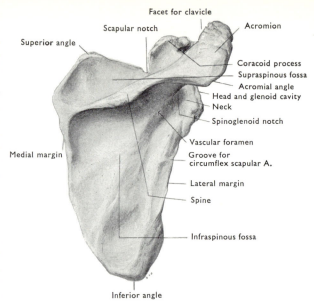

FIG. 33   Dorsal surface of right scapula.

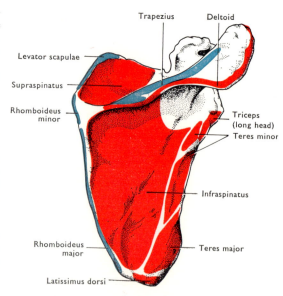

FIG. 34   Muscle attachments to dorsal surface of right scapula.

the **axillary nerve**. Action: it is an adductor and lateral rotator of the arm (see also subscapularis).

Teres Major

This is an elongated, rounded muscle that arises from the oval surface on the dorsum of the scapula close to the inferior angle [FIG. 34]. It is inserted into the crest of the lesser tubercle of the humerus [FIG. 40]. Nerve supply: the **lower subscapular nerve**. Action: it is an adductor, a medial rotator and an extensor of the arm. The triple relation of the latissimus dorsi to the teres major was explained on page 41.

Subscapularis

The subscapularis is a thick, wide muscle that arises from the subscapular fossa, except near the neck of the scapula, but including the groove along the lateral border [FIG. 19]. Like the deltoid, the subscapularis is a multipennate muscle, many fibres arising from tendinous intersections attached to the ridges on the scapula. The fleshy fibres converge upon a stout tendon which is adherent to the capsule of the shoulder joint, and is inserted into the lesser tubercle of the humerus; a few of the lower fleshy fibres, however, gain independent insertion into the shaft below the tubercle [FIG. 40].

The muscle passes to its insertion under an arch formed by the coracoid process and the conjoined origin of the short head of the biceps and the coracobrachialis. Nerve supply : the **upper** and **lower subscapular nerves**. Action : it is an adductor and medial rotator of the arm. The attachments of teres minor and subscapularis to the humerus lie on the axis of abduction ; thus they are able to prevent the deltoid drawing the humerus up against the coraco-acromial arch without interfering with abduction, and are therefore synergists of this movement.

DISSECTION. Pull the long head of the biceps out of the intertubercular groove. Separate the tendon

of the latissimus dorsi from the anterior surface of the teres major, looking for an occasional small bursa between them and noting the fibrous slip which passes from the latissimus to the long head of the triceps [Fig. 10]; then, follow the tendon of the latissimus to its insertion.

The insertions of pectoralis major, latissimus dorsi and teres major are now fully exposed, and the student should review their insertions [see pp. 20, 40 and 41]. The fibrous slip that connects the lower margin of the latissimus to the fascia on the long head of the triceps is of interest as it represents a muscle, called the dorso-epitrochlearis, which is present in certain animals.

DISSECTION. Depress the upper border of the subscapularis as it passes below the coracoid process, and expose the subscapular bursa. Inflate the bursa with a blowpipe, and notice that, as air is blown in, the capsule of the shoulder joint it distended. Open the bursa and examine the interior.

Subscapular Bursa. This is a prolongation of the synovial membrane of the shoulder joint through a large aperture in the upper and anterior part of the fibrous capsule [FIGS. 47, 48]. It extends laterally between the subscapularis and the medial part of the capsule, and medially in front of the neck of the scapula and the root of the coracoid process. It facilitates the movement of the subscapularis over these parts.

DISSECTION. Cut through the subscapularis vertically below the coracoid process, and detach the bursa from its deep surface. Turn the medial part of the muscle towards the medial border of the scapula, and note the anastomosis between the arteries on its deep surface. Turn the lateral portion towards the humerus, detaching it carefully from the capsule of the shoulder, and examine its insertion.

Divide the supraspinatus medial to the coracoid process. Turn the medial part towards the medial border of the scapula, and dissect its nerve of supply. Turn the lateral part towards the humerus, forcing it beneath the coraco-acromial arch, but avoiding injury to the suprascapular nerve and vessels, which lie beneath it. As its tendon crosses the top of the shoulder joint, it must be carefully detached from the capsule.

Divide the infraspinatus medial to the lateral border of the spine of the scapula. Turn the medial part medially and dissect out the vessels and nerves from its deep surface. Follow the lateral part to its insertion, and, as it is displaced, take care not to injure the suprascapular nerve and vessels and the circumflex scapular vessels, which lie between it and the bone. As you separate it from the capsule of the shoulder joint, avoid injury to the capsule. If there is a bursa under the tendon, see whether it communicates with the joint or not.

Divide the teres minor where the circumflex scapular artery passes between it and the bone; turn its lateral part towards the insertion, avoiding injury to the capsule as you divide the adhesion between them.

Now look for the suprascapular ligament, which bridges across the notch on the upper border of the scapula. Find there the suprascapular nerve and vessels. Clean them, following them down into the infraspinous fossa; but be careful not to injure the branches of the nerve.

in the dissection of the back [p. 42].

The **suprascapular artery** arises in the root of the neck, runs laterally behind the clavicle, and descends to the upper border of the scapula under cover of the trapezius. It then passes backwards over the suprascapular ligament, gives branches to the supraspinatus muscle, and descends through the spino-glenoid notch to end by ramifying in the infraspinatus.

The **subscapular artery** has been traced in the dissection of the axilla [p. 28]. Its largest branch is the **circumflex scapular artery**, which sends branches into the subscapular fossa, and then runs under cover of the teres minor into the infraspinous fossa to ramify and anastomose there.

This complete arterial anastomosis ensures an adequate blood supply to the highly

Superior Transverse Scapular Ligament

This ligament is a firm fibrous band that passes from the upper border of the scapula to the root of the coracoid process. It bridges across the scapular notch, converting it into a foramen; sometimes it is ossified. The suprascapular nerve passes backwards through the foramen, and the suprascapular vessels lie above the ligament.

DISSECTION. Revise the arteries that run in relation with the borders and surfaces of the scapula, and dissect out the anastomoses between their branches.

Anastomosis around the Scapula

An important and free anastomosis takes place between the branches of three arteries which lie in close relation with the scapula and send branches to both its surfaces [FIG. 35].

The relation of the **deep branch of the transverse cervical artery** to the medial border of the scapula has been seen already

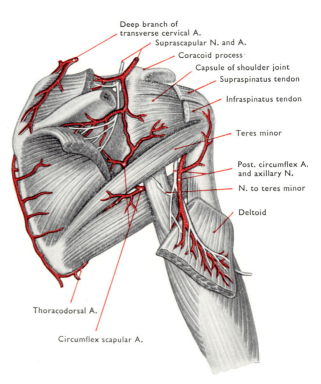

Deep branch of transverse cervical A.
Suprascapular N. and A.
Coracoid process
Capsule of shoulder joint
Supraspinatus tendon
Infraspinatus tendon
Teres minor
Post. circumflex A. and axillary N.
N. to teres minor
Deltoid
Thoracodorsal A.
Circumflex scapular A.

FIG. 35   Anastomosing arteries around the scapula.

movable scapula, and, being fed by branches of the first part of the subclavian and third part of the axillary arteries, forms a route through which the limb can be supplied with blood if the main artery is blocked or has to be ligated between these two parts.

Suprascapular Nerve

This nerve arises from the fifth and sixth cervical nerves where they unite to form the upper trunk of the brachial plexus. It runs downwards and backwards in the neck, above the brachial plexus, passes under cover of the trapezius a little above the clavicle, and descends, in company with the suprascapular vessels, to the upper border of the scapula. It then passes downwards and backwards through the scapular notch, below the superior transverse scapular ligament which separates it from the suprascapular vessels.

Having entered the supraspinous fossa it gives one or two branches to the supraspinatus and filaments to the capsules of the acromioclavicular and shoulder joints; it then descends through the spinoglenoid notch, under cover of a loose fascial band that stretches across it, to end in the infraspinatus, having given additional twigs to the shoulder joint.

LIGAMENTS THAT CONNECT THE
CLAVICLE WITH THE SCAPULA

DISSECTION. **Lift up the medial end of the clavicle to put tension on the coracoclavicular ligament. Remove any parts of the deltoid and trapezius that conceal the ligament. Clean its surfaces and borders. Note that it is divisible into two parts. Look for a bursa between the two parts.**

Next, remove the remains of the deltoid and trapezius muscles from the capsule of the acromioclavicular joint, and clean the external surface of the capsule. Open the joint, and see if there is an articular disc inside it.

Coracoclavicular Ligament

This is a powerful ligament which binds the lateral part of the clavicle to the coracoid process. It is incompletely divided into conoid and trapezoid parts that meet at an angle; the angle is open anteriorly, and often contains a small bursa that diminishes the friction between the parts when the ligament is twisted during movement of the shoulder girdle.

The **conoid part** lies behind and medial to the trapezoid part. Its thick end is attached to the conoid tubercle of the clavicle [FIG. 7]. The pointed end is attached to the upper surface of the coracoid process where the process bends forwards from its root. The **trapezoid part** is flat, thick and obliquely placed. It is attached to the trapezoid ridge of the clavicle and to the upper surface of the coracoid process.

The coracoclavicular ligament helps to prevent dislocation of the acromial end of the clavicle, and, to a certain extent, it limits the movements of the acromioclavicular joint. It is therefore an accessory ligament of that joint. It is also the main medium by which the scapula and, indirectly, the other parts of the upper limb are suspended from the clavicle and through which forces applied to the upper limb are transmitted to the trunk. If the clavicle is broken medial to the attachment of the ligament, the upper limb, as a whole, at once falls—a characteristic sign of this common variety of fracture.

Acromioclavicular Joint

This is a synovial joint. The fibrous capsule is attached to the margins of the articular surfaces, and its upper part is thickened to form the **acromioclavicular ligament**. The cavity is usually partially divided by a wedge-shaped **articular disc** whose base is attached to the upper part of the capsule [FIG. 45].

The surfaces of the joint are ovoid and flat, and each slopes obliquely downwards and medially. The clavicle tends therefore to glide on to the upper surface of the acromion. The tendency is counteracted by the acromioclavicular ligament but more particularly by the coracoclavicular ligament.

The capsule of the joint is supplied by filaments from the circumflex, suprascapular and pectoral nerves.

Movements. The only movements are slight gliding and rotatory movements. They occur in association with pivotal movements of the shoulder girdle as a whole at the sternoclavicular joint, and allow the scapula to remain in apposition with the chest wall in different positions of the girdle. [*See also* Movements at the Shoulder Joint, p. 80].

THE UPPER ARM

THE FRONT OF THE UPPER ARM

The deep fascia is already exposed and has been partly examined. Before proceeding to investigate the deeper connexions of the deep fascia, it may be well to review its general characters [p. 54] and the surface anatomy of the upper arm and the elbow [p. 43].

DISSECTION. (1) Cut through the deep fascia along the borders of the bicipital aponeurosis, so as to leave the aponeurosis in position. (2) Make a longitudinal incision through the deep fascia along the middle line of the biceps. (3) At the level of the epicondyles, make a transverse incision. (4) Reflect each of the two longitudinal flaps to its own side. As the reflexion proceeds it will become evident that four septa pass

from the deep surface of the deep fascia between the various muscles.

Septa of Deep Fascia. A loose septum passes transversely from side to side between the biceps and the muscle that lies behind it —the brachialis [FIGS. 36, 37]; the musculocutaneous nerve is embedded in it. Another septum dips backwards to separate the brachialis from the muscles that spring from the lateral supracondylar ridge; embedded in it there are the radial nerve and a small artery. But the strongest and most important septa are the **lateral** and **medial intermuscular septa,** which connect the investing layer of the deep fascia with the margins of the humerus, and,

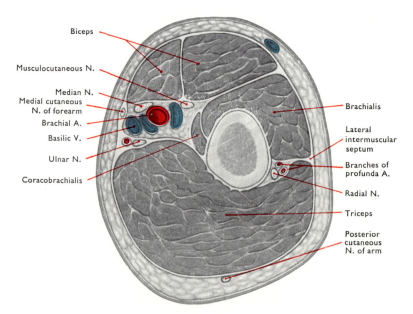

Biceps
Musculocutaneous N.
Median N.
Medial cutaneous N. of forearm
Brachial A.
Basilic V.
Ulnar N.
Coracobrachialis
Brachialis
Lateral intermuscular septum
Branches of profunda A.
Radial N.
Triceps
Posterior cutaneous N. of arm

FIG. 36 Section through the middle of right arm. Note positions of neurovascular bundles and intermuscular septa.

together with the humerus, divide the upper arm into two osteofascial compartments—an anterior and a posterior [Figs. 36, 37]. These two septa will be examined more fully after the back of the upper arm has been dissected [p. 74].

Anterior Compartment of Upper Arm. The **biceps brachii** is the most anterior muscle ; the **brachialis**, under cover of its distal half is closely applied to the front of the humerus ; and the **coracobrachialis** lies along the medial side of the proximal half of the biceps. The **brachioradialis** and the **extensor carpi radialis longus** lie in the distal part of the compartment along the lateral side of the brachialis, to which they are closely applied ; the brachioradialis is the upper and the anterior of the two. The **brachial vessels** traverse the whole length of the compartment, in relation with the medial border of the biceps. The **median nerve** also runs through the whole length of the compartment, lying lateral to the brachial artery in the proximal half, and medial to it in the distal half. The **basilic**

vein enters the compartment at the middle of the upper arm, where it pierces the deep fascia ; it then ascends along the medial side of the brachial artery.

DISSECTION. Clean the brachial artery and its branches, its venae comitantes, the proximal part of the basilic vein, and the accompanying nerves.

The artery should be disturbed as little as possible before its relations are studied. Therefore clean the nerves and the veins first, and take care not to injure the branches of the artery.

Begin with the medial cutaneous nerves of arm and forearm and trace them to the points where they pierce the deep fascia.

Clean the basilic vein and push it forwards. Pick up the ulnar nerve, and follow it downwards till it pierces the medial intermuscular septum. Next, follow the median nerve to the front of the elbow, and then clean the venae comitantes of the brachial artery, following them up to the axillary vein. At the same time clean the brachial artery, dividing the cross-channels that connect its venae comitantes as required.

Push the upper part of the brachial artery forwards to get at the radial nerve. Follow the nerve to the upper end of the radial groove of the humerus, and follow the

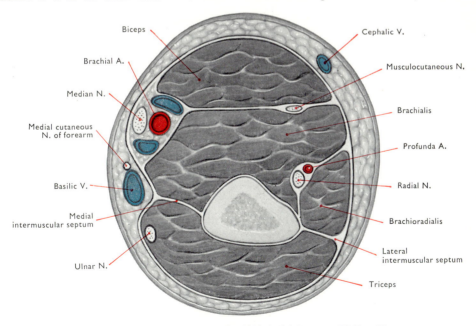

Fig. 37   Section through the distal third of right arm. Cf. Fig. 36.

branches which it gives off before it disappears.

Now identify the branches of the brachial artery; those named spring from its medial side or from the back of it.

Median Nerve

The median nerve arises in the axilla by two roots—one from the medial cord of the brachial plexus and one from the lateral cord. The nerve descends along the lateral side of the distal part of the axillary artery and the proximal half of the brachial artery as far as the insertion of the coracobrachialis ; there it crosses in front of the brachial artery (sometimes behind) and descends along its medial side to the bend of the elbow, where it enters the forearm. It gives off no branches either in the axilla or in the upper arm.

Ulnar Nerve

The ulnar nerve is the largest branch of the medial cord of the brachial plexus ; occasionally the lateral cord contributes a slender root (passing behind the medial root of the median nerve) which brings fibres of the seventh cervical nerve to the ulnar nerve. Like the other large nerves that spring from the plexus, it arises opposite the lower border of the pectoralis minor, near the coracoid process. It descends, along the medial side of the third part of the axillary artery and of the proximal half of the brachial artery, to the insertion of the coracobrachialis. It then leaves the brachial artery and, accompanied by the superior ulnar collateral artery, passes downwards and backwards through the medial intermuscular septum into the posterior compartment [FIG. 37] where it descends, on the medial head of the triceps, to the back of the medial epicondyle. Do not follow it into the posterior compartment at present ; it will be dissected there at a later period. Like the median nerve, it gives off no branches while it is in the axilla and the upper arm.

Brachial Artery

The brachial artery is the direct continuation of the axillary artery at the lower border of the teres major. It passes downwards and slightly laterally to the cubital fossa, where, at the level of the neck of the radius, it divides into the radial and the ulnar arteries [FIGS. 41, 53, 78]. In its proximal part it lies to the medial side of the humerus, with the medial head of the triceps behind it [FIG. 36], but as it approaches the elbow it passes to the front of the bone and lies on the brachialis [FIG. 37]. Thus pressure applied to the vessel in order to control the flow of blood through it must be directed laterally and backwards to the proximal part, and directly backwards in the distal part.

The neurovascular bundle on the medial aspect of the arm, containing the brachial artery, its venae comitantes and the median nerve, lies immediately deep to the fascia throughout its length, but is overlapped by coracobrachialis and biceps brachii [FIGS. 12, 36]. Superior to the insertion of coracobrachialis it is joined by the basilic vein and the medial cutaneous nerves of the arm and forearm from the superficial fascia, and by the ulnar nerve from the posterior compartment of the arm. In the proximal 2–3 cm. of the artery the radial nerve joins it from the radial groove of the humerus, emerging from between the medial and lateral heads of triceps.

Branches of the Brachial Artery. Several branches arise from the brachial artery. Those which arise from its lateral side are irregular and are distributed to the muscles and skin of the front of the arm. The named branches from the medial side and back are as follows.

The **profunda brachii artery** is the largest branch. It takes origin high up and accompanies the radial nerve to the back of the arm. Consequently, only a short part of the vessel is seen in the present dissection.

The **superior ulnar collateral artery** is a long, slender artery that accompanies the ulnar nerve to the back of the elbow.

The **nutrient artery** arises near the insertion of the coracobrachialis and very soon disappears into the nutrient foramen of the humerus.

The **inferior ulnar collateral artery** arises about 5 cm. above the bend of the elbow, runs medially on the brachialis and divides into an anterior branch and a larger posterior branch. These pass inferiorly towards the forearm anterior and posterior to the medial epicondyle of the humerus.

DISSECTION. Clean the biceps brachii, but do not injure the bicipital aponeurosis. Clean the coraco-brachialis; separate it carefully from the short head of the biceps to find the musculocutaneous nerve as it leaves the coracobrachialis; follow the nerve to the point where it emerges from behind the biceps, noting its branches to the biceps and brachialis and the

main arteries of supply that accompany them into the muscles. Clean the brachialis as far as the bend of the elbow.

Musculocutaneous Nerve

This nerve arises from the lateral cord of the brachial plexus and inclines laterally to enter the deep surface of the coracobrachialis a little below the pectoralis minor. It perforates the coracobrachialis and descends obliquely between the biceps and the brachialis until it approaches the bend of the elbow, where it pierces the deep fascia at the lateral border of the tendon of the biceps. From that point it

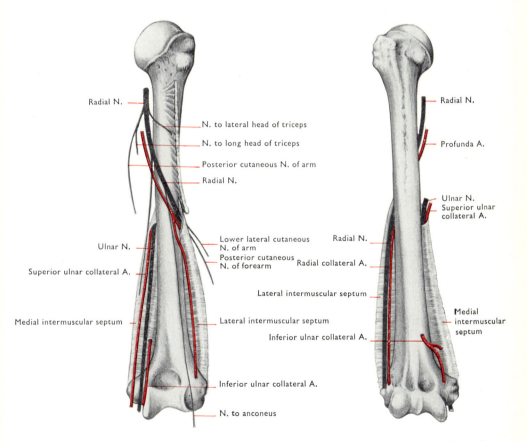

FIG. 38 Diagram to show relation of radial nerve to humerus, and of vessels and nerves (black) to the intermuscular septa.

has already been traced as the **lateral cutaneous nerve of the forearm** [p. 52].

The musculocutaneous nerve supplies branches to the coracobrachialis, the biceps and the brachialis. The first is given off before the parent trunk enters the muscle; the branch to the biceps springs from the trunk as it emerges from the coracobrachialis, and the branch to the brachialis arises as the trunk passes between that muscle and the biceps.

Coracobrachialis

This fairly slender, rounded muscle takes origin from the tip of the coracoid process in conjunction with the short head of the biceps brachii. It descends along the medial margin of the biceps, and is inserted into the medial margin of the humerus about its middle. Action: it is a flexor and adductor of the upper arm.

Biceps Brachii

The biceps muscle arises from the scapula by two heads. The short, medial head springs from the tip of the coracoid process in conjunction with the coracobrachialis [FIG. 19, p. 35]. The long, lateral head has a rounded tendon which occupies the intertubercular sulcus of the humerus. Its origin (from the supraglenoid tubercle of the scapula) cannot be studied at this stage, because it is within the shoulder joint. Both heads swell out into elongated fleshy bellies which are united in the distal third of the upper arm. Towards the bend of the elbow the fleshy fibres converge upon a stout, short tendon which is inserted into the posterior part of the tuberosity of the radius. A synovial bursa is interposed between the tendon and the anterior part of the radial tuberosity, which is smooth in consequence.

The **bicipital aponeurosis** [p. 54], already separated, artificially, from the deep fascia, springs from the tendon of the biceps, and also from the lower end of the short head. Tendinous fibres from each of the heads can be traced into it, and it is, in effect, an additional insertion of the muscle.

Nerve supply : the **musculocutaneous nerve** by a branch that divides to supply each head separately. Action: it is a powerful supinator [p. 123] and, with the brachialis, a flexor of the elbow. It contracts also in flexion at the shoulder joint, but the principal function of the tendon of the long head is to assist other muscles in retaining the head of the humerus in the glenoid cavity.

Brachialis

The brachialis is a strong muscle that arises from the front of the distal half of the

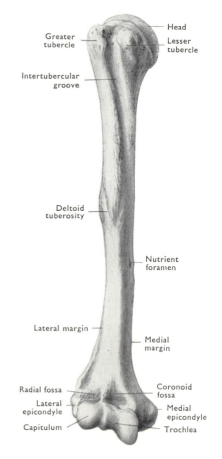

FIG. 39 Right humerus (anterior aspect).

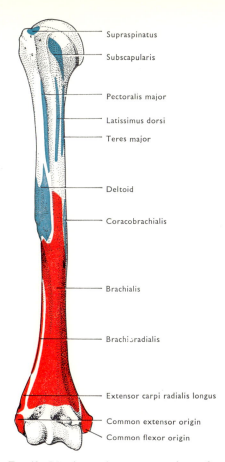

Supraspinatus

Subscapularis

Pectoralis major

Latissimus dorsi

Teres major

Deltoid

Coracobrachialis

Brachialis

Brachioradialis

Extensor carpi radialis longus

Common extensor origin

Common flexor origin

FIG. 40 Muscle attachments to anterior surface of right humerus.

shaft of the humerus (embracing the insertion of the deltoid) and from the intermuscular septa. The fibres converge to be inserted into the front of the coronoid process of the ulna by a short, thick tendon. The muscle lies partly under cover of the biceps brachii but is seen also on each side of it. It is overlapped on its medial side by the pronator teres, and on the lateral side by the brachioradialis and extensor carpi radialis longus. Its deep surface is closely connected to the anterior part of the capsule of the elbow joint.

Nerve supply: the **musculocutaneous**, enters

by several twigs near the medial border, but the muscle receives also one or two small, sensory (afferent) twigs from the radial nerve given off under cover of the brachioradialis. Action : the brachialis is the primary flexor of the elbow joint.

DISSECTION. **Separate the brachioradialis from the brachialis muscle, and dissect out the radial nerve and its accompanying artery, which lie deeply in the interval between the muscles. Look also for the branches given by the nerve to the brachialis, brachioradialis and extensor carpi radialis longus.**

THE CUBITAL FOSSA

The cubital fossa is the hollow in front of the elbow. It corresponds to the popliteal fossa at the back of the knee.

It is triangular in outline, with the base above. The **roof** is the deep fascia strengthened by the bicipital aponeurosis [FIGS. 28, 41]; it is pierced by a communication between the deep veins and the median cubital vein. It is covered by superficial fascia which contains portions of the cephalic and basilic veins, the median cubital vein, the anterior branch of the medial cutaneous nerve of the forearm, and the lateral cutaneous nerve of the forearm.

The **base** is an imaginary line drawn between the two epicondyles. The **medial border** is the pronator teres muscle. The **lateral border** is the brachioradialis. Those two muscles meet at the **apex,** where the brachioradialis overlaps the pronator teres. The **floor** is formed by the distal part of the brachialis muscle and the anterior part of the supinator muscle, which is wrapped round the proximal third of the shaft of the radius.

The contents of the fossa are shown in FIGURE 41.

The ulnar artery leaves the space by passing under cover of the pronator teres ; the radial artery descends through the apex of the fossa, overlapped by the brachioradialis. The median nerve, having given off branches to the muscles on its medial side, disappears between the two heads of the pronator teres. The tendon of the biceps brachii inclines

69

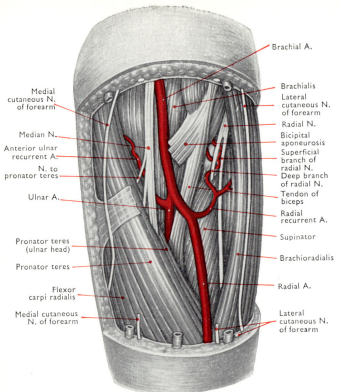

Brachial A.

Brachialis
Lateral cutaneous N. of forearm
Radial N.
Bicipital aponeurosis
Superficial branch of radial N.
Deep branch of radial N.
Tendon of biceps
Radial recurrent A.
Supinator
Brachioradialis

Radial A.

Lateral cutaneous N. of forearm

Medial cutaneous N. of forearm

Median N.
Anterior ulnar recurrent A.
N. to pronator teres

Ulnar A.

Pronator teres (ulnar head)

Pronator teres

Flexor carpi radialis

Medial cutaneous N. of forearm

FIG. 41   Dissection of left cubital fossa.
The fat has been removed and the bicipital aponeurosis cut away with the rest of the deep fascia.

To facilitate the cleaning of the floor and to expose structures which are not strictly contents of the fossa but lie under cover of its boundaries, bend the elbow slightly, and pull the boundaries of the fossa still wider apart. Find the radial nerve, and the radial collateral branch of the profunda artery at the level of the lateral epicondyle, between the brachioradialis and the brachialis. Follow the nerve and its deep branch, which disappears into the substance of the supinator, a muscle that is wrapped round the proximal part of the radius [Fig 41]. The superficial branch descends into the forearm between the brachioradialis and the supinator.

After the contents of the cubital fossa have been cleaned and their relative positions noted, turn to the dissection of the back of the upper arm.

THE BACK OF THE UPPER ARM

Revise the cutaneous nerves before proceeding with the dissection [see p. 50].

backwards, between the two bones of the forearm, to reach its insertion.

DISSECTION. Cut across the bicipital aponeurosis near the biceps [Fig. 41], open up the fossa by pulling aside its boundaries with hooks, and then proceed to clean its contents.

Follow the median nerve to the point where it disappears between the heads of the pronator teres, and secure the branches arising from its medial side. Clean the brachial, radial and ulnar arteries ; if their venae comitantes are in the way, remove them. Secure and clean the branches that arise from the radial and ulnar arteries in the fossa. Clean the tendon of the biceps brachii and follow it to its insertion. Look for its bursa and open it [p. 68].

DISSECTION. Make a longitudinal incision through the deep fascia as far as the olecranon, and a transverse incision from one epicondyle to the other, taking care not to injure the posterior cutaneous nerve of the forearm. Reflect the flaps of deep fascia until their continuity with the medial and lateral intermuscular septa is demonstrated. As the medial flap is reflected, avoid injury to the ulnar nerve and the artery which accompanies it. Clean the triceps muscle and define its attachments.

Triceps Brachii

The triceps muscle occupies the entire posterior osteofascial compartment of the arm. It arises by a long head from the scapula, and by two shorter heads—lateral and medial

—from the humerus. The fleshy fibres of the three heads join a common tendon which is inserted into the olecranon.

The superficial part of the muscle is, for the most part, formed by the long and lateral heads. The medial head is deeply placed, but a very small portion of it appears superficially, above the elbow, on each side of the common tendon of insertion.

The **long head** of the triceps arises, by a flattened tendon, from the infraglenoid tubercle of the scapula [FIG. 34].

The **two humeral heads** take origin from the back of the humerus. If it is borne in mind that no fibres arise from the radial groove and that the groove intervenes between the origins of the two heads, their relations will be easily understood.

The **lateral head** of the triceps arises from a rough strip that descends from the back of the greater tubercle to the groove—and also from the fascial sheet that bridges across the groove and the radial nerve.

The **medial head** of the triceps arises from

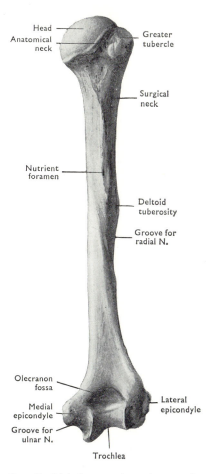

FIG. 42   Right humerus (posterior aspect).

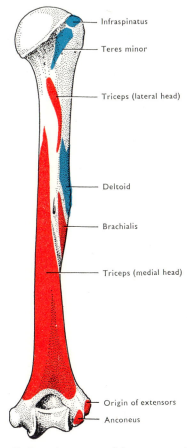

FIG. 43 Posterior aspect of humerus to show muscular attachments.

the whole of the back of the humerus below the radial groove, and from the intermuscular septa. The upper end of the origin, which is narrow and pointed, reaches the insertion of the teres major and is seen better on the front of the limb than on the back. The origin gradually widens as the groove passes towards the lateral border of the humerus, and in its distal third it covers the whole width of the back of the humerus. The medial head of the triceps, therefore, has very much the same origin from the back of the bone that the brachialis has from the front [cf. FIGS. 40 and 43].

The **common tendon** is inserted into the posterior part of the superior surface of the olecranon and into the fascia that covers the anconeus muscle, which lies at the lateral side of the olecranon. Some of the short, fleshy fibres of the medial head are attached directly to the olecranon, and a few of them are inserted into the posterior part of the capsule of the elbow joint. A small bursa, which lies on the top of the olecranon, separates the common tendon from the capsule of the elbow joint.

Nerve supply : the **radial nerve**. Action : it is a powerful extensor of the elbow joint and, by virtue of its long head, takes part also in movements at the shoulder joint.

DISSECTION. To expose the radial nerve and the profunda brachii artery fully, divide the lateral head of the triceps. The handle of a seeker thrust along the radial groove deep to the muscle will give the direction in which it should be severed. Beyond cleaning the nerve and its branches and the profunda brachii artery, as they lie in the groove, no further dissection is necessary.

Radial Nerve

The radial nerve is a terminal branch of the posterior cord of the brachial plexus. It is the thickest branch of that plexus and, like the ulnar and median nerves, it extends from the axilla to the hand. The radial nerve at first descends behind the third part of the axillary artery and the proximal part of the brachial artery. But it soon leaves the front of the arm in the interval between the long and the medial heads of the triceps, and enters a

shallow groove on the back of the humerus. In that groove, **sulcus n. radialis,** it passes round the back of the humerus, under cover of the lateral head of the triceps and, on the lateral side of the limb, it pierces the lateral intermuscular septum and passes into the anterior compartment of the arm, where it has been dissected already. There it lies deeply, in the interval that separates the brachialis from the brachioradialis and extensor carpi radialis longus. At the level of the lateral epicondyle of the humerus it gives off its deep branch, and then descends (superficial branch), in front of the lateral part of the elbow joint, into the forearm.

Branches. The branches which proceed from the radial nerve are muscular, cutaneous, and articular.

The **cutaneous branches** have already been traced. They are : (1) the posterior cutaneous nerve of the arm; (2) the lower lateral cutaneous nerve of the arm; and (3) the posterior cutaneous nerve of the forearm.

The superficial branch of the radial nerve which is continued into the forearm is cutaneous, but it does not pierce the deep fascia till it approaches the wrist. Its distribution is to the skin of the back of the hand and the digits [p. 53].

The **muscular branches** are distributed to the three heads of the triceps, to the anconeus, to the brachioradialis, and to the extensor carpi radialis longus, and give sensory fibres to brachialis. The branches to the three last-named muscles spring from the trunk of the nerve after it has pierced the lateral intermuscular septum. The branch to the long head of the triceps arises in the axilla [p. 25] and pierces its anterior surface ; those to the other heads of the triceps arise as the main nerve enters the radial groove. In addition, the medial head receives on its anteromedial surface a long, slender branch that runs with the ulnar nerve in the upper arm. The branch to the anconeus, also long and slender, reaches the muscle through the substance of the medial head of the triceps [FIG. 41].

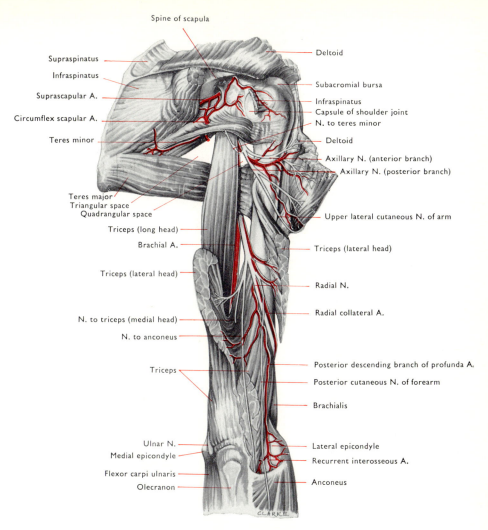

Spine of scapula

Supraspinatus

Infraspinatus

Suprascapular A.

Circumflex scapular A.

Teres minor

Teres major
Triangular space
Quadrangular space

Triceps (long head)

Brachial A.

Triceps (lateral head)

N. to triceps (medial head)

N. to anconeus

Triceps

Ulnar N.

Medial epicondyle

Flexor carpi ulnaris

Olecranon

Deltoid

Subacromial bursa

Infraspinatus

Capsule of shoulder joint

N. to teres minor

Deltoid

Axillary N. (anterior branch)

Axillary N. (posterior branch)

Upper lateral cutaneous N. of arm

Triceps (lateral head)

Radial N.

Radial collateral A.

Posterior descending branch of profunda A.

Posterior cutaneous N. of forearm

Brachialis

Lateral epicondyle

Recurrent interosseous A.

Anconeus

CLARKE

FIG. 44 Dissection of back of shoulder and arm. The lateral head of triceps has been divided and turned aside to expose the spiral groove on the humerus for the radial nerve.

The **articular branches** arise near the elbow, and supply the capsule of the elbow joint.

The deep branch, continuing as the **posterior interosseous nerve** has an extensive distribution to the muscles on the back of the forearm and

to the radiocarpal and carpal joints. It will be dissected later.

Profunda Brachii Artery

The profunda artery [p. 66] accompanies the radial nerve through the radial groove.

Before it reaches the lateral intermuscular septum it divides into two descending terminal branches—an anterior (**radial collateral artery**) and a posterior—which take part in the anastomoses around the elbow joint.

The other branches are distributed chiefly to the triceps; but a **nutrient artery** often springs from the profunda and enters the humerus through the floor of the radial groove. An ascending or **deltoid branch,** which runs upwards between the long and lateral heads of the triceps to anastomose with the **posterior circumflex humeral artery,** is more important as it forms a link between the axillary and brachial systems of branches, and

sometimes replaces the posterior circumflex [p. 59].

DISSECTION. Trace the ulnar nerve and the superior ulnar collateral artery to the medial epicondyle. Clean also the posterior branch of the inferior ulnar collateral artery. Raise the tendon of the triceps, and look for the bursa that lies under cover of it.

Review the intermuscular septa, which are now fully exposed.

Intermuscular Septa

The **medial intermuscular septum** is the stronger. It connects the investing deep fascia with the medial border of the humerus, and

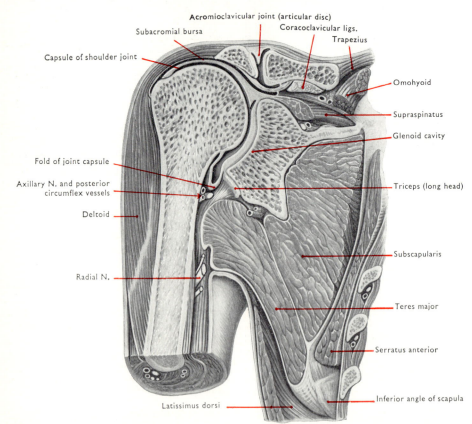

FIG. 45 Coronal section through right shoulder joint. The inferior part of serratus anterior has been cut away. (Viewed from the front. Cf. FIG. 49.)

separates the medial head of the triceps from the brachialis, giving attachment to both muscles. It extends, as a strong membrane, from the medial epicondyle to the insertion of the coracobrachialis. At the level of the insertion of the coracobrachialis, it is pierced by the **ulnar nerve** which then descends behind it to the medial epicondyle, covered by a thin layer of fleshy fibres that belong to the medial head of the triceps [FIGS. 36, 38].

The **lateral intermuscular septum** connects the deep fascia with the lateral border of the humerus. It extends from the lateral epicondyle to the insertion of the deltoid muscle. It separates the lateral part of the medial head of the triceps, which arises from its posterior surface, from three muscles that spring from its anterior surface — the brachialis, brachioradialis and extensor carpi radialis longus. At the junction of the middle and distal thirds of the upper arm, it is pierced by the **radial nerve** [FIGS. 36, 38].

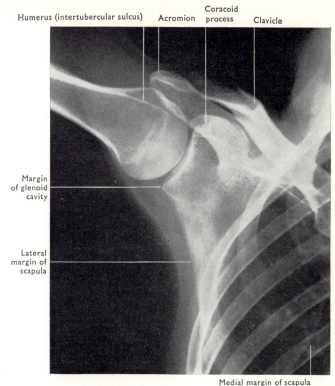

Humerus (intertubercular sulcus) Acromion Coracoid process Clavicle

Margin of glenoid cavity

Lateral margin of scapula

Medial margin of scapula

FIG. 46   Radiograph of the shoulder with the arm abducted. Note that the humerus lies in line with the spine of the scapula, and that the scapula has rotated so that the glenoid cavity faces upwards and laterally, and the lateral end of the clavicle has been elevated. Cf. FIG. 51.

THE SHOULDER JOINT

This is the time to dissect the shoulder joint, in order that the ligaments may be examined before they have become too dry.

The shoulder joint belongs to the ball-and-socket group of synovial joints. The socket is the glenoid cavity of the scapula, and the ball is the head of the humerus.

In no joint in the body are the movements so free and so varied as in the shoulder joint. This is necessary owing to the many functions performed by the upper limb. Freedom of movement is provided for in two ways: (1)

by the large size of the head of the humerus, in comparison with the small, shallow glenoid cavity; (2) by the great laxity of the capsule of the joint. These provisions for allowing an extensive range of movement might, at first sight, lead one to doubt the security of the joint. Its strength certainly does not lie in the adaptation of the bony surfaces to each other, nor in the strength of its ligaments. It lies in: (1) the powerful muscles by which it is closely surrounded; (2) the coraco-acromial arch, which overhangs it and forms a secondary socket for the head of the humerus, and effectually prevents upward displacement;

and (3) atmospheric pressure, which exercises a powerful influence in keeping the opposed surfaces in contact with each other.

On all aspects, except over a small area below, the capsule is supported by muscles, the tendons of which are more or less adherent to it. **Above,** it is covered by the supraspinatus; **behind,** the infraspinatus and teres minor are applied to it; **in front,** there is the subscapularis—which is also below the capsule near the scapula [FIG. 48]. **Below,** the capsule is otherwise unsupported by muscles, and there, in the ordinary dependent position of the limb, it bulges downwards, in the form of a fold, into the upper part of the quadrangular space [FIGS. 45, 49]. When, however, the arm is abducted, the fold is obliterated and the head of the bone rests upon the inferior part of the capsule, which now receives partial support from the long head of the triceps and the teres major which are stretched

under it. Nevertheless, this is the weakest part of the joint, and dislocation of the head of the humerus downwards into the axilla, through the inferior part of the capsule, is consequently an occurrence of considerable frequency. When the dislocation occurs, the circumflex vessels and axillary nerve may be injured as they are close to the capsule [FIGS. 45, 49].

DISSECTION. The capsule of the shoulder joint was to a large extent exposed by the reflexion of the muscles inserted into the tubercles of the humerus; and the subscapular bursa has been examined.

To expose the capsule more fully: Cut through the combined tendon of the coracobrachialis and biceps, and displace the muscles downwards. Cut through the teres major about its middle, and the long head of the triceps about 2 cm. below its origin, and turn both muscles aside. Turn aside the reflected subscapularis, supraspinatus, infraspinatus and teres minor muscles, and note whether or not there is an aperture in

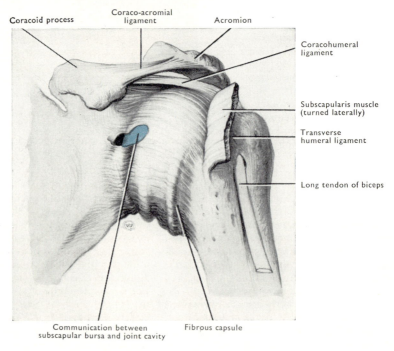

Coracoid process — Coraco-acromial ligament — Acromion — Coracohumeral ligament — Subscapularis muscle (turned laterally) — Transverse humeral ligament — Long tendon of biceps — Communication between subscapular bursa and joint cavity — Fibrous capsule

FIG. 47 Anterior aspect of left shoulder joint.

76

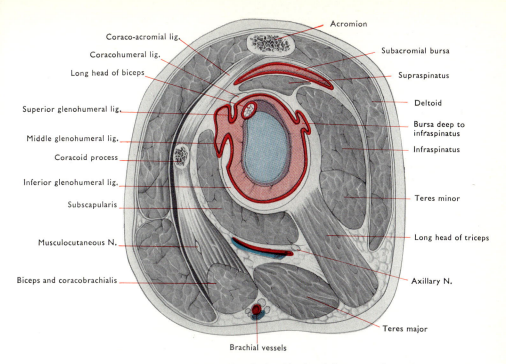

FIG. 48   Dissection of sagittal section through left shoulder (semi-diagrammatic).   The subscapular bursa protrudes between the superior and middle glenohumeral ligaments.

the capsule between subscapularis and supraspinatus through which the subacromial bursa communicates with the joint.

Re-examine the subscapular bursa, and note that its aperture of communication with the joint is situated near the root of the coracoid process. Clean the outer surface of the capsule thoroughly. Note its laxity, and define its attachments.

Fibrous Capsule

The fibrous capsule is a thin but fairly dense and strong tubular membrane which envelops the joint on all sides. It is attached to the scapula around the margin of the glenoid cavity, fusing with the outer surface of a fibrocartilaginous ring, called the labrum glenoidale, which is attached to the margin of the cavity and increases its depth. Laterally, the capsule is attached to the anatomical neck of the humerus and to the transverse ligament, which bridges across the top of the inter-

tubercular groove. Superiorly this attachment is close to the articular surface of the head, but inferiorly it is 1·5 cm. or more from the articular surface; consequently, a considerable part of the medial surface of the surgical neck is inside the fibrous part of the capsule, and is covered with the synovial membrane [FIG. 49]. This cannot be seen until the capsule has been opened.

Apertures in Fibrous Capsule. The fibrous capsule is not complete at all points. Its continuity is always broken by one aperture and sometimes by two more; and where its lateral margin is attached to the transverse ligament, there is an aperture below the margin. Prolongations of the synovial membrane protrude through all the apertures.

The largest opening is in the antero-medial part near the root of the coracoid process; and the protruding synovial membrane

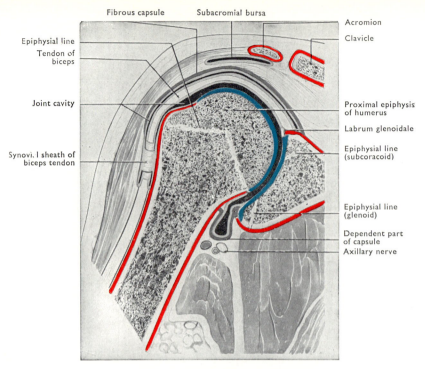

Fibrous capsule · Subacromial bursa · Acromion · Clavicle · Epiphysial line · Tendon of biceps · Joint cavity · Synovi. l sheath of biceps tendon · Proximal epiphysis of humerus · Labrum glenoidale · Epiphysial line (subcoracoid) · Epiphysial line (glenoid) · Dependent part of capsule · Axillary nerve

FIG. 49   Coronal section through the right shoulder joint. The parietal and visceral layers of the synovial sheath of the biceps tendon have been partially left in place.

forms the **subscapular bursa,** which separates the subscapularis from the capsule and the neck of the scapula anteriorly. When the joint is dislocated, the head of the humerus is occasionally driven through this opening instead of through the lower part of the capsule. A second opening is sometimes found in the posterolateral part of the capsule, the synovial membrane protruding to form a bursa under the infraspinatus muscle [FIG. 48]. Still more rarely, the subacromial bursa communicates with the cavity of the joint through an opening opposite the interval between the supraspinatus and subscapularis muscles.

Transverse Humeral Ligament. This ligament bridges across the intertubercular groove which contains the tendon of the long head of biceps surrounded by a tubular prolongation of the synovial membrane. The tendon and

its sheath escape from beneath the free lower border of the ligament at the level of the epiphysial line [FIG. 49].

Accessory Bands. The fibrous capsule is thickened by bands of fibres which pass from the scapula to the humerus. One of them— the **coracohumeral ligament** [FIG. 47]—can be seen from the exterior; it is a wide, strong band on the upper surface of the joint, and is more or less completely incorporated in the capsule. The other three—the **glenohumeral ligaments** [FIG. 50]—can be seen only from the inside, where they may raise ridges of synovial membrane.

The pectoralis minor occasionally sends a slip through the coraco-acromial ligament to fuse with the coracohumeral ligament and, through it, to gain attachment to the humerus.

78

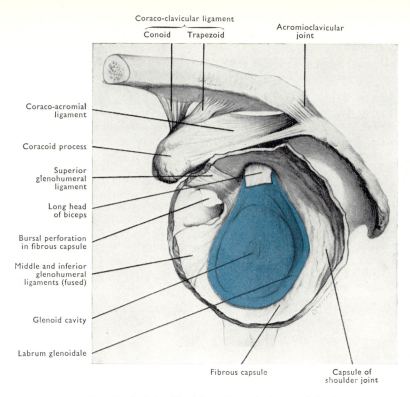

Coraco-clavicular ligament

Conoid   Trapezoid

Acromioclavicular joint

Coraco-acromial ligament

Coracoid process

Superior glenohumeral ligament

Long head of biceps

Bursal perforation in fibrous capsule

Middle and inferior glenohumeral ligaments (fused)

Glenoid cavity

Labrum glenoidale

Fibrous capsule

Capsule of shoulder joint

FIG. 50 Left shoulder joint. The articular capsule has been cut across and the humerus removed together with the surrounding muscles.

DISSECTION. **Make a vertical incision through the posterior part of the capsule. Turn the head of the humerus aside and note the glenohumeral ligaments, if visible. Then complete the division of the capsule, cut the long tendon of the biceps, and pull the humerus and scapula apart.**

Labrum Glenoidale

The labrum is the dense, fibrocartilaginous lip which is attached to the rim of the glenoid cavity and serves to deepen and widen the socket.

Tendon of Long Head of Biceps. This tendon is an important factor in the mechanism of the shoulder joint. Traced from below, it enters the joint through the opening between the two tubercles of the humerus, and is prolonged over the head of the bone to the apex of the glenoid cavity, where it is attached chiefly to the bone but partly blends with the labrum. By its position within the capsule and in the deep sulcus between the tubercles of the humerus, it prevents upward displacement of the head of the humerus and steadies it during movement.

Synovial Membrane

The synovial membrane lines the fibrous capsule, and is reflected from it on to the labrum and on to the neck of the humerus as far as the articular margin of the head. It envelopes the tendon of biceps in the joint and forms a number of protrusions [p. 77, FIG. 48].

Articular Surfaces

The cartilage of the head of the humerus is thickest in the centre and thins towards the edges. In the glenoid cavity the reverse of this will be seen if the cartilage is incised.

Movements at the Shoulder Joint

The shoulder is a ball-and-socket joint, and consequently movement in every direction is permitted, viz.: (1) **Flexion,** or forward movement; (2) **extension,** or backward movement; (3) **abduction;** (4) **adduction.** By combination of the angular movements, **circumduction** is produced. The muscles inserted into the tubercles act mainly in steadying and preventing displacement of the head of the humerus, while the main effectors of these movements are inserted further from the joint. **Rotation** of the humerus around its long axis, to the extent of quarter of a circle, occurs also.

The range of movement of the limb as a whole depends upon movements of the shoulder girdle, which are invariably associated with movements at the shoulder joint. In abducting the arm to the horizontal position, for example, and then raising it above the head, the movements at shoulder joint and of shoulder girdle are associated throughout. Radiographs taken in different phases of the action [FIG. 51] demonstrate this association, and it has been shown that there is continuous movement of the scapula on the chest wall, and of the humerus at the shoulder joint. Abduction of the humerus includes considerable lateral rotation if the arm is raised in the coronal plane. If it is raised in the plane of the scapula—a combination of pure flexion and abduction relative to the trunk—there is no rotation; and in that plane the arm can be easily raised much higher above the head.

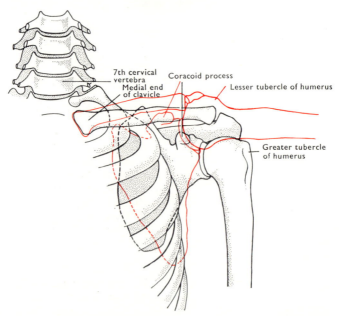

FIG. 51 A diagram prepared from tracings of two radiographs of the same individual to show the change in position of the various bones during abduction of the arm to the horizontal. Note the rotation of the scapula. the elevation of the clavicle, and the elevation and rotation of the humerus laterally.

THE FOREARM AND HAND

Before proceeding with the dissection, review the surface anatomy of the forearm and hand [p. 43], the arrangement of the superficial veins [p. 46], and the cutaneous nerves [p. 52].

THE FLEXOR COMPARTMENT OF THE FOREARM

In this dissection the structures to be displayed are the radial and ulnar arteries, the median, ulnar and radial nerves, and the group of pronator and flexor muscles.

DISSECTION. Make two incisions through the deep fascia: (1) a transverse incision along the upper border of the flexor retinaculum; (2) a longitudinal incision from the apex of the cubital fossa to the transverse incision.

As the transverse incision is made, be careful not to injure the structures that are immediately subjacent to the deep fascia.

Turn the two flaps aside, dividing the septa which pass from their deep surfaces between the adjacent muscles. Both flaps can be reflected to the posterior border of the ulna, but, for the present, do not reflect the lateral flap beyond the radial border of the forearm. Near the elbow, where the muscles gain additional origin from the fascia, leave the fascia in situ, for attempts to remove it will result only in laceration of the muscles.

MUSCLES OF THE FRONT OF FOREARM

These muscles are the flexors of the wrist and digits and the pronators of the forearm,

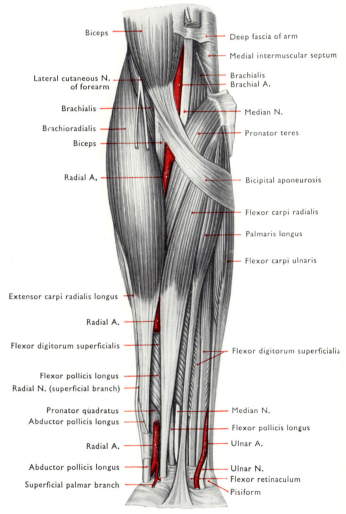

FIG. 52   Dissection of superficial muscles, arteries, and nerves of front of forearm.   Part of the radial artery was removed to show the muscles deep to it.

and are arranged in a superficial and a deep group.

The **superficial group** consists of the pronator teres, the flexor carpi radialis, the palmaris longus, and the flexor carpi ulnaris (from the lateral to the medial side), and also the flexor digitorum superficialis, which is in a deeper plane, and comes to the surface only partially.

Identify these five muscles by reference to

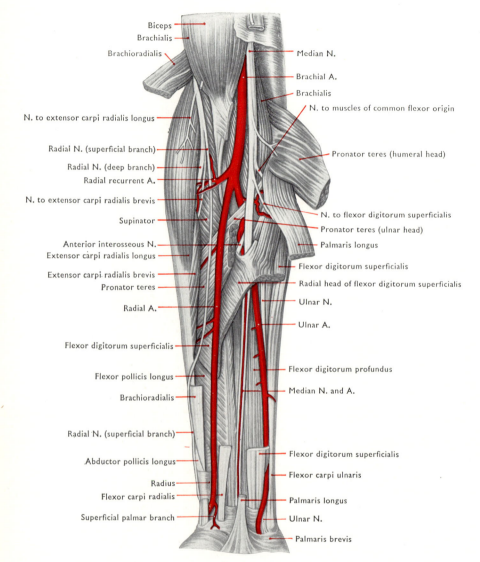

FIG. 53 Deep dissection of muscles, and nerves of front of forearm. The division of the brachial artery is slightly lower than usual.

FIGURE 52; they extend distally from the medial epicondyle. The pronator teres ends at the middle of the radius, the remainder reach the hand.

The **deep group** is composed of three muscles, placed in contact with the bones and interosseous membrane [FIG. 59].

The **brachioradialis** muscle, though it belongs to the extensor group, lies in the lateral part of the **front** of the forearm and is functionally a flexor of the elbow. It extends from the lateral supracondylar ridge of the humerus to the distal end of the radius and it should be dissected at this stage with the radial artery and the radial nerve. Its description will be found with the other members of its group.

DISSECTION. Clean the brachioradialis from end to end. Two muscles overlie its distal part—the abductor pollicis longus and extensor pollicis brevis. Push them aside, taking care not to injure the superficial branch of the radial nerve. Having cleaned the brachioradialis, pull it aside and clean the radial nerve and the radial artery and its branches.

Radial Artery

This, the smaller of the two terminal branches of the brachial artery, is a direct continuation of the parent trunk in the forearm. It takes origin in the cubital fossa opposite the neck of the radius, and it descends in the lateral part of the front of the limb to the distal end of the radius. There, it turns round the lateral border of the wrist and leaves the present dissection [FIG. 68].

Relations in Forearm. Throughout its whole length it is closely accompanied by **venae comitantes.** Deeply placed in the upper half of the forearm it becomes superficial between the tendons of brachioradialis and flexor carpi radialis in the lower half [FIG. 52]. It lies on the muscles attached to the anterior surface of the radius and, distally, on the radius itself [FIG. 53] against which its pulsations (the radial pulse) can be felt readily just lateral to the tendon of flexor carpi radialis. The superficial branch of the radial nerve lies lateral to it in the upper two-thirds

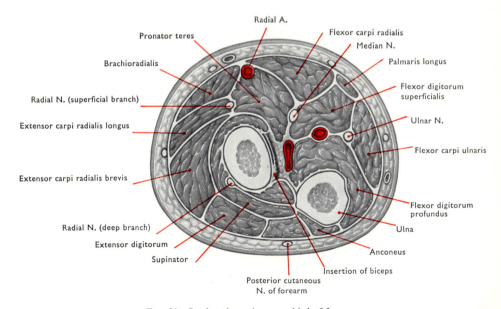

FIG. 54   Section through upper third of forearm.

of the forearm, then turns round the lateral aspect of the forearm under the tendon of brachioradialis.

Branches in Forearm. The **muscular branches** are numerous; they arise at irregular points, mainly in the upper part of its course in the forearm [FIG. 53].

The **radial recurrent artery** takes origin close to the beginning of the radial artery. It runs upwards to anastomose with the radial collateral branch of the profunda brachii artery in front of the lateral epicondyle.

The **superficial palmar artery,** small and variable, arises a short distance above the wrist, and ends in the thenar muscles. It may, however, continue into the palm and take part in forming the superficial palmar arch.

The **anterior carpal artery** is a small branch that runs medially on the distal end of the radius.

BRANCHES OF THE RADIAL NERVE

The **deep branch** of the radial nerve springs from the main trunk at the level of the lateral epicondyle of the humerus and descends in front of the capitulum and lateral part of the head of the radius under cover of the brachioradialis. It gives branches to the extensor carpi radialis brevis and the supinator, and then disappears into the supinator to reappear in the back of the forearm as the **posterior interosseous nerve.**

The **superficial branch** leaves the upper arm by descending in front of the lateral part of the elbow joint. In the forearm it lies for a great part of its course under cover of the brachioradialis, coming into relation with the lateral side of the radial artery in the middle third of the forearm. In the distal third it leaves the artery, inclines backwards, appears at the posterior border of the tendon of the brachioradialis, pierces the deep fascia about 5 cm. above the wrist, and descends across the abductor pollicis longus and extensor pollicis brevis into the hand, where it has been examined already. It gives off no branches in the forearm.

DISSECTION. Before you begin to clean the superficial flexor muscles, make an attempt to demonstrate the synovial sheaths of the flexor tendons; their upper parts are under cover of the deep fascia above the flexor retinaculum. They are: the common sheath of the superficial and deep flexors of the fingers, the sheath of the flexor pollicis longus and the sheath of the flexor carpi radialis.

If the sheaths are uninjured they can be distended with air by means of a blowpipe, or by liquid forced in through a syringe. If they have been injured, explore them with a blunt probe.

Examine, first, the common sheath of the flexor tendons of the fingers. Pick up a fold of the medial part of its anterior wall with the forceps, and introduce the blowpipe or the needle of the syringe into the base of the fold. As the air or liquid enters the sheath, note that it is distended at first upwards as far as 2·5 cm. above the flexor retinaculum. The swelling then passes downwards, behind the retinaculum to the middle of the palm and along the little finger, as far as the terminal phalanx.

The sheath of the flexor carpi radialis is not easily distended because it is enclosed for the greater part of its extent in an osteofibrous canal. Open it at the upper border of the retinaculum and investigate it with a blunt probe.

Pull the tendon of the flexor carpi radialis medially, find the tendon of the flexor pollicis longus behind it, and either distend its sheath in the manner indicated or examine it with a probe.

SYNOVIAL SHEATHS OF FLEXOR TENDONS

Synovial sheaths surround tendons where they pass through fascial or osteofascial canals. They consist of two concentric tubes of smooth synovial membrane joined together at the ends and separated by a capillary interval (the cavity of the sheath) which contains only sufficient synovia to lubricate their opposing surfaces, and to allow them to slide on each other. The inner tube surrounds and is adherent to the tendon (or tendons), the outer tube lines the fibrous or bony canal and is fused with it. Tendons may be completely enclosed in the synovial sheath in this way or appear to be invaginated into the sheath from one side and suspended in it by a fold of synovial membrane. In the latter case blood vessels can reach the tendon at any point along the length of the sheath, but in the

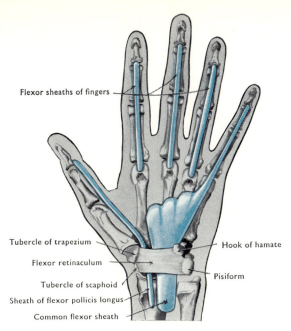

Flexor sheaths of fingers

Tubercle of trapezium

Flexor retinaculum

Tubercle of scaphoid

Sheath of flexor pollicis longus

Common flexor sheath

Hook of hamate

Pisiform

FIG. 55 Synovial sheaths of flexor tendons of digits.

FIG. 56 Drawing of transverse section through distal row of carpal bones to show position of long flexor tendons and their synovial sheaths (red). At this level the tendons to the index and middle fingers are leaving the common synovial sheath, which still surrounds those to the ring and little fingers.

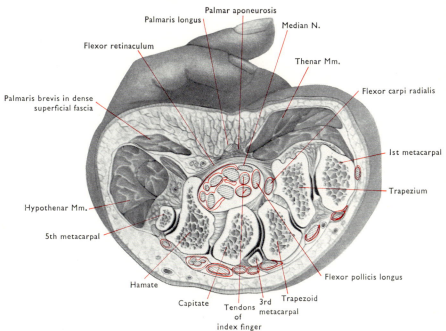

Palmar aponeurosis

Palmaris longus

Median N.

Flexor retinaculum

Thenar Mm.

Palmaris brevis in dense superficial fascia

Flexor carpi radialis

1st metacarpal

Trapezium

Hypothenar Mm.

5th metacarpal

Flexor pollicis longus

Hamate

Capitate

Tendons of index finger

3rd metacarpal

Trapezoid

former they must enter from the ends or run across the cavity of the sheath in a tubular sleeve of synovial membrane (see vincula). When inflamed, the cavity of the sheath becomes distended with fluid, tense and painful [p. 102].

As the tendons pass behind the flexor retinaculum, accompanied by the median nerve, the flexor pollicis longus is surrounded by one sheath, and the flexors of the fingers by a single **common flexor sheath** into which they are invaginated from the lateral side [FIGS. 56 and 66]. These sheaths, which may communicate, line the carpal tunnel, are prolonged for 2–3 cm. or more into the forearm, and reach distally to the terminal phalanx only in the case of the thumb and little finger [FIG. 55]; the other fingers have separate synovial sheaths within their fibrous flexor sheaths. Other tendons entering the hand are also surrounded by their own synovial sheaths.

DISSECTION. Clean the muscles that arise from the medial epicondyle, and be careful not to damage their nerves, which enter them (with the exception of the flexor carpi ulnaris) from the median nerve in the cubital fossa.

Begin with the pronator teres. Clean it from end to end, pushing aside the muscles that cover its insertion, and be careful not to injure the radial origin of the flexor digitorum superficialis, which lies deep to its lower part. Separate the pronator teres from the flexor carpi radialis. Cut the head of the pronator that arises from the medial epicondyle. Turn the lower part downwards and find the deep head, a slender slip behind the median nerve arising from the coronoid process of the ulna.

Clean the flexor carpi radialis down to the flexor retinaculum, and clean the palmaris longus down to its insertion into the palmar aponeurosis. (The palmaris longus is sometimes absent.)

Now clean the flexor carpi ulnaris—first down to the pisiform bone, and then upwards. In addition to its epicondylar origin it has a thin, wide head that arises from the posterior, subcutaneous border of the ulna. Find the ulnar nerve between the two heads at the elbow and, by separating the muscle from the palmaris longus and flexor digitorum superficialis, trace the nerve into the forearm and onwards to the wrist. Secure its branches to the flexor carpi ulnaris, which arise just below the elbow, and to the flexor digitorum

profundus a little lower down; also the cutaneous branches (dorsal branch and palmar cutaneous branch, p. 53) that arise from it in the lower half of the forearm. Clean the lower half of the ulnar artery (and its branches) as far as the wrist; its carpal branches, given off near the wrist, are very liable to injury.

To get a good view of the flexor digitorum superficialis: Divide the palmaris longus and the flexor carpi radialis at the middle of the forearm; turn their proximal parts upwards and separate them from the pronator teres and the superficial flexor by splitting the intervening intermuscular septa; trace the median nerve to the point at which it disappears behind the flexor digitorum superficialis. Then clean the muscle and its four tendons, being careful not to injure the part of it that arises from the radius. Pull upon the tendons and note the results. Do not follow them farther than the flexor retinaculum at present.

SUPERFICIAL FLEXOR MUSCLES

These five muscles have a **common origin** from the front of the medial epicondyle, from which they diverge as a narrow fan; the lateral muscles running an oblique course across the forearm tend to cause pronation [p. 124] as well as flexion.

Pronator Teres

This muscle crosses the proximal half of the front of the forearm obliquely. It arises by two heads.

The **humeral head** constitutes the chief bulk of the muscle. It springs from the medial epicondyle and from the distal part of the medial supracondylar ridge. The **ulnar head** is a small slip which arises from the medial border of the coronoid process of the ulna [FIG. 40], passes between the median nerve and the ulnar artery, and joins the deep surface of the humeral head.

The muscle descends obliquely and ends by a tendon in a rough impression on the middle of the lateral surface of the radius [FIG. 59]. This attachment is on the summit of the chief curve of the radius—an arrangement which enables the muscle to exercise its pronating action at great advantage. Nerve supply: the **median nerve.** Action: it is a pronator and a flexor of the elbow.

Flexor Carpi Radialis

The radial flexor of the wrist arises chiefly from the medial epicondyle. A short distance below the middle of the forearm, its fleshy belly gives place to a long tendon which, at the wrist, traverses the groove on the front of the trapezium in a special compartment at the lateral end of the flexor retinaculum [Fig. 56]. It is inserted chiefly into the base of the metacarpal bone of the index.

Nerve supply: **median.** Action: It is a flexor of the wrist and elbow, an abductor of the hand, and assists pronation.

Palmaris Longus

This long, slender muscle is not always present. Its tendon pierces the deep fascia immediately above the wrist, and then crosses the flexor retinaculum, adhering to it, to be inserted into the apex of the palmar aponeurosis. Nerve supply: **median.** Action: a flexor of the wrist and elbow joints.

Flexor Carpi Ulnaris

The ulnar flexor of the wrist arises by : (1) The **humeral head** from the medial epicondyle ; (2) the **ulnar head** from the olecranon and, by a wide **aponeurosis,** from the upper two-thirds of the posterior border of the ulna. The two heads of origin bridge across the interval between the medial epicondyle and the olecranon, and under this arch the ulnar nerve passes into the forearm. The tendon appears on the anterior border of the muscle, and is inserted into the pisiform bone.

Nerve supply: **ulnar.** Action: flexor and adductor of the hand and a flexor of the elbow.

Flexor Digitorum Superficialis

This muscle receives its name because it is superficial to the flexor profundus, but for the most part it lies deeper than the other superficial muscles [Fig. 52]. It is a powerful muscle which arises by : (1) The **humero-ulnar head** chiefly from the medial epicondyle and the coronoid process. (2) The **radial head,** a thin sheet that arises from the upper half of the anterior border of the radius [Fig. 59].

The four tendons enter the palm by passing under cover of the flexor retinaculum and go to the medial four digits to be inserted into the middle phalanx. Note that for 2–3 cm. above the wrist, they are enveloped by the synovial sheath, and also that they lie in pairs—the tendons to the ring and middle fingers being placed in front of those for the index and little fingers.

Nerve supply : **median.** Action : a flexor of the proximal interphalangeal joints of the fingers, the metacarpo-phalangeal joints, and the wrist joint.

DISSECTION. Divide the radial head from the main mass of the flexor digitorum superficialis and separate the two portions. Detach the median nerve from the deep surface of the muscle, and trace it downwards. Secure its palmar cutaneous branch near the wrist, and look for a branch it may give to the lower part of the superficial flexor.

Clean the flexor pollicis longus and the flexor digitorum profundus, taking care of their nerves, and complete the cleaning of the ulnar artery.

Return to the median nerve in the cubital fossa. Trace its branches to neighbouring muscles. Follow it downwards and secure the anterior interosseous nerve, which springs from the median as it passes between the heads of the pronator teres. Find the common interosseous artery, which arises from the ulnar 2–3 cm. below its origin, and soon divides into the anterior and posterior interosseous arteries. The posterior branch passes backwards out of this dissection. Separate the flexor pollicis and flexor profundus, and trace the anterior interosseous artery and nerve downwards to the pronator quadratus—taking care of the branches of the nerve. Clean the pronator quadratus.

THE ULNAR ARTERY

This is the larger of the two terminal branches of the brachial trunk. It takes origin, in the cubital fossa, at the level of the neck of the radius [Fig. 78]. In the upper third of the forearm it passes obliquely downwards and medially, and then proceeds straight down to the wrist. It is accompanied by two venae comitantes and lies on the brachialis and flexor digitorum profundus [Fig. 53] deep to the superficial flexor muscles of the forearm, and crossed by the median nerve. A short distance above the wrist it becomes superficial between the tendons of flexor carpi ulnaris and flexor digitorum superficialis and, piercing the deep fascia just proximal to the flexor retinaculum, passes on to its superficial surface. Here it gives off a deep palmar branch and continues as the superficial palmar arch.

Branches of the Ulnar Artery in Forearm

In addition to **muscular branches,** there are several that are named.

The **ulnar recurrent arteries,** anterior and posterior, arise near the elbow and anastomose with branches of the brachial artery on the front and back of the medial epicondyle.

The **common interosseous artery** is a short wide trunk which takes origin below the recurrent branches, about 2 cm. from the commencement of the ulnar artery. It passes backwards to the upper margin of the interosseous membrane, where it divides.

The **posterior interosseous artery** passes backwards above the interosseous membrane to the back of the forearm, where it will be dissected at a later period.

The **anterior interosseous artery** descends over the front of the interosseous membrane, between the flexor pollicis longus and the flexor digitorum profundus. At the upper border of the pronator quadratus, it pierces the interosseous membrane and passes to the back of the forearm, where it will be seen later. In addition to **muscular** twigs, it supplies **nutrient arteries** to the radius and the ulna,

and gives off the **median artery**—long and slender—which accompanies the median nerve.

The **carpal branches** of the ulnar artery are small arteries that arise near the wrist. They anastomose with corresponding branches of

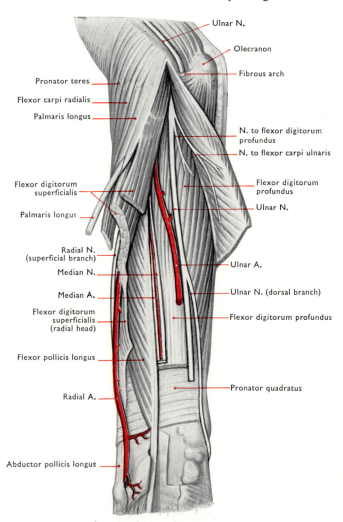

Fig. 57   Deep dissection of front of forearm.
The elbow is partially flexed, the forearm semi-pronated. The superficial muscles are cut short and turned aside. The deeper parts are still further displayed by the separation of the flexor digitorum superficialis from the flexor carpi ulnaris.

88

the radial artery in the formation of **anterior** and **posterior carpal arches.**

THE ULNAR NERVE

The ulnar nerve arises in the axilla from the medial cord of the brachial plexus, descends through the medial part of the upper arm to the back of the medial epicondyle, and passes between the heads of the flexor carpi ulnaris to enter the forearm.

Course in Forearm. It descends in the medial part of the front of the forearm, lying upon the flexor digitorum profundus, under cover of the flexor carpi ulnaris. Near the pisiform bone, it pierces the deep fascia at the lateral side of the flexor carpi ulnaris, and leaves the forearm by passing on to the front of the flexor retinaculum, where it ends by dividing into two terminal branches—a superficial and a deep.

At the elbow the ulnar nerve is separated from the ulnar artery by a wide interval but, as they descend in the upper third of the forearm, the artery approaches the nerve, and, in the lower two-thirds, is closely applied to its lateral side.

Branches in Forearm. The ulnar nerve gives off no branches until it reaches the forearm, where it supplies **articular branches** to the elbow joint; **muscular branches** which arise near the elbow for the flexor carpi ulnaris and the medial half of the flexor digitorum profundus; and the **dorsal** and **palmar cutaneous branches** [p. 53].

The ulnar nerve frequently receives a communication from the median nerve in the forearm; by this path, or through the slender contribution already noted [p. 66] from the lateral cord of the brachial plexus in the axilla, it obtains fibres derived from the seventh cervical nerve.

THE MEDIAN NERVE

The median nerve arises in the axilla by two roots that spring from the lateral and medial cords of the brachial plexus. It descends through the upper arm, at first on the medial side and then passes anterior to the elbow joint into the forearm [p. 66].

Course in Forearm. In the cubital fossa, the median nerve lies in front of the brachialis at the medial side first of the brachial and then of the ulnar artery. It leaves the fossa by passing between the two heads of the pronator teres, crossing anterior to the ulnar artery. It then descends through the middle of the front of the forearm, adhering to the deep surface of the superficial flexor, and near the wrist it winds round the lateral side of its tendons to lie anterior to them opposite the interval between the tendons of the palmaris longus and flexor carpi radialis [FIG. 52].

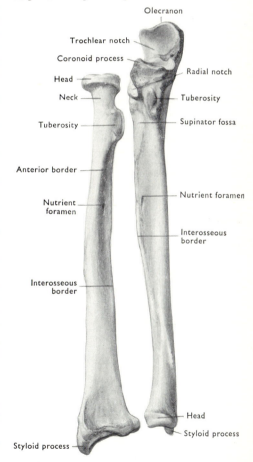

FIG. 58   Right radius and ulna (anterior surface).

It leaves the forearm with the tendons of the flexor superficialis by entering the carpal tunnel behind the flexor retinaculum, near the distal border of which it ends by dividing into lateral and medial branches.

Branches in Forearm. Like the ulnar nerve, the median nerve gives off no branches in the upper arm. In the cubital fossa, it sends branches from its medial side to **pronator teres, flexor carpi radialis, palmaris longus** and **flexor digitorum superficialis.** As it leaves the fossa, it gives off the **anterior interosseous nerve.** In the distal half of the forearm, it may give another branch to the flexor superficialis, and, near the wrist, its **palmar cutaneous branch** springs from it [p. 53].

DISSECTION. The anterior interosseous nerve has been traced down to the pronator quadratus. Now divide the pronator quadratus by a vertical cut through its middle, and turn the two parts aside. Secure the branches that the anterior interosseous nerve gives to the muscle, and then trace the nerve down to the front of the wrist joint.

DEEP STRUCTURES OF THE FRONT OF FOREARM

These are the anterior interosseous vessels [p. 88] and nerve, the flexor digitorum profundus, the flexor pollicis longus, and the pronator quadratus.

Anterior Interosseous Nerve

This is a branch that arises from the median nerve as it emerges from between the two heads of the pronator teres. It descends over

90

the front of the interosseous membrane between the flexor profundus and the flexor pollicis longus, passes behind the pronator quadratus and runs on to the front of the wrist joint. It gives **muscular** branches to those three muscles, and **articular** branches to the inferior radio-ulnar and wrist joints.

Flexor Digitorum Profundus

The deep flexor of the fingers is a long, thick muscle that lies deeply in the front of

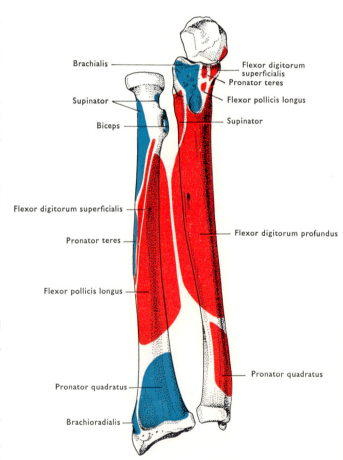

FIG. 59   Muscle attachments to anterior surface of right radius and ulna.

the forearm, but more superficially on the medial border and the back of the forearm, for it is on the medial side of the ulna as well as on the front of it [FIG. 54]. Examine the back of your forearm, and identify the groove that marks the posterior, subcutaneous border of the ulna. The fleshy mass at the medial side of the groove is the flexor profundus covered with the aponeurosis of the flexor carpi ulnaris. In this situation it can be felt to harden when it is made to contract by clenching the fist.

The chief origin of the muscle is from the upper three-fourths of the medial and anterior surfaces of the ulna. The fleshy belly becomes a thick tendinous mass which divides into four tendons—one for each finger—but only the tendon for the forefinger becomes separate and distinct in the forearm. The tendons pass through the carpal tunnel into the palm, and each is inserted into the terminal phalanx of a finger.

Nerve supply: lateral half by the **anterior interosseous nerve,** medial half by the **ulnar nerve.** Action: it flexes the wrist and all the joints of the fingers.

Flexor Pollicis Longus

The long flexor of the thumb lies deeply in the forearm, taking origin chiefly from the upper two-thirds of the front of the radius. A rounded tendon issues from the fleshy belly, proceeds through the carpal tunnel into the palm, and runs to the thumb to be inserted into its terminal phalanx.

Nerve supply: the **anterior interosseous nerve.** Action: it flexes all the joints of the thumb and the wrist.

Pronator Quadratus

The pronator quadratus lies deeply in the distal fourth of the forearm, taking origin from the front of the ulna, and passing across to be inserted into the radius. Nerve supply: **anterior interosseous nerve.** Action: pronation.

THE WRIST AND PALM

Before proceeding with the dissection of the palm, the student should revise its surface anatomy [p. 44], the superficial nerves [pp. 52–54], and the deep fascia [p. 55].

Palmaris Brevis

This is a thin, subcutaneous muscle that lies across the proximal 2-3 cm. of the hypothenar eminence, concealing the termination of the ulnar artery and nerve. It arises from the flexor retinaculum and the palmar aponeurosis, and is inserted into the skin of the ulnar border of the hand. Nerve supply: the superficial terminal branch of the **ulnar nerve.** Action: it deepens the cup of the palm, and enables the hand to take a firmer

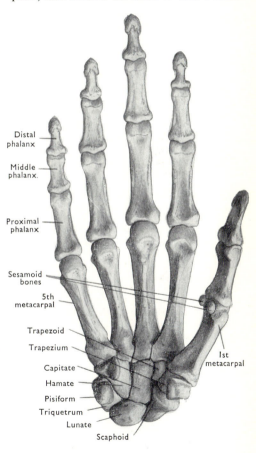

Distal phalanx

Middle phalanx.

Proximal phalanx

Sesamoid bones

5th metacarpal

Trapezoid

Trapezium

Capitate

Hamate

Pisiform

Triquetrum

Lunate

Scaphoid

1st metacarpal

FIG. 60   Palmar aspect of bones of right hand.

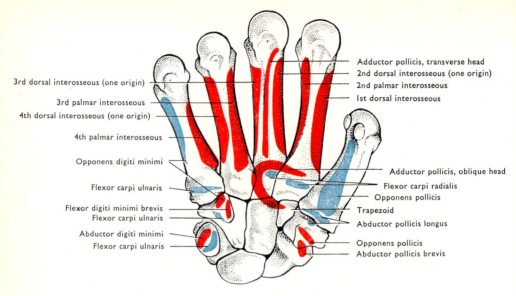

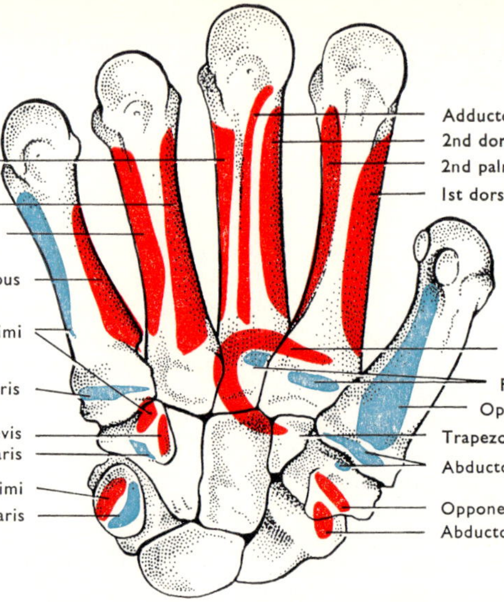
3rd dorsal interosseous (one origin)
3rd palmar interosseous
4th dorsal interosseous (one origin)
4th palmar interosseous
Opponens digiti minimi
Flexor carpi ulnaris
Flexor digiti minimi brevis
Flexor carpi ulnaris
Abductor digiti minimi
Flexor carpi ulnaris
Adductor pollicis, transverse head
2nd dorsal interosseous (one origin)
2nd palmar interosseous
1st dorsal interosseous
Adductor pollicis, oblique head
Flexor carpi radialis
Opponens pollicis
Trapezoid
Abductor pollicis longus
Opponens pollicis
Abductor pollicis brevis

FIG. 61 Muscle attachments to palmar surfaces of carpus and metacarpus.

grip by raising a cushion of skin and fascia against which the handle of a tool can be pressed and held steady.

DISSECTION. Reflect the palmaris brevis towards its origin, and secure its nerve of supply. Remove the deep fascia from the hypothenar muscles. Clean the ulnar artery till it disappears behind the palmar aponeurosis and secure its deep palmar branch, which sinks backwards between the hypothenar muscles. Trace the terminal branches of the ulnar nerve—the superficial to its subdivision into the palmar digital branches (dissected already) and the deep branch into the cleft between the two superficial muscles of the hypothenar eminence. Secure its branches to those two muscles and to the deeper muscle of the eminence. Then separate and clean those three muscles, avoiding injury to the nerves.

Short Muscles of Little Finger

These muscles make up the hypothenar eminence or ball of the little finger. The abductor and the flexor lie superficially side by side and the opponens is deep to both. They are all supplied by the deep branch of the **ulnar nerve.**

These muscles have a more or less common origin from the pisiform bone (abductor), the hook of the hamate and the medial part of the flexor retinaculum (flexor and opponens). The **abductor digiti minimi** is inserted into the medial side of the base of the proximal phalanx of the little finger. The **flexor digiti minimi** is variable in size, and is inserted with the abductor. It is partly fused with the abductor, and may not be easily separated from the opponens. The **opponens digiti minimi** lies on a deeper plane, and is inserted into the whole length of the medial part of the front of the fifth metacarpal bone.

These muscles should be compared with the corresponding short muscles of the thumb.

DISSECTION. Separate the apex of the palmar aponeurosis from the tendon of the palmaris longus and from the flexor retinaculum, and define the distal margin of the retinaculum. Then, reflect the aponeurosis towards the roots of the fingers. Do not fail to note that, from its medial and lateral margins, septa pass backwards into the palm. Divide these septa, and continue the reflexion until the deep surfaces of the processes which pass to the fingers are fully exposed.

Note that, at the roots of the fingers, each process divides into two slips. Clean these two slips and note their connexions with the fibrous flexor sheath and with the more deeply placed ligaments.

Palmar Aponeurosis

This dense, strong fibrous sheet underlies the superficial fascia of the middle part of the palm, and protects the tendons and the chief vessels and nerves which are proceeding to the fingers. It is composed of strong longitudinal fibres mixed with transverse fibres which bind them together.

It is triangular in outline. Its **apex** is situated at the distal border of the flexor retinaculum. There its deeper fibres fuse with the retinaculum, while the superficial fibres are continuous with the tendon of the palmaris longus.

Its **lateral** and **medial margins** are continuous with the deep fascia that covers the thenar and hypothenar muscles and, from each margin, a septum is sent backwards into the palm to fuse with the fascia on the muscles that lie deeply in the palm. These two septa separate the thenar and hypothenar muscles from the long flexor tendons of the fingers, the lateral septum crossing the anterior surface of

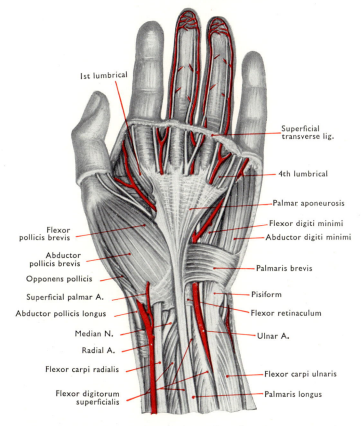

1st lumbrical

Superficial transverse lig.

4th lumbrical

Palmar aponeurosis

Flexor digiti minimi

Flexor pollicis brevis

Abductor digiti minimi

Abductor pollicis brevis

Palmaris brevis

Opponens pollicis

Pisiform

Superficial palmar A.

Flexor retinaculum

Abductor pollicis longus

Median N.

Ulnar A.

Radial A.

Flexor carpi radialis

Flexor carpi ulnaris

Flexor digitorum superficialis

Palmaris longus

FIG. 62   Superficial dissection of palm to show the palmar aponeurosis. The deep fascia has been removed from the thenar and hypothenar eminences. Cf. FIG. 64.

adductor pollicis to reach the middle metacarpal bone.

The **base** of the aponeurosis is opposite the distal parts of the metacarpal bones. It divides into four processes—one for each finger. Each process passes towards the root of a digit and divides into two slips. The slips diverge from each other and curve dorsally. Their distal borders are continuous with the fibrous flexor sheath of the digit, but are separated from it where the digital vessels and nerves and the lumbrical muscle enter the finger; their ends fuse with the deep fascia on the back of the digit and with strong bands called the deep transverse metacarpal ligaments.

A progressive shortening of the medial part of the palmar aponeurosis is known as Dupuytren's contraction; it produces flexion of the ring and little fingers, and is a chronic condition that requires surgical treatment.

Fascial Planes and Compartments of Palm [FIG. 63]

The two septa which pass from the margins of the palmar aponeurosis into the depths of the palm join the fascia on the medial interosseous muscles and the adductor of the thumb; and the two heads of the adductor are separated from the interossei of the lateral two interosseous spaces by another layer of fascia. There are, therefore, four main fascial compartments in the palm:

1. A lateral compartment which contains the thenar muscles.

2. A medial compartment which contains the hypothenar muscles.

3. An intermediate compartment, separated into (*a*) a superficial part which contains the superficial palmar arch and its branches and branches of the median and ulnar nerves, and (*b*) a deeper part enclosing the flexor tendons and their sheaths.

4. An adductor compartment which contains the adductor pollicis.

When wounds of the fingers or hand become infected, there may be effusion of serum or the formation of pus in the fascial plane deep to the flexor tendons [FIG. 63]. That plane then becomes loosened to form the 'fascial spaces' recognized by the surgeon.

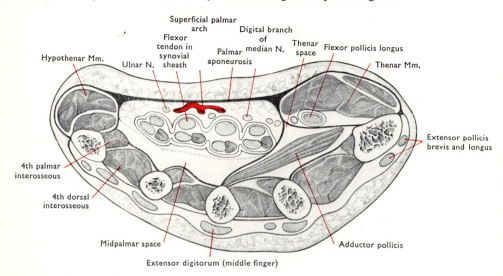

FIG. 63   Diagram of an oblique section through the hand to show the fascial layers and spaces of the palm. The thenar and midpalmar spaces are shown distended, and the thickness of the fascial layers is exaggerated.

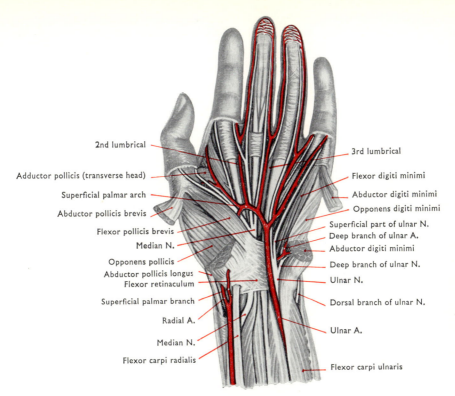

2nd lumbrical

Adductor pollicis (transverse head)

Superficial palmar arch

Abductor pollicis brevis

Flexor pollicis brevis

Median N.

Opponens pollicis

Abductor pollicis longus
Flexor retinaculum

Superficial palmar branch

Radial A.

Median N.

Flexor carpi radialis

3rd lumbrical

Flexor digiti minimi

Abductor digiti minimi

Opponens digiti minimi

Superficial part of ulnar N.
Deep branch of ulnar A.

Abductor digiti minimi

Deep branch of ulnar N.

Ulnar N.

Dorsal branch of ulnar N.

Ulnar A.

Flexor carpi ulnaris

FIG. 64   Structures in palm displayed by removal of palmar aponeurosis.   In this specimen the radialis indicis and the princeps pollicis arteries took origin from the superficial palmar arch.

DISSECTION.   Clean the superficial palmar arch and the four digital branches which it gives to the fingers.

Find the terminal branches of the median nerve at the lower border of the flexor retinaculum.   Follow the lateral branch first.   Secure the stout branch that it gives to the thenar muscles, and then trace the digital nerves to the thumb and forefinger, and find the branch of the latter to a slender slip of muscle called the first lumbrical muscle.   Now follow the two digital nerves into which the medial branch divides.   Do so with care, for the lateral one gives a branch to the second lumbrical muscle, and the other communicates with the nearest digital branch of the ulnar nerve.

Superficial Palmar Arch

This is an arterial arcade which lies immediately subjacent to the palmar aponeurosis, its most distal point being situated at the level of the distal border of the fully extended thumb.   It is the continuation of the ulnar artery after that artery has given off its deep branch.   It begins on the flexor retinaculum immediately distal to the pisiform bone, crosses the hook of the hamate bone deep to palmaris brevis, and turning laterally, pierces the medial septum of the palm.   It continues deep to the palmar aponeurosis to join one or other of the branches of the radial artery [FIGS. 64, 68].   The arch lies on the digital branches of the median nerve and the flexor tendons.

Branches.   The arch gives off small twigs to the adjacent tendons and fascia, but its chief branches are the **four digital arteries**

95

which spring from its convexity. The first of the four remains undivided. It runs to the medial border of the little finger, along which it passes to the terminal phalanx. The other three—common palmar digital arteries—pass towards the interdigital clefts, and each divides, at the level of the bases of the first phalanges, into two branches, which supply the adjacent sides of two fingers [FIGS. 62, 64, 68].

Opposite the terminal phalanx, the two arteries of each finger join to form an arch from which a great number of fine branches are distributed to the pulp of the finger and to the bed upon which the nail rests.

At the interdigital clefts the digital arteries are joined by the corresponding **palmar metacarpal arteries** from the deep palmar arch.

Median Nerve

The median nerve descends into the palm of the hand behind the flexor retinaculum, in front of the tendons of the flexor digitorum superficialis, or along their lateral margin [FIG. 56], and in close relation with their synovial sheath. Near the distal border of the retinaculum, it splits into a lateral and a medial division.

The **lateral division** is the smaller. It gives off a branch which supplies the abductor brevis, the opponens and the flexor brevis of the thumb. It then divides into three digital branches. Two of them go to the sides of the thumb; the third runs to the radial side of the index finger and, on its way, it gives a twig to the first lumbrical muscle.

The **medial division** divides into two branches. One runs towards the cleft between the index and middle fingers, gives a branch to the second lumbrical muscle, and divides to supply the adjacent sides of those fingers. The other gives a communicating twig to the lateral digital branch of the ulnar nerve, and divides to supply the adjacent sides of the middle and ring digits. It sometimes gives a branch to the third lumbrical muscle.

In the palm, the digital branches of the median nerve are deep to the superficial palmar arch and its digital branches but, as they approach the fingers, they cross the digital arteries to lie in front of them on the fingers. Note also that the digital nerves divide more proximally than the arteries do. Their distribution in the digits is described on page 54.

Ulnar Nerve

The ulnar nerve enters the hand by passing on to the front of the flexor retinaculum close to the lateral side of the pisiform bone; it divides there into two terminal branches.

The **deep branch** passes to the medial side of the hook of the hamate bone, and then dips deeply into the palm, with the deep branch of the ulnar artery, through the cleft between the abductor and the flexor of the little finger. It supplies the short muscles of the little finger as it passes between them, and afterwards gives branches to numerous other muscles. Its further course and distribution will be seen when the deep part of the palm is dissected.

The **superficial branch** descends deep to the palmaris brevis, supplies it, and divides into two digital branches. The medial of the two branches passes to the medial side of the little finger. The lateral branch, joined by a communicating branch from the nearest digital branch of the median nerve, divides into two branches which supply the adjacent sides of the ring and little fingers [p. 53].

DISSECTION. Remove the deep fascia from the muscles of the thenar eminence, but preserve their nerve of supply. Two muscles are then exposed—the abductor and flexor pollicis brevis. The abductor is the lateral muscle. Pass the handle of the scalpel behind its lateral border and lift it from the opponens pollicis. Then divide the abductor, and turn the two parts upwards and downwards. The opponens is then exposed, and must be cleaned.

Next divide the short flexor at its middle and reflect it towards its ends. That will bring into view part of the adductor pollicis, emerging from behind the flexor tendons. Along the medial border of the opponens pollicis, the tendon of the flexor pollicis longus will be seen; do not injure its synovial sheath.

At this stage, re-examine the synovial sheaths of the flexor tendons by inflation or with a blunt probe [see p. 84].

Flexor Retinaculum

This is a thick, dense, fibrous band which stretches across the concavity of the carpus and converts it into an osteofibrous tunnel for the passage of the flexor tendons into the palm. It acts as a pulley against which the tendons run on flexion of the wrist. At the sides, it is attached to the piers of the carpal arch, viz. on the **lateral side** to the tubercle of the scaphoid bone and the front of the trapezium; on the **medial side** to the pisiform and the hook of the hamate. The attachment to the trapezium is chiefly to the tubercle at the lateral side of the groove on the front of the bone, but it sends a process also to the medial margin of the groove. In that way it converts the groove into a canal which transmits the flexor carpi radialis tendon and is lined with its synovial sheath.

The proximal margin of the retinaculum is continuous with the deep fascia of the fore- arm, and its distal border is connected with the palmar aponeurosis.

The retinaculum is partly concealed by the thenar and hypothenar muscles that arise from it, and by structures that run on to its surface: (1) the **ulnar nerve** and **vessels,** close to the pisiform bone; (2) the **palmar cutaneous branch of the ulnar nerve,** lateral to the vessels; (3) **palmaris longus tendon,** at the middle of the retinaculum; and (4) the **palmar cutaneous branch of the median nerve,** at the lateral side of the tendon.

The tunnel which the flexor retinaculum forms with the concavity of the carpus transmits the tendons of the superficial and deep flexors of the digits, flexor pollicis longus and the median nerve.

DISSECTION. Clean the fibrous sheaths of the flexor tendons of the fingers and the thumb.

Fibrous Flexor Sheaths

The fibrous flexor sheaths are simply the deep fascia of the fronts of the digits greatly

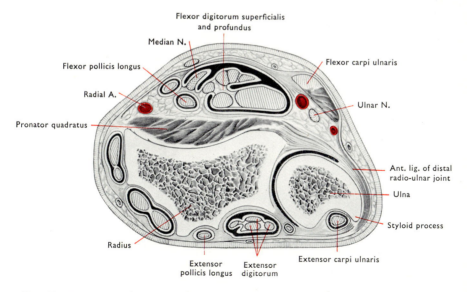

FIG. 65   Transverse section through forearm above flexor retinaculum showing the relation of the synovial sheaths to the tendons.

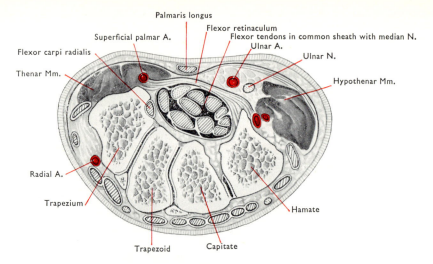

FIG. 66   Transverse section at the level of distal row of carpal bones. The flexor pollicis longus, the median nerve, and the tendons of the two flexors (superficial and deep) of the digits are seen in the carpal tunnel. The sheath of flexor pollicis longus is continuous with the common sheath at this level.

condensed in order to hold the flexor tendons in contact with the palmar surfaces of the phalanges and the joints, during flexion of the digits. Each sheath is an elongated plate curved round the front and sides of the flexor tendons. Its edges are attached to the margins of the phalanges and the margins of the palmar ligaments of the metacarpo-phalangeal and interphalangeal joints. Its distal end is attached to the palmar surface of the distal phalanx immediately beyond the insertion of the flexor profundus tendon. At its proximal end it is continuous with the corresponding slip or process of the palmar aponeurosis. It consists chiefly of transverse fibres and it is very dense opposite the phalanges, but is thinner and weaker opposite the joints and thus does not interfere with flexion.

Each sheath, together with the phalanges and the palmar ligaments of the joints, forms an osteofibrous canal which lodges the flexor tendons enclosed in a synovial sheath. In a finger, the tendons are the flexor superficialis and profundus; in the thumb, it is flexor pollicis longus alone.

DISSECTION. Leave the fibrous sheath of the middle finger intact for revision. Open the other sheaths by longitudinal incisions. Evert the two halves of the fibrous sheath, and examine the extent and arrangement of the synovial sheath. Lift up the tendons and separate them. Examine their insertions; note their relations to each other, and examine also the slender bands called vincula, which connect the tendons to the phalanges.

Synovial Sheaths in the Digits

Each synovial sheath extends to the insertion of the tendon into the base of the terminal phalanx. The sheath of the thumb extends from the interphalangeal joint up into the forearm 2–3 cm. above the crease at the wrist. The sheath of the little finger is continuous with the common flexor sheath in the palm. The sheaths of the other digits extend almost to the middle of the palm, but are not continuous with the large sheath [FIG. 58, p. 85]. For structure of sheaths see page 84.

Vincula Tendinum. These are thin fibrous structures that pass between the bones and the tendons. They carry blood vessels to the tendons and they are covered with synovial

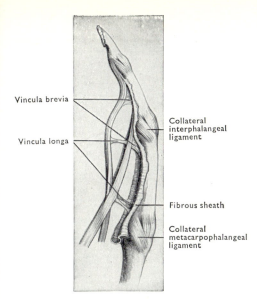

Vincula brevia

Vincula longa

Collateral
interphalangeal
ligament

Fibrous sheath

Collateral
metacarpophalangeal
ligament

FIG. 67 Flexor tendons of finger with vincula tendinum.

membrane. They are of two kinds—long and short. The **vincula brevia** are triangular sheets set between the bones and the tendons at their insertion. The **vincula longa** are very slender bands situated nearer the root of the finger [FIG. 67].

DISSECTION. Open the carpal tunnel by making a vertical incision through the middle of the flexor retinaculum. Clean the synovial sheaths from the flexor tendons. Separate the tendons carefully from one another, and clean the slender slips—the lumbrical muscles—which spring from the tendons of the flexor digitorum profundus, taking care not to injure their nerves.

Examine the arrangement of the flexor tendons and the origins and insertions of the lumbrical muscles.

Tendon of Flexor Pollicis Longus

This tendon occupies the lateral part of the carpal tunnel, turns laterally in the palm and runs towards the thumb along the distal margin of the thenar eminence between the flexor pollicis brevis and adductor pollicis. It enters the fibrous flexor sheath at the base

of the proximal phalanx, and then runs to the base of the terminal phalanx, into which it is inserted.

Flexor Tendons of Fingers

Deep to the flexor retinaculum, the four tendons of the **flexor digitorum superficialis** are arranged in pairs ; those for the little finger and the index lie behind those for the ring and middle fingers. Of the tendons of the **flexor digitorum profundus**, only that for the index finger is distinct and separate ; the other three, as a rule, remain united until the tendinous mass emerges from the distal border of the retinaculum.

In the palm, the flexor tendons diverge ; and two—one from each flexor—go to each of the four fingers. The lumbrical muscles and the palmar digital nerves and arteries run in the intervals between the tendons as they approach the fingers.

In the **fingers,** the two flexor tendons run along the palmar surfaces of the phalanges, and are held in position by the fibrous flexor sheaths. On the palmar surface of the first phalanx, the tendon of the flexor superficialis becomes flattened and folded round the subjacent tendon of the flexor profundus. It then splits into two parts which pass behind the tendon of the flexor profundus, where their reversed edges fuse together and partially decussate ; they then diverge again to be inserted into the borders of the shaft of the second phalanx. By this special arrangement the tendon of the flexor superficialis forms a short tubular passage, which cannot be obliterated by tension, through which the tendon of the flexor profundus proceeds onwards to the base of the terminal phalanx. In each of the four fingers the same arrangement is found.

Lumbrical Muscles

The lumbrical muscles are four slender fleshy bellies which arise from the radial or adjacent sides of the tendons of the flexor digitorum profundus as they traverse the palm. Each of them ends in a delicate tendon which passes backwards across the radial

99

surface of a metacarpo-phalangeal joint, is connected with the expansion of the extensor tendon, and is inserted, with the tendon of an interosseous muscle, into the dorsum of a terminal phalanx. Their action is explained on page 109.

The lateral two lumbrical muscles are supplied on their superficial surface by twigs from the digital branches of the **median nerve** for the index finger; the medial two on their deep surface by the deep branch of the **ulnar nerve**; the third lumbrical often receives an additional twig from the most medial digital branch of the median nerve.

DISSECTION. Divide the flexor digitorum profundus in the forearm, and turn the distal part towards the fingers. As the tendons and the lumbrical muscles are raised, secure the fine twigs of supply which pass to the medial two lumbricals.

Now clean the deep palmar arch and the deep branch of the ulnar nerve, and trace the branches of the nerve to the interosseous muscles and to the adductor pollicis.

Deep Palmar Arch

Two arteries take part in the arch—the radial and the deep palmar branch of the ulnar.

The radial plays the chief part. It enters the palm through the proximal end of the first interosseous space, between the two heads of the first dorsal interosseous muscle. In the present stage of dissection it appears through the cleft between the oblique and transverse heads of the adductor pollicis (or through the transverse head), and runs medially to join the deep branch of the ulnar artery at the base of the fifth metacarpal bone.

The arterial arcade, so formed, lies across the metacarpal bones immediately distal to their bases. The deep arch is therefore about a finger's breadth nearer the wrist than the superficial arch. The convexity of the deep arch is directed towards the fingers, and the deep branch of the ulnar nerve lies in its concavity [Fig. 68].

Its chief branches are three **palmar metacarpal arteries,** which run towards the interdigital clefts and unite with digital branches of the superficial arch. Sometimes these metacarpal arteries are large and take the place of the corresponding palmar digital arteries.

Deep Branch of Ulnar Nerve

This branch springs from the parent trunk on the front of the flexor retinaculum, and at once gives off a branch to the three short muscles of the little finger. Accompanied by the deep branch of the ulnar artery, it passes

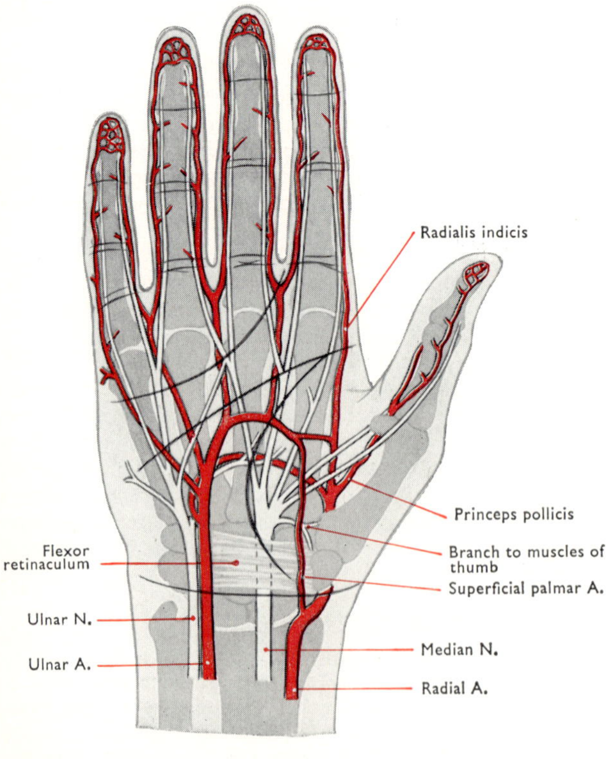

Radialis indicis

Princeps pollicis

Branch to muscles of thumb

Superficial palmar A.

Flexor retinaculum

Ulnar N.

Ulnar A.

Median N.

Radial A.

Fig. 68 Diagram of nerves and vessels of hand in relation to bones and skin markings.

deeply between the abductor and flexor digiti minimi, and turns laterally across the palm, deep to the flexor tendons. Near the lateral border of the palm, it breaks up into terminal twigs which supply the adductor pollicis and the first dorsal interosseous muscle. In its course across the palm it lies along the proximal border of the deep palmar arch, and sends a fine branch downwards in front of each of the medial three interosseous spaces. They supply the interosseous muscles in these spaces and the medial two give branches to the corresponding lumbrical muscles.

The deep branch of the ulnar nerve therefore supplies all the muscles of the palm which are medial to the tendon of the flexor pollicis longus, except the lateral two lumbrical muscles, which are supplied by the median nerve. It is of some clinical importance, however, to note that the flexor pollicis brevis often receives a branch from the ulnar nerve in addition to its branch from the median nerve, or even as the sole supply of the muscle.

DISSECTION. Clean the adductor of the thumb and then examine the other short muscles of the thumb.

Short Muscles of Thumb

The abductor, the flexor brevis and the opponens are lateral to the tendon of the flexor pollicis longus and form the ball of the thumb; they are supplied by the **median nerve.** The adductor is medial to that tendon and is supplied by the deep branch of the **ulnar nerve,** which may supply the flexor brevis also.

The **abductor pollicis brevis** forms the antero-lateral part of the ball of the thumb. The **flexor pollicis brevis** is immediately medial to the abductor. The **opponens pollicis** is deep to both of them and is exposed when they are pulled apart or reflected [FIGS. 62, 64]. All three arise from the lateral part of the flexor retinaculum with some of the more lateral and deeper fibres gaining origin from the tubercles of the scaphoid and the trapezium [FIG. 61].

The abductor and the flexor are inserted together into the lateral side of the base of the proximal phalanx of the thumb. The abductor, however, produces its major movement at the carpometacarpal joint, drawing the thumb anteriorly away from the index finger. The fibres of the opponens spread out to be inserted into the lateral half of the palmar surface of the first metacarpal bone. The main action of the opponens is to pull the thumb towards the centre of the palm and rotate it medially at the carpo-metacarpal joint, so that its palmar surface, which normally faces medially, is rotated to face the palmar surfaces of the fingers.

Adductor Pollicis. The adductor is a fan-shaped muscle that lies deeply in the palm; it is incompletely divided into upper oblique and lower transverse heads. The **oblique head** arises from the bases of the second and third metacarpals and the adjacent carpal bones. The **transverse head** arises from the front of the third metacarpal bone [FIG. 61]. The two heads converge, unite, and are inserted into the medial side of the base of the proximal phalanx of the thumb. Action: it draws the thumb posteriorly towards the palm and can act as a flexor of the metacarpo-phalangeal joint in the fully opposed thumb.

These muscles should be compared with the corresponding short muscles of the little finger [see p. 92].

Sesamoid Bones. A small sesamoid bone is developed in the tendon of the adductor pollicis and another in the common tendon of the abductor and flexor [FIG. 60]. One surface of each of these little bones is covered with cartilage and plays upon the palmar surface of the head of the first metacarpal bone, which is grooved to articulate with them.

DISSECTION. To display the branches of the palmar part of the radial artery, cut through the two parts of the adductor pollicis midway between their origins and insertions, and turn the separated portions aside. The first dorsal interosseous muscle is now exposed; the radial artery will be found entering the palm between its two heads, and giving off its last two branches—the princeps pollicis and the radialis indicis. At the same time, look for a slender slip of muscle—

the first palmar interosseous — that lies along the ulnar side of the first metacarpal bone.

Radial Artery in Palm

The radial artery enters the palm through the proximal end of the first intermetacarpal space between the two heads of the first dorsal interosseous muscle. In the palm, it lies at first between that muscle and the adductor pollicis, where it gives off the radialis indicis and princeps pollicis arteries; it then passes through the adductor to become the deep palmar arch [FIG. 68].

The **radialis indicis artery** descends between the transverse head of the adductor pollicis and the first dorsal interosseous muscle to the lateral border of the index as its lateral palmar digital artery.

The **princeps pollicis artery** runs laterally, under cover of the oblique head of the adductor, to the metacarpal bone of the thumb. Here it lies deep to the long flexor tendon, and divides into two branches which run along the sides of the tendon as the palmar digital arteries of the thumb.

THE SURGICAL ANATOMY OF
THE FINGERS AND PALM

The fingers are a common site of minor injuries which are often followed by infection. The inflammatory process which ensues is associated with much swelling and the development of considerable pressure within the dense fibrous tissues of the finger. This may be either in the pulp of the finger distal to the termination of the fibrous flexor sheath, or contained within the sheath. The pressure tends to interfere with the local circulation and may lead to death of the terminal phalanx if in the pulp, or to the degeneration of the tendons if in the fibrous flexor sheath. It is essential, therefore, that such inflammatory processes, or whitlows, should be relieved early by adequate incision, and in the case of the thumb and little finger is even more urgent because the synovial sheath of the little finger is usually continuous, and that of the thumb frequently continuous, with the common

sheath of the flexor tendons to which the infection can spread [FIGS. 55, 66].

When an abscess (*i.e.*, a collection of pus) forms in the superficial intermediate compartment of the palm, early surgical interference is called for. The dense palmar aponeurosis effectually prevents the passage of the pus to the surface of the palm, and it tends to spread deeply into the synovial sheath of the flexor tendons. It is necessary, therefore, that before this can occur the surgeon should make openings by means of which the pus can escape; such openings must take account of the position of the superficial palmar arch and of the palmar digital arteries that spring from it.

The synovial sheath which envelops the flexor tendons has been seen to extend upwards into the distal part of the forearm, and downwards into the palm. When the sheath is attacked by inflammation, it is liable to become distended with fluid which may become purulent, and the anatomical arrangement of the parts at once offers an explanation of the appearance which is presented. There is a bulging in the proximal part of the palm and in the distal part of the forearm, but no swelling at all opposite the carpus. There, the flexor retinaculum resists the expansion of the synovial sheath.

There is no complete agreement about the arrangement of the palmar fascia, but in general the hand consists of three main compartments: the thenar and hypothenar, each containing the corresponding short muscles and enclosed in its own layer of fascia; and a central compartment containing the long flexor tendons of the fingers, the lumbricals, and most of the blood vessels and nerves. This is covered by the palmar aponeurosis which fuses at its edges with the fascia covering the thenar and hypothenar compartments, and sends a number of septa into the loose connective tissue which separates the flexor tendons and their synovial sheaths from the fascia covering the interossei. The most lateral of these septa passes deeply along the line of the lateral longitudinal palmar crease and, curving medially dorsal to the tendons, converges with the adductor pollicis on the third metacarpal to which it is attached. This septum divides the loose fatty tissue dorsal to the tendons into a lateral compartment, anterior to the adductor pollicis, the **thenar space**, and a medial compartment over the third and fourth interosseous spaces, the **midpalmar space.** The latter is separated from the long tendons by the rather dense fascia which surrounds them and separates them anteriorly from the palmar aponeurosis [FIG. 63].

When an abscess forms in the palm it is usually found either in the thenar or the midpalmar space, and it is the presence of such an abscess which splits apart the loose fascia and forms these artificial 'fascial spaces' recognized by the surgeon.

THE EXTENSOR COMPARTMENT OF THE FOREARM AND HAND

Before this dissection is begun, revise the surface anatomy [pp. 43–45], and re-examine the superficial veins, the cutaneous nerves and the deep fascia [pp. 46, 52, 53, 55].

DISSECTION. Leave the extensor retinaculum [p. 55] in situ until the dissection of the back of the forearm and hand is completed. To secure its retention, isolate it by cutting carefully through the deep fascia parallel with its upper border—avoiding injury to the synovial sheaths of the extensor tendons, which lie immediately subjacent to the deep fascia.

When the front of the forearm was dissected, the lateral flap of deep fascia was reflected only as far as the radial border of the forearm. Now continue the reflexion until the attachment of the flap to the posterior border of the ulna is reached. As the reflexion proceeds, divide the intermuscular septa.

MUSCLES OF THE BACK OF THE FOREARM

These muscles are more numerous than on the front, and, like them, are arranged in a superficial and a deep group.

Named from the lateral to the medial border of the forearm, the **superficial muscles** are:

1. Brachioradialis.
2. Extensor carpi radialis longus.
3. Extensor carpi radialis brevis.
4. Extensor digitorum.
5. Extensor digiti minimi.
6. Extensor carpi ulnaris.
7. Anconeus.

This group therefore comprises one flexor of the elbow, the brachioradialis [see p. 83], three extensors of the wrist, two extensors of the fingers, and a feeble extensor of the elbow (the anconeus). Identify them at once from their relative positions and by reference to FIGURE 69. They are all long muscles except the anconeus, which is the small, triangular muscle on the lateral side of the upper part of the ulna.

The **deep muscles** are:

1. Supinator.
2. Abductor pollicis longus.
3. Extensor pollicis brevis.
4. Extensor pollicis longus.
5. Extensor indicis.

They also are long muscles, except the supinator which is wrapped round the upper third of the radius.

Though deeply placed for most of their course, the abductor pollicis longus and the two extensors of the thumb become superficial as they move towards the lateral border of the forearm in its distal part. Here they lie between the tendons of extensor digitorum and extensor carpi radialis and will cross the latter before reaching their insertions [FIGS. 69, 75]. The tendon of the fourth long muscle of the deep group—the extensor indicis—will be found under cover of the extensor digitorum near the wrist.

DISSECTION. Introduce a blowpipe into each sheath [Figs. 70, 71] immediately above the retinaculum, and inflate the sheath. A better demonstration may be made by a thin mixture of coloured starch injected through a large hypodermic syringe. If the sheaths have been injured, and it is not possible to distend them, then open each and examine its extent with the aid of a blunt probe.

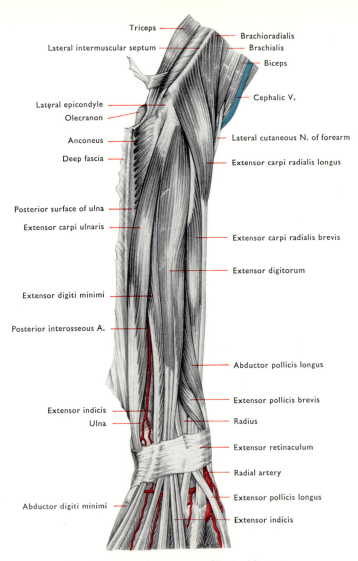

Triceps

Lateral intermuscular septum

Brachioradialis

Brachialis

Biceps

Cephalic V.

Lateral epicondyle

Olecranon

Anconeus

Deep fascia

Lateral cutaneous N. of forearm

Extensor carpi radialis longus

Posterior surface of ulna

Extensor carpi ulnaris

Extensor carpi radialis brevis

Extensor digitorum

Extensor digiti minimi

Posterior interosseous A.

Abductor pollicis longus

Extensor pollicis brevis

Extensor indicis

Ulna

Radius

Extensor retinaculum

Radial artery

Extensor pollicis longus

Abductor digiti minimi

Extensor indicis

FIG. 69   Superficial dissection of back of forearm.

Extensor Retinaculum

This thickened portion of the deep fascia, about 2·5 cm. wide, lies obliquely across the back of the limb at the junction of the forearm and wrist. It extends from the triquetral bone and styloid process of the ulna on the medial side, to the sharp edge between the lateral and anterior surfaces of the distal part of the radius on the lateral side, an arrangement which prevents it interfering with the free movement of the

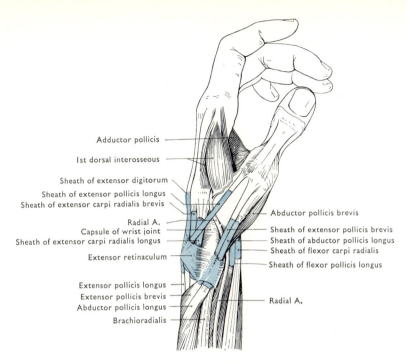

Adductor pollicis
1st dorsal interosseous
Sheath of extensor digitorum
Sheath of extensor pollicis longus
Sheath of extensor carpi radialis brevis
Radial A.
Capsule of wrist joint
Sheath of extensor carpi radialis longus
Extensor retinaculum
Extensor pollicis longus
Extensor pollicis brevis
Abductor pollicis longus
Brachioradialis

Abductor pollicis brevis
Sheath of extensor pollicis brevis
Sheath of abductor pollicis longus
Sheath of flexor carpi radialis
Sheath of flexor pollicis longus
Radial A.

FIG. 70   Dissection of lateral side of left wrist and hand showing synovial sheaths of tendons.

radius during pronation and supination. In addition to these attachments it sends five septa inwards to be attached to the head of the ulna and the ridges on the posterior surface of the distal end of the radius, thus splitting up the space deep to it into six compartments each of which contains one or more tendons in their synovial sheaths [Figs. 65, 70, 71].

DISSECTION. Slit the retinaculum at each compartment. Examine the tendons and synovial sheaths that lie in them.

The **first compartment** is on the lateral side of the distal end of the radius. It contains the tendons of the abductor pollicis longus and the extensor pollicis brevis.

The **second compartment** corresponds with the most lateral groove on the back of the radius. It holds the tendons of the two radial extensors of the carpus.

The **third compartment** is formed over the narrow, deep, oblique groove on the distal end of the radius. It contains the tendon of the extensor pollicis longus.

The **fourth compartment** is placed over the wide, shallow groove which marks the medial part of the back of the distal end of the radius. It is traversed by tendons of the extensor digitorum and extensor indicis and, deep to their sheath, by the terminal parts of the posterior interosseous nerve and anterior interosseous artery.

The **fifth compartment** is situated over the interval between the distal ends of the radius and ulna. It contains the tendon of the extensor digiti minimi.

The **sixth** and **most medial compartment,** which corresponds with the groove on the

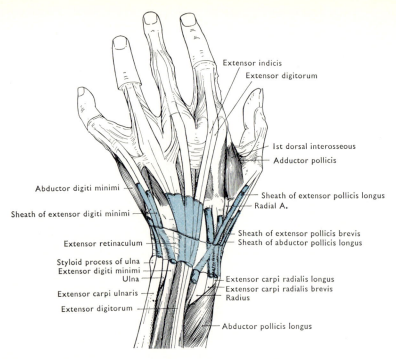

Extensor indicis
Extensor digitorum

Ist dorsal interosseous
Adductor pollicis

Abductor digiti minimi

Sheath of extensor pollicis longus
Radial A.

Sheath of extensor digiti minimi

Extensor retinaculum

Sheath of extensor pollicis brevis
Sheath of abductor pollicis longus

Styloid process of ulna
Extensor digiti minimi
Ulna

Extensor carpi radialis longus
Extensor carpi radialis brevis
Radius

Extensor carpi ulnaris

Extensor digitorum

Abductor pollicis longus

FIG. 71   Dissection of back of forearm, wrist, and hand showing synovial sheaths of tendons.

dorsum of the distal end of the ulna, encloses the tendon of the extensor carpi ulnaris.

Synovial Sheaths of Extensor Tendons
[FIGS. 65, 70, 71]

Eight synovial sheaths surround the tendons which pass through the six compartments under cover of the extensor retinaculum— each of the nine tendons having its own sheath, except the extensor digitorum and extensor indicis, which have a common sheath.

The upper ends of the sheaths are deep to the extensor retinaculum or slightly above it. The sheaths of the abductor pollicis longus and the three extensors of the carpus extend to the insertions of those muscles. The sheaths of the extensors of the digits usually end about the mid-length of the hand [FIGS. 70, 71]. Occasionally the abductor pollicis longus and the extensor pollicis brevis have

a common sheath, and sometimes a single sheath encloses the radial extensors of the wrist.

SUPERFICIAL MUSCLES

DISSECTION. Clean the brachioradialis to its insertion and the other superficial muscles, separating them from one another. Their proximal parts are united by fascial septa. Split the septa with the knife, up to the bony origins of the muscles.

Anconeus

The anconeus is a short, triangular muscle that lies at the lateral part of the back of the elbow. It arises, by a tendon, from the lateral epicondyle, and spreads out to be inserted into the lateral border of the olecranon [FIG. 69] and the upper third of the back of the shaft of the ulna [FIG. 77]. Nerve supply: a long slender branch of the **radial nerve** that

106

reaches the muscle through the medial head of the triceps [p. 72 and Fig. 44]. Action : it slews the ulna laterally during pronation.

Brachioradialis

This muscle lies more on the front of the forearm than on the back. It takes origin from the upper two-thirds of the lateral supracondylar ridge of the humerus. Near the middle of the forearm a flat tendon emerges from its fleshy belly and proceeds downwards to gain insertion into the lateral surface of the distal end of the radius, under cover of the tendons of the abductor pollicis longus and extensor pollicis brevis. Nerve supply : a branch of the **radial nerve** enters the muscle above the elbow. Action : it can help to initiate supination of the prone forearm and pronation of the supine forearm, but its main action is flexion of the elbow. Flex your own elbow against resistance in the semi-prone position, and note how the muscle stands out.

Extensor Carpi Radialis Longus

This muscle is placed behind the brachioradialis, and arises from the distal third of the lateral supracondylar ridge. From the fleshy portion of the muscle a long tendon arises, which passes under cover of the extensor retinaculum and is inserted into the base of the second metacarpal bone. Nerve supply : **radial nerve** above the elbow. Action : it extends and abducts the hand at the wrist joint [Figs. 70, 71, 86].

The four remaining superficial extensor muscles arise by a **common extensor tendon** from the lower anterior part of the lateral epicondyle of the humerus.

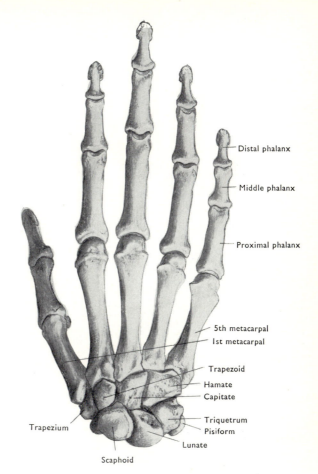

Distal phalanx

Middle phalanx

Proximal phalanx

5th metacarpal
1st metacarpal

Trapezoid
Hamate
Capite

Triquetrum
Pisiform
Trapezium
Lunate
Scaphoid

Fig. 72   Dorsal aspect of bones of right hand.

Extensor Carpi Radialis Brevis

The short radial extensor of the wrist is immediately posterior to the long extensor; its tendon accompanies that of the long extensor under cover of the extensor retinaculum, and is inserted into the base of the third metacarpal bone. Nerve supply: usually from the **deep branch of the radial nerve** before that nerve pierces the supinator muscle, but it may be direct from the superficial division of the radial nerve. Action : extensor and abductor of the wrist.

107

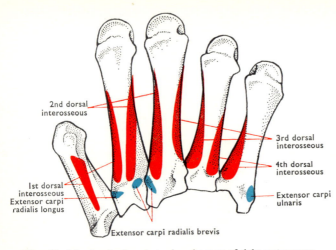

2nd dorsal interosseous

3rd dorsal interosseous

4th dorsal interosseous

Extensor carpi ulnaris

1st dorsal interosseous

Extensor carpi radialis longus

Extensor carpi radialis brevis

FIG. 73   Muscle attachments to dorsal aspect of right metacarpus.

Extensor Carpi Ulnaris

The ulnar extensor of the wrist gains additional origin from the strong fascia that binds it to the posterior border of the ulna. The tendon does not become free from the fleshy fibres until it is near the wrist. It occupies the groove on the back of the distal end of the ulna, and, escaping from the extensor retinaculum, it is inserted into the base of the fifth metacarpal bone. Nerve supply : the **posterior interosseous nerve.** Action : it is an extensor of the wrist and elbow ; and it aids the flexor carpi ulnaris in adducting the hand.

DISSECTION. Remove the deep fascia of the back of the hand. Clear away the synovial sheaths of the tendons, and clean the tendons as far as their insertions, but do not remove (1) the extensor retinaculum, (2) the blood vessels which lie deep to the tendons and in the intervals between them, (3) the slips which connect the tendons to one another.

Note that the extensor tendon expands on the back of the first phalanx of a finger, but is not inserted into that phalanx. Lift up the expansion, clean its edges, and find the tendons of the lumbrical and interosseous muscles, which are connected with those edges.

On at least one finger, define the three slips into which the extensor tendon splits, and trace them to their insertions.

Extensor Digitorum

The extensor of the fingers arises from the common extensor origin and the surrounding fascia. In the distal part of the forearm it forms a tendon which splits to pass to each finger, the separation of the medial two parts occurring distally in the hand so that independent movement of the ring and little fingers by means of these tendons is impossible. The tendons may be linked by oblique bands which further limit the amount of separate movement. Insertion is into the bases of the middle and distal phalanges through the extensor expansion which the tendons form. Nerve supply : **posterior interosseous nerve.**

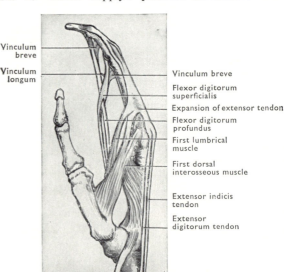

Vinculum breve

Vinculum longum

Vinculum breve

Flexor digitorum superficialis

Expansion of extensor tendon

Flexor digitorum profundus

First lumbrical muscle

First dorsal interosseous muscle

Extensor indicis tendon

Extensor digitorum tendon

FIG. 74   The tendons attached to the index finger.

Action : extensor of the wrist and fingers.

Extensor Expansion. As the extensor tendon approaches the metacarpo-phalangeal joint, it spreads out to form the dorsal part of the joint capsule and covers the dorsal surface of the proximal phalanx where it divides into three slips.

The middle slip passes across the joint and carries the main insertion of the extensor into the base of the middle phalanx. The two collateral slips converge over the middle phalanx, and unite to be inserted into the base of the terminal phalanx [FIGS. 71, 74]. The collateral slips are joined by parts of the tendons of the interossei and, on the radial side, by the tendon of the lumbrical muscle, both of which are inserted into the terminal phalanx through them.

Extensor Digiti Minimi

This slender muscle arises in common with the extensor digitorum, lies along its medial side, and appears at first sight to be a part of it, but its tendon passes through a special compartment in the extensor retinaculum. The tendon splits into two parts [FIG. 71]. The medial part takes the main share in forming the expansion on the first phalanx. The lateral part, before it joins the expansion, is joined by the tendon from the extensor digitorum. Nerve supply : **posterior interosseous nerve**. Action : extension of little finger and wrist ; it allows the separate extension of the little finger.

MOVEMENTS OF THE FINGERS

The dissector should now note the movements he can make with his own fingers.

1. He can flex all three joints of the fingers —the metacarpo-phalangeal, and the proximal and distal interphalangeal joints as in 'making a fist'.

2. He can extend all three joints.

3. He can flex the interphalangeal joints with the fingers extended at the metacarpo-phalangeal joints ; but he will find increasing difficulty in performing this movement with individual fingers as he proceeds from the index to the little finger.

4. He can also flex the metacarpo-phalangeal joints and extend the interphalangeal joints. The last combination of movements is called 'putting the fingers in the writing position'. It is due mainly to the actions of the lumbricals and interossei which pass from the front to the back across the metacarpo-phalangeal joints, and so are enabled to flex those joints ; through their attachments to the extensor expansions they are able directly to extend the interphalangeal joints.

5. Close the fist, and note that, though the fingers are unequal in length, their tips come into line and meet the palm with equal pressure. Note also that, as the fist is closed, the hand bends backwards—i.e., it becomes extended at the wrist joint. This is due to the extensors of the wrist preventing the flexors from bending the wrist forward and thus enabling the flexors to exert their full range of action on the fingers, which they can do only when the wrist is extended. It is because of this fact that, if the wrist joint has to be fixed owing to disease, it is put up in the extended position in order that the fingers may retain their full grasping power. To test more fully how flexion of the fingers may be hampered by the position of the hand, flex the wrist joint as far as possible and then try to close the fist ; it cannot be done, for the extensors will not stretch enough ('passive insufficiency') to allow complete flexion at all the joints. This fact explains the common trick by which one can force a person to release the grasp by suddenly flexing the wrist joint.

6. Note, further, that, as the fist is closed, the fingers come together owing to the line of pull of the flexor tendons. It is impossible to keep them apart, and they cannot be separated while the fist is closed ; though this is easily done (by the dorsal interossei) with the fingers extended, or even partly flexed, so long as both flexors are not fully in action.

7. Flex one finger (*e.g.*, the middle finger) at the metacarpo-phalangeal joint and proximal interphalangeal joint. The distal phalanx is now quite lax : you can neither flex it nor extend it, for the flexor profundus cannot act easily on one finger separately, and the

extensors cannot act on the distal phalanx without extending the middle phalanx at the same time. The surgeons take advantage of this when the extensor tendon is ruptured at the base of the distal phalanx. They splint the finger in the flexed position to prevent the flexor profundus from bending the distal phalanx and thus increasing the interval between the torn ends of the extensor tendon, and they set the distal phalanx in the fully extended position to make the interval between the torn ends as small as possible.

DEEP STRUCTURES OF THE BACK OF FOREARM
[Figs. 69, 75, 77]

The deep structures are the posterior interosseous nerve and vessels, the terminal part of the anterior interosseous vessels and the five deep muscles named on page 103. The supinator will be recognized from the close manner in which it is applied to the upper part of the radius [Fig. 75]; its attachments will be seen at a later stage. The other muscles are recognized by means of their tendons, already identified.

DISSECTION. Reflect the extensor digitorum and the extensor digiti minimi by dividing them about their middle and turning them upwards and downwards ; as the muscles are reflected, secure their nerves. Pull aside the extensor carpi ulnaris. The greater parts of the posterior interosseous vessels and nerve and of the deep muscles will then be exposed.

Find the posterior interosseous nerve as it emerges from the supinator; follow it downwards among the

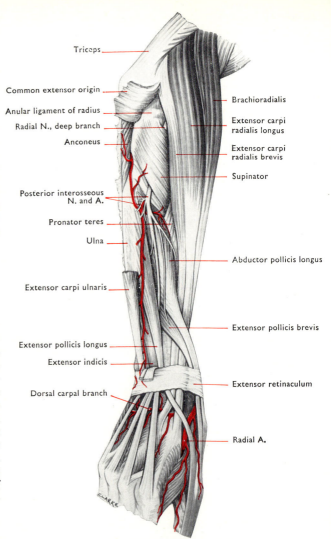

Triceps

Common extensor origin

Anular ligament of radius

Radial N., deep branch

Anconeus

Posterior interosseous N. and A.

Pronator teres

Ulna

Extensor carpi ulnaris

Extensor pollicis longus

Extensor indicis

Dorsal carpal branch

Brachioradialis

Extensor carpi radialis longus

Extensor carpi radialis brevis

Supinator

Abductor pollicis longus

Extensor pollicis brevis

Extensor retinaculum

Radial A.

Fig. 75   Deep dissection of back of forearm.

muscles, and trace its branches to the muscles. In the lower part of the forearm, it lies very deeply and is joined by the anterior interosseous artery. Follow them to the level of the retinaculum; open the compartment through which the extensor digitorum and extensor indicis pass, and trace the nerve and artery to the back of the wrist.

110

Return to the posterior interosseous artery as it emerges between the supinator and the abductor pollicis longus, and follow it downwards.

Then clean the muscles; define their origins; note where their tendons pass under the retinaculum, and trace the tendons to their insertions.

Abductor Pollicis Longus

The long abductor of the thumb arises from the back of the interosseous membrane and both bones of the forearm. The muscle

proceeds downwards and laterally, and comes to the surface in the interval between the extensor digitorum and the extensor carpi radialis brevis. It then crosses the two radial extensors, closely accompanied by the extensor pollicis brevis. Its tendon continues downwards, over the lateral side of the distal end of the radius and under cover of the extensor retinaculum, and is inserted into the base of the metacarpal bone of the thumb.

Nerve supply: the **posterior interosseous nerve**. Action: abductor of the thumb, and of the hand; and it may become important as a flexor of the wrist when the flexor muscles of the forearm are paralysed.

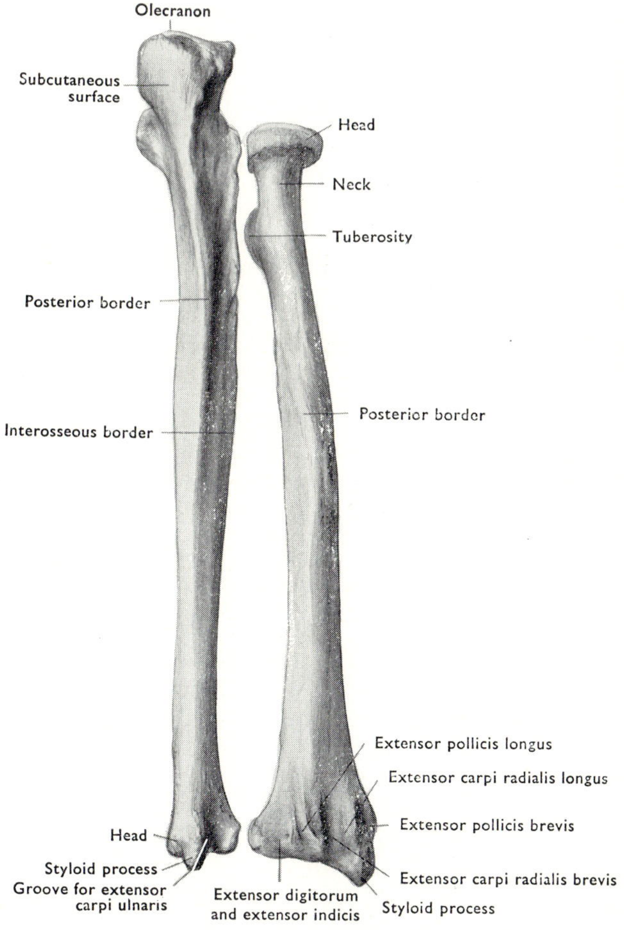

Extensor Pollicis Brevis

The short extensor, arising from a small portion of the posterior surface of the radius, and also from the interosseous membrane is placed along the distal border of the preceding muscle. The two tendons, closely applied to each other, cross the wrist in the same compartment of the extensor retinaculum; the tendon of the extensor pollicis brevis then passes along the back of the metacarpal bone of the thumb, to be inserted into the base of the proximal phalanx.

Nerve supply: the **posterior interosseous nerve**. Action: extension of the carpometacarpal and metacarpo-phalangeal joints of the thumb.

Extensor Pollicis Longus

This takes origin from the posterior surface of the middle third of the ulna, and also from the interosseous membrane. It overlaps the preceding muscle to some extent, and its tendon passes under cover of the extensor

Olecranon
Subcutaneous surface
Head
Neck
Tuberosity
Posterior border
Posterior border
Interosseous border
Extensor pollicis longus
Extensor carpi radialis longus
Extensor pollicis brevis
Head
Extensor carpi radialis brevis
Styloid process
Groove for extensor carpi ulnaris
Extensor digitorum and extensor indicis
Styloid process

FIG. 76   Right radius and ulna (posterior surface).

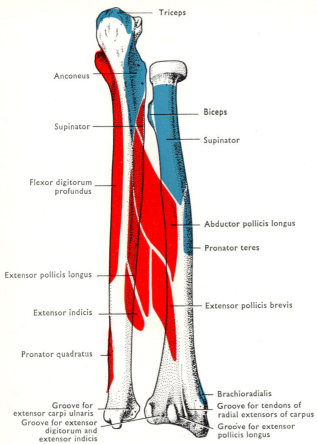

Triceps

Anconeus

Supinator

Flexor digitorum
profundus

Biceps

Supinator

Abductor pollicis longus

Pronator teres

Extensor pollicis longus

Extensor indicis

Pronator quadratus

Extensor pollicis brevis

Brachioradialis
Groove for
extensor carpi ulnaris
Groove for extensor
digitorum and
extensor indicis

Groove for tendons of
radial extensors of carpus
Groove for extensor
pollicis longus

Fig. 77 Muscle attachments to posterior surface of right radius and ulna.

retinaculum in a deep narrow groove on the back of the distal end of the radius, medial to the dorsal tubercle of the radius which acts as a sort of pulley for the tendon, enabling it to alter its direction and take an oblique course on the carpus. After crossing the tendons of the two radial extensors and the radial artery, it proceeds along the back of the thumb, and is inserted into the base of its distal phalanx.

Nerve supply : the **posterior interosseous nerve**. Action : extension of all the joints of the thumb.

112

Extensor Indicis

It arises from a limited area on the back of the ulna and the interosseous membrane distal to the preceding muscle. Its tendon accompanies the tendons of the extensor digitorum under the extensor retinaculum, in the same synovial sheath. On the dorsum of the hand, it lies along the medial side of the most lateral tendon of the common extensor, and it terminates in the expansion of that tendon on the dorsum of the first phalanx of the index finger.

Nerve supply: the **posterior interosseous nerve.**

Posterior Interosseous Nerve

This is the continuation, on the posterior surface of the forearm, of the deep branch of the radial nerve. The deep branch of the radial nerve arises opposite the lateral epicondyle of the humerus [p. 84], descends between the elbow joint and the brachioradialis muscle, gives branches to the extensor carpi radialis brevis, and to the supinator, and then disappears into the supinator. It reaches the back of the forearm by traversing the substance of the supinator obliquely, and at the same time winding round the lateral side of the shaft of the radius. It emerges from the supinator, as the posterior interosseous nerve, a short distance above the lower border of the muscle, and passes downwards, with the posterior interosseous vessels, across the surface of the abductor pollicis longus, under cover of the extensor digitorum.

It leaves the vessels by passing under cover of the extensor pollicis longus, and is joined by the anterior interosseous artery on the back of the interosseous membrane. Together they pass over the back of the distal end of the radius, deep to the synovial sheath of the extensor digitorum, to the back of the wrist joint. There the nerve ends in a slight swelling which sends branches to the wrist joint and to the intercarpal joints.

The branches of the deep branch of the radial nerve and the posterior interosseous nerve are very numerous, and they supply muscles and joints.

The **articular** branches are distributed to the elbow, distal radio-ulnar, wrist and intercarpal joints.

The **muscular** branches that arise in front of the elbow supply the extensor carpi radialis brevis and supinator; those that arise in the back of the forearm supply all the other muscles there, including an occasional additional twig to the anconeus.

Posterior Interosseous Artery

This artery arises, in the front of the forearm, from the common interosseous branch of the ulnar artery, and proceeds backwards at once between the two bones of the forearm immediately proximal to the interosseous membrane. It appears in the back of the forearm between the supinator and the abductor pollicis longus, and then runs downwards between the superficial and deep muscles. It reaches the back of the wrist, but its lower part is so slender that it can seldom be traced below the middle of the forearm unless it is exceptionally well injected. It gives off branches to the adjacent muscles, and takes part in the anastomosis around the elbow through the **interosseous recurrent artery** [FIGS. 75, 78].

Terminal Part of Anterior Interosseous Artery

It perforates the interosseous membrane about 5 cm. above the distal end of the radius, and is at once joined by the posterior interosseous nerve. It descends, with the nerve, to the dorsum of the carpus, where it joins the **posterior carpal arch**.

Tendons at the Wrist in the Living Limb

First make sure that you can identify the bony landmarks at the wrist [pp. 43–45] and then proceed to identify the tendons at the wrist and the distal part of the forearm in your own limb :

1. Palmaris longus, at the middle in front, with flexor carpi radialis immediately lateral to it. (The palmaris longus may be absent.)

2. Flexor carpi ulnaris, along the medial margin of the front of the distal part of forearm, ending in the pisiform bone.

3. The tendons of flexor superficialis rise into view, between the flexor carpi ulnaris and the palmaris longus, when the fist is clenched and the wrist is flexed ; relax the tension of the fingers and the tendon of the flexor carpi radialis springs forward.

4. Abductor pollicis longus and extensor pollicis brevis lie close together in the anterior boundary of the 'snuff-box', and form a prominent ridge when the thumb is extended. Extensor pollicis longus, running obliquely towards the thumb, lies in the posterior boundary of the 'snuff-box' [p. 44].

5. Extensor carpi radialis longus and brevis are crossed and partly hidden by the extensor pollicis longus, but they rise better into view when the fist is closed, for they then contract to prevent the flexors of the fingers from flexing the wrist also ; the brevis stands out more prominently than the longus.

6. Extensor indicis and extensor digitorum lie at the middle of the back of the wrist ; the diverging tendons of digitorum are seen best when the flexed fingers are extended at the metacarpo-phalangeal joints.

7. Extensor digiti minimi lies close to the radial side of the head of the ulna, but is not visible till it enters the hand.

8. Extensor carpi ulnaris, escaping from the groove between the head and the styloid process of the ulna, forms a thick, indistinct ridge at the ulnar margin of the back of the wrist.

DISSECTION. Clean the part of the radial artery that lies on the radial side of the wrist with its branches, displacing the tendons as required.

Radial Artery

Only a small portion of the radial artery is seen in this dissection. At the distal end of the radius, the vessel leaves the front of the forearm, turns backwards distal to the styloid process of the radius, and then descends over the scaphoid and trapezium to reach the proximal end of the first interosseous space. There it turns forwards through the space, between the two heads of the first dorsal interosseous muscle, to enter the palm [p. 102 and Fig. 75].

As it turns backwards distal to the radius, it lies on the lateral ligament of the wrist joint, and is crossed by the tendons of the abductor pollicis longus and extensor pollicis brevis. It crosses the carpus in the floor of the 'anatomical snuff-box', where it can be felt pulsating. Note in your own hand that the commencement of the cephalic vein overlies it, and may be seen through the skin. Before the artery disappears it is crossed by the extensor pollicis longus and digital branches of the radial nerve.

In this part of its course it supplies the structures on the back of the hand and digits by small branches.

The posterior carpal artery joins the similar branch of the ulnar artery to form the posterior carpal arch, from which two dorsal metacarpal arteries run towards the clefts between the medial three fingers, where each divides into two small dorsal digital arteries for the adjacent sides of the fingers. The first dorsal metacarpal artery may arise in common with the posterior carpal artery, and goes to the cleft between the forefinger and middle finger.

Each dorsal metacarpal artery sends two perforating arteries forwards through the interosseous space to connect it with the deep palmar arch and with a palmar digital artery.

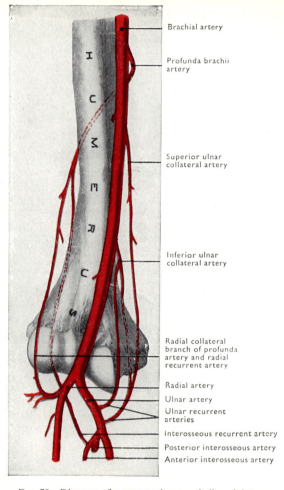

FIG. 78   Diagram of anastomosis around elbow joint.

Brachial artery

Profunda brachii artery

Superior ulnar collateral artery

Inferior ulnar collateral artery

Radial collateral branch of profunda artery and radial recurrent artery

Radial artery

Ulnar artery

Ulnar recurrent arteries

Interosseous recurrent artery

Posterior interosseous artery

Anterior interosseous artery

The dorsal digital arteries for the thumb and radial side of the forefinger arise independently from the radial artery before it disappears into the palm.

DISSECTION. Detach the anconeus from its origin, turn it downwards and trace the interosseous recurrent artery to the back of the lateral epicondyle.

Anastomosis around the Elbow Joint [Fig. 78]. Small vessels that arise from the brachial,

114

radial and ulnar arteries have already been traced to the elbow where they ramify and anastomose to form a rich network around the elbow. The branches that arise from the network supply the bones, ligaments and synovial membrane of the elbow and proximal radio-ulnar joints, and also the structures around the joints.

The vessels of the lateral and medial sides communicate freely, and the chief transverse anastomosis arches across the back of the humerus immediately above the olecranon fossa.

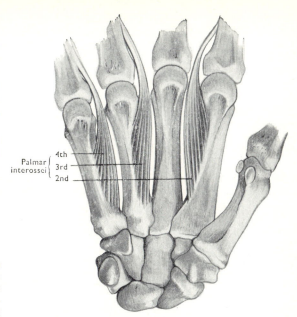

Palmar interossei
4th
3rd
2nd

FIG. 79   The second, third, and fourth palmar interosseous muscles (right side). See FIG. 80 for first palmar interosseous muscle.

DEEPEST STRUCTURES IN THE PALM AND FOREARM

DISSECTION. Complete the dissection of the palm by defining the deep transverse ligaments. They are found in the spaces between the heads of the medial four metacarpal bones by displacing the lumbrical muscle and the digital nerves and artery.

Deep Transverse Metacarpal Ligaments

This name is given to the three strong, flat bands attached to the margins of the palmar ligaments of the metacarpo-phalangeal joints of the fingers. The slips of the palmar aponeurosis gain partial attachment to their palmar surfaces. The lumbrical muscles and digital vessels and nerves lie in front of them. The interosseous muscles lie behind them. Though they are not directly fixed to bones, their connexion with the palmar ligaments of the joints (which are very strong) enables them to prevent excessive separation of the metacarpal bones from one another.

DISSECTION. The interosseous muscles have been partly exposed already. To expose them fully, draw the flexor tendons, the lumbricals and the digital nerves and vessels out of the way, remove the transverse head of the adductor pollicis from the third metacarpal bone, and divide the deep transverse metacarpal ligaments. Clean the interosseous muscles, define their margins, and follow their tendons backwards to their insertions.

Interosseous Muscles

The interosseous muscles [FIGS. 63, 79, 80] occupy the intervals between the metacarpal bones, and extend on to their palmar aspects. There are four **palmar interossei** which arise from the palmar aspect of the metacarpal of the finger on which they act; they are found on all the metacarpals except that of the middle finger. There are also four **dorsal interossei** which arise from the adjacent sides of the metacarpals forming each of the four interosseous spaces, and each converges on its tendon in bipennate (herringbone) form.

The tendons of all the interossei behave in the same way: they enter the finger posterior to the deep transverse metacarpal ligament, are bound to the capsule of the metacarpo-phalangeal joint (except the first palmar interosseous) and are lightly attached to the base of the proximal phalanx. The main part of the tendon inclines posteriorly to join the edge of the extensor expansion,

115

through which it is inserted into the dorsal surface of the base of the terminal phalanx. These attachments allow the interossei to flex the metacarpo-phalangeal joints and extend the interphalangeal joints [see p. 109]. Because they pass either to the radial or the ulnar side of the metacarpo-phalangeal joints (whose configuration allows of lateral movements) and lie in the plane of the fingers, their main action is to spread the fingers. *i.e.* abduct or draw them away from the middle metacarpal (action of dorsal interossei), and draw them together, *i.e.* adduct or draw them towards the middle metacarpal (action of palmar interossei).

In their function as abductors and adductors, the interossei act with the named abductors of the thumb and little finger and the adductor of the thumb. They are so arranged that each digit has an abductor and an adductor. FIGURES 79 and 80 show the arrangement clearly and the following points should be noted: The little finger has a special abductor and a palmar interosseous to its radial side. The ring finger has a dorsal interosseous on its ulnar side and a palmar to its radial side. The middle finger has two dorsal interossei, one on each side, which act alternately as abductors and adductors. The index finger has a palmar interosseous on its ulnar side and the first dorsal interosseous on its radial side. This is the largest dorsal interosseous and its belly forms the bulge in the dorsal part of the space between thumb and index finger. It can be seen and felt to contract either when the index finger is abducted or when it is flexed at the metacarpo-phalangeal joint and extended at the interphalangeal joints. The thumb has a special adductor and two special abductors (longus and brevis), but frequently it has also a slender first palmar interosseous muscle placed between the

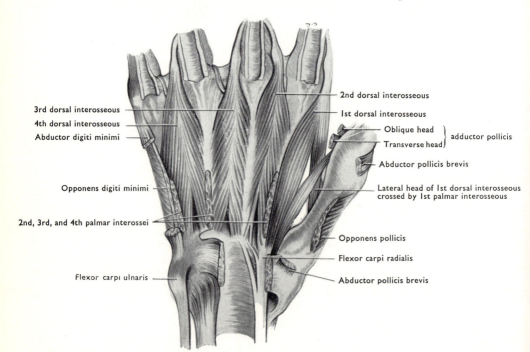

3rd dorsal interosseous
4th dorsal interosseous
Abductor digiti minimi

Opponens digiti minimi

2nd, 3rd, and 4th palmar interossei

Flexor carpi ulnaris

2nd dorsal interosseous
1st dorsal interosseous
Oblique head ⎫
Transverse head ⎭ adductor pollicis
Abductor pollicis brevis
Lateral head of 1st dorsal interosseous crossed by 1st palmar interosseous
Opponens pollicis
Flexor carpi radialis
Abductor pollicis brevis

FIG. 80   Dorsal interosseous muscles of right hand (seen from the palmar aspect).

adductor pollicis and the first dorsal interosseous muscle.

The interossei are all supplied by the **deep branch of the ulnar nerve** (T. 1); and, since they act as extensors and flexors of different joints of the fingers, the hand assumes a peculiar shape in ulnar paralysis. When the interossei are paralysed, the balanced action of the opposing sets of muscles is upset. Through the loss of the action of the interossei on the metacarpo-phalangeal joints, the extensors bend the fingers backwards at those joints. But, at the same time, the flexors bend the fingers forward at the interphalangeal joints, which the interossei usually extend. The result is the *main en griffe* or claw-hand.

DISSECTION. Clear away the thenar muscles from the flexor retinaculum; displace the tendon of the flexor pollicis longus and remove the oblique head of the adductor pollicis from its origin. Pull on the tendon of the flexor carpi radialis, and cut through the part of the retinaculum that covers it. Examine the synovial sheath of the tendon, and clean it down to its insertion.

Tendon of Flexor Carpi Radialis

This tendon crosses in front of the tubercle of the scaphoid bone, descends in the groove on the front of the trapezium covered by the retinaculum and by the origins of the thenar muscles, and passes to its insertion into the base of the second metacarpal bone covered by a prolongation of the retinaculum and by a part of the origin of the adductor pollicis. The tendon of the flexor pollicis longus has a double relation to it: that tendon crosses behind it at the wrist joint, and in front of it near its insertion.

DISSECTION. All the muscles around the elbow joint should be removed. As the brachialis and the triceps are raised, some care is required to avoid injury to the anterior and posterior parts of the capsule. Leave the supinator to the last, because it is only when it is completely isolated that a proper idea of its attachments and mode of action can be obtained.

Supinator

This muscle envelops the neck and the proximal part of the shaft of the radius, covering it completely, except on its medial side [FIGS. 54, 75, 77]. It arises chiefly from the floor of the deep depression below the radial notch of the ulna. From their origin, the fibres sweep round the radius, and clothe its shaft as far down as the insertion of the pronator teres. Nerve supply: the **deep branch of the radial nerve** which traverses its substance, and partially separates it into two layers. Action: supination.

THE JOINTS OF THE UPPER LIMB

THE ELBOW JOINT

Ligaments

This joint is formed by the articulation of the trochlea and capitulum of the humerus with the trochlear notch of the ulna and the head of the radius respectively. It is essentially a hinge joint, and has, therefore, strong radial and ulnar collateral ligaments, while the anterior and posterior parts of the fibrous capsule are weak and contain many oblique fibres which allow the full range of movement.

The **anterior ligament** passes from the epicondyles and the upper margins of the radial and coronoid fossae of the humerus, to the coronoid process of the ulna and the anular ligament of the radius.

The **posterior ligament** is weak, especially medially. It stretches from a line joining the epicondyles across the floor of the olecranon fossa, where its attachment is very loose, to the articular margin of the olecranon.

The **radial collateral ligament** is a strong, short band which is attached to the lower surface of the lateral epicondyle, and spreads out inferiorly to be fixed to the lateral and posterior parts of the anular ligament.

The **ulnar collateral ligament** radiates from the lower border of the medial epicondyle to the medial margins of the coronoid process

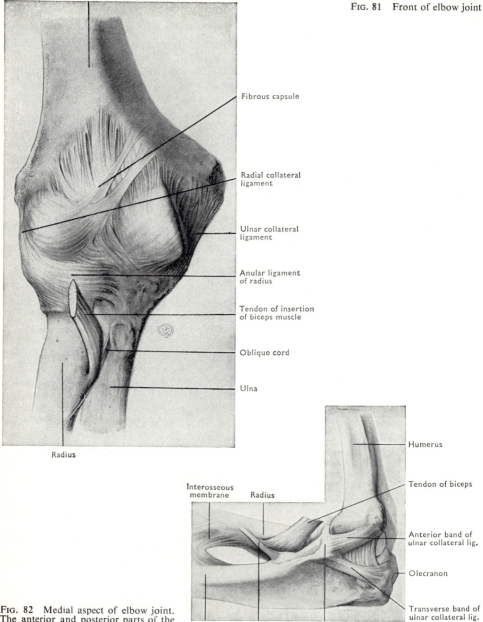

Humerus

FIG. 81 Front of elbow joint

Fibrous capsule

Radial collateral
ligament

Ulnar collateral
ligament

Anular ligament
of radius

Tendon of insertion
of biceps muscle

Oblique cord

Ulna

Radius

Humerus

Tendon of biceps

Anterior band of
ulnar collateral lig.

Olecranon

Transverse band of
ulnar collateral lig.

Interosseous
membrane   Radius

FIG. 82 Medial aspect of elbow joint.
The anterior and posterior parts of the
articular capsule were removed.

Ulna   Oblique cord   Coronoid process

118

and olecranon and to an oblique band that bridges across the interval between those margins. The anterior and posterior parts of this radiating ligament are thick; the middle part, which is attached to the oblique band, is thin. The ulnar nerve, as it descends from the back of the medial epicondyle into the forearm, lies on the posterior and middle parts of the ligament, and the posterior ulnar recurrent artery ascends close to the nerve.

Synovial Membrane

The synovial membrane lines the deep surface of the fibrous capsule. **Superiorly,** it is reflected on to the humerus to cover the non-articular part of the bone enclosed within the fibrous capsule. As it passes over the floor of the olecranon fossa it is separated from the bone by a little soft fat. Beside the olecranon fossa and the coronoid and radial fossae it is separated from the fibrous capsule by pads of fat [FIG. 83] which bulge it into the fossae when the bony processes are withdrawn. **Inferiorly,** at the back, at the front and at the medial side, it passes off the fibrous

capsule to overlap the articular margins of the coronoid process and the olecranon; but, at the lateral side, it is directly continuous with the synovial membrane of the proximal radio-ulnar joint.

The nerve supply of the joint is derived from the median, musculocutaneous, ulnar, radial, and posterior interosseous.

The **structures related** to the surfaces of the joint are shown in section in FIGURE 83.

Movements at the Elbow Joint

The movements at the elbow joint are distinct from those that take place at the proximal radio-ulnar joint. The elbow joint is essentially a hinge joint, but since its surfaces of articulation between the humerus and ulna are in the nature of a modified saddle joint, some slight adduction and abduction of the ulna is possible. Its main movements are flexion, or forward movement of the forearm, and extension or backward movement of the forearm; in full extension the arm is straight.

The **muscles** which are chiefly concerned in flexing the forearm are the biceps, brachialis, brachioradialis and pronator teres, assisted, to a slight extent, by the other muscles attached to the medial epicondyle. The

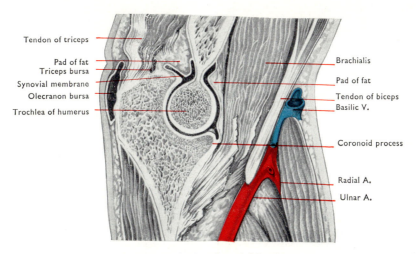

Tendon of triceps

Pad of fat
Triceps bursa
Synovial membrane
Olecranon bursa
Trochlea of humerus

Brachialis

Pad of fat

Tendon of biceps
Basilic V.

Coronoid process

Radial A.

Ulnar A.

FIG. 83   Sagittal section of right elbow.

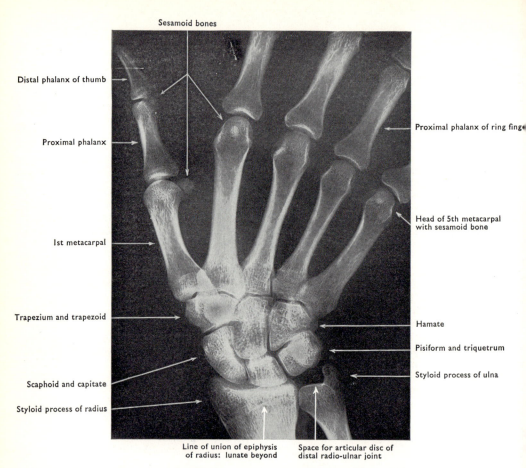

Sesamoid bones

Distal phalanx of thumb

Proximal phalanx

1st metacarpal

Trapezium and trapezoid

Scaphoid and capitate

Styloid process of radius

Proximal phalanx of ring finger

Head of 5th metacarpal with sesamoid bone

Hamate

Pisiform and triquetrum

Styloid process of ulna

Line of union of epiphysis of radius: lunate beyond

Space for articular disc of distal radio-ulnar joint

FIG. 84   Radiograph of wrist and palm of girl aged 17. The hand is in position of adduction (ulnar deviation).

muscle which extends the forearm is the triceps, aided slightly by the muscles which spring from the lateral epicondyle.

DISSECTION. Cut away the remains of the thenar and hypothenar muscles. Remove the flexor and extensor retinacula and the flexor and extensor tendons from the wrist—but do not detach the tendons from the digits.

THE WRIST JOINT

This **radiocarpal** joint consists of the articulation between the convex proximal

surface of the carpus (formed by the scaphoid, lunate, and triquetral bones and their interosseous ligaments) and the concave socket formed by the extremity of the radius, extended medially by the triangular **articular disc** which joins the distal end of the radius to the styloid process of the ulna, and separates the ulna from the joint. In the normal position of the hand only the scaphoid and part of the lunate articulate with the radius, the surface of which shows two shallow fossae to receive these. The remainder of the lunate articulates with the articular disc, and the

120

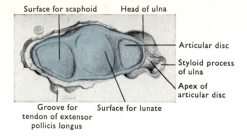

Surface for scaphoid   Head of ulna

Articular disc

Styloid process
of ulna

Apex of
articular disc

Groove for   Surface for lunate
tendon of extensor
pollicis longus

FIG. 85   Proximal articular surface of wrist joint.

triquetrum with the capsule of the joint. The direction of the radiocarpal joint is oblique, the lateral and dorsal parts of the radius extending further distally, with a corresponding extension of the articular surface on the carpus.

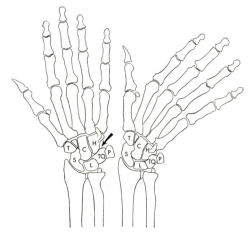

FIG. 86 Outline tracings of the bones of the hand taken from radiographs of the same individual in abducted and fully adducted positions of the wrist. Note how, in adduction, the proximal row of carpal bones slides laterally on the radius to bring the lunate fully into contact with the distal end of the radius, and the triquetrum against the disc on the distal end of the ulna. The distal row of carpal bones slides in the concavity of the proximal row, so as to bring the hamate into contact with the lunate, and the whole of its medial aspect against the triquetrum ; the capitate sliding laterally off the lunate on to the scaphoid, and the trapezium gliding medially on the distal surface of the scaphoid.

C. Capitate   S. Scaphoid
H. Hamate   T. Trapezium
L. Lunate   TQ. Triquetrum
P. Pisiform

Fibrous Capsule

This extends from the margins of the distal ends of the radius and ulna and the articular disc, to the proximal row of carpal bones, excluding the pisiform. It is thickened to form **radial** and **ulnar collateral ligaments** attached to the styloid processes of these bones, while the anterior and posterior parts are strengthened by fibres which pass obliquely downwards and medially. It is lined by synovial membrane which also covers the interosseous ligaments of the carpus and may be continuous with that of the distal radioulnar joint if the articular disc is incomplete.

Nerve supply: anterior and posterior interosseous nerves and the dorsal branch of the ulnar nerve.

Movements

A wide range of movements is possible at the wrist joint and these are associated with movements at the intercarpal joints. Extension and adduction have the greatest range, while abduction occurs mainly at the intercarpal joints, the styloid process of the radius riding against the scaphoid early in the movement. Flexion has a smaller range than extension, but with the flexion at the intercarpal joints added, appears to be greater. In adduction, the carpal bones slide laterally, the lunate passing entirely on to the radius, while the triquetrum articulates with the disc [FIG. 86].

The muscles which produce the various movements are : Flexion, all tendons passing anterior to the joint, but especially the radial and ulnar carpal flexors and palmaris longus. Extension, all tendons passing posterior to the joint, but especially the carpal extensors. Abduction, the radial flexor and extensors of the carpus, abductor pollicis longus and extensor pollicis brevis. Adduction, the ulnar flexor and extensor of the carpus.

DISSECTION. Divide the anterior, medial and lateral ligaments by a transverse incision across the front of the joint. Bend the hand backwards to expose the articular surfaces.

THE RADIO-ULNAR JOINTS

Proximal Radio-ulnar Joint

This joint is between the head of the radius and the radial notch of the ulna; and its **ligaments** are the anular and the quadrate.

Anular Ligament of Radius. This is a strong, fibrous collar (*anulus* = a ring) which encircles the head of the radius and retains it in the radial notch of the ulna. It forms four-fifths of a circle, and is attached by its extremities to the anterior and posterior margins of the notch. It is slightly narrower below than above, and prevents the head of the radius being pulled downwards out of it. The ligament is braced tightly towards the elbow and also strengthened by the anterior and lateral ligaments of the elbow, which are attached to its upper border. Its lower border is attached, loosely, to the neck of the radius by a thin layer of fibrous tissue which closes the joint inferiorly—except at the medial side, where the closure is completed by the **quadrate ligament,** a small, loose, weak sheet of fibres that connects the neck of the radius to the lower margin of the radial notch of the ulna.

Synovial Membrane. The synovial membrane of the proximal radio-ulnar joint is a prolongation downwards of the synovial membrane of the elbow joint; it lines the deep surface of the anular ligament and the upper surface of the quadrate ligament. As it is reflected upwards to reach the articular cartilage around the head of the radius, it encloses the intracapsular part of the neck in a tubular sheath.

Distal Radio-ulnar Joint

At this joint the head of the ulna is received into the ulnar notch of the radius and the bones are united by a fibrous capsule and the articular disc.

Articular Disc. The disc is the true bond of union at this joint. It has already been noticed in connexion with the radiocarpal joint, where it extends the radial articular surface in a medial direction. It separates the distal end of the ulna from the lunate and triquetrum and intervenes, therefore, between the cavities of the wrist joint and distal radio-ulnar joint [Fig. 89]. It is a thick, firm, fibrocartilaginous plate of triangular outline, attached by its base to the distal margin of the ulnar notch of the radius, and by its apex to the depression at the root of the styloid process of the ulna.

Fibrous Capsule. The fibrous capsule consists of lax fibres which can have little influence in retaining the distal ends of the bones in apposition. It is attached to the anterior and posterior borders of the articular disc, and to the front and back of both bones of the forearm, extending upwards to the lower ends of their interosseous borders to enclose an upward prolongation of the cavity of the joint called the **recessus sacciformis.**

The **synovial membrane** lines the fibrous capsule, and covers the upper surface of the disc.

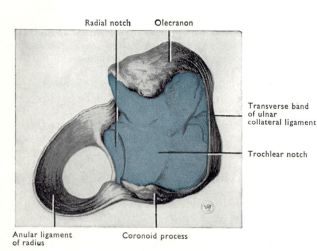

Radial notch   Olecranon

Transverse band of ulnar collateral ligament

Trochlear notch

Anular ligament of radius   Coronoid process

Fig. 87   Anular ligament of radius and proximal articular surfaces of ulna.

In addition to the ligaments of the two joints, the bones are held together by the interosseous membrane.

DISSECTION. To expose the interosseous membrane, remove the muscles from the back and the front of the forearm.

Interosseous Membrane of Forearm

The interosseous membrane is a fibrous sheet that stretches across the interval between the two bones of the forearm, and is attached to the interosseous border of each. Its upper border is situated about 2·5 cm. below the tuberosity of the radius. Distally, it blends with the capsule of the distal radio-ulnar joint. The posterior interosseous vessels pass backwards, above its upper margin, between the two bones of the forearm, and the anterior interosseous vessels pierce it about 5 cm. from its distal end.

Its fibres run for the most part obliquely downwards and medially from the radius to the ulna, although several strands may be noticed taking an opposite direction. The membrane therefore braces the two bones together in such a manner that forces, passing upwards from the hand through the radius, are transmitted from the radius to the ulna. It also extends the surface of origin for the muscles of the forearm. By its anterior surface it gives origin to the flexor digitorum profundus and the flexor pollicis longus muscles, whilst from its posterior surface spring fibres of the two extensor muscles of the thumb, the abductor pollicis longus, and the extensor indicis.

DISSECTION. Cut through the anular ligament, divide the interosseous membrane from above downwards, open the capsule of the distal radio-ulnar joint, and draw the radius laterally. Examine the connexions of the capsule and articular disc.

Movements at the Radio-ulnar Joints

The movements of pronation and supination take place at the radio-ulnar joints. When the limb is in the position of complete **supination**, the thumb is directed laterally and the two bones of the forearm are parallel. In the movement of **pronation**, the radius describes a segment of a cone the apex of which lies at the centre of the head of the radius, and the centre of the base is the attachment of the

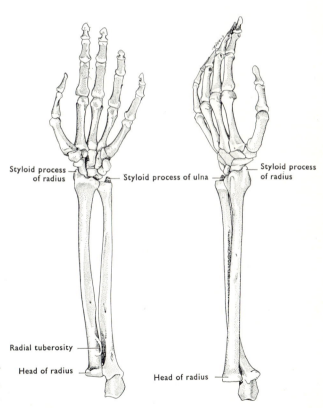

Styloid process of radius — Styloid process of ulna — Styloid process of radius

Radial tuberosity —

Head of radius —

Head of radius —

FIG. 88 Outline drawing of the position of the forearm and hand bones in supination (left) and pronation (right). Note that the ulna remains stationary and that the distal end of the radius rotates around it carrying the hand. The head of the radius rotates in the radial notch of the ulna.

123

articular disc of the distal radio-ulnar joint to the base of the styloid process of the ulna. Thus the head of the radius, resting against the capitulum of the humerus, rotates in the anular ligament, while the distal end turns around the stationary ulna carrying the hand and the articular disc with it. The styloid process of the radius, describing an arc of a circle, passes from the lateral to the medial side of the ulna, so that the dorsal surfaces of the radius and hand face anteriorly in pronation, and the thumb comes to lie on the medial side. The head of the radius remaining in the same position while its distal end is turned over to the medial side, the shaft of the radius comes to lie obliquely across the anterior surface of the ulna.

Pronation is produced by muscles on the anterior surface of the forearm which run from the medial to the lateral side either directly, pronator quadratus, or obliquely, pronator teres and flexor carpi radialis. Pronator teres has the maximum mechanical advantage by being attached to the point of maximum lateral curvature of the radius. Brachioradialis has a weak pronating action on the fully supinated forearm.

Supination. Biceps is the most powerful supinator. Its tendon sweeps round the medial side of the radius to be inserted into the dorsal part of the radial tuberosity, so that it forcibly rotates the radius laterally on contraction. Supination is also produced by muscles which run from medial to lateral on the dorsal surface of the forearm, *i.e.*, supinator and abductor pollicis longus. Brachioradialis can also assist in starting supination of the fully pronated forearm. The supinators are more powerful than the pronators, as can be seen from the greater force which a right handed person can apply to a screwdriver when inserting a screw than

when removing it ; a feature for which biceps is responsible.

When the elbow is extended, the range of pronation and supination appears to be increased because of the addition of rotation of the humerus. For this reason, clinical tests for the range of movement at the radio-ulnar joints are always carried out with the elbow flexed.

THE INTERCARPAL, CARPO-METACARPAL AND INTERMETA-CARPAL JOINTS

In the carpus there are only two joint cavities.

At the **pisiform joint,** the pisiform bone articulates with the palmar surface of the triquetrum, to which it is attached by an articular capsule. The pisiform is held in position, against the pull of flexor carpi ulnaris which is inserted into it, by the **pisohamate** and the **pisometacarpal ligaments** attached respectively to the hook of the hamate and the base of the fifth metacarpal bone.

The other **intercarpal joints** [FIG. 89] share one complex cavity which is also common to the carpometacarpal and intermetacarpal joints of the fingers, but does not communicate either with any of the joints of the thumb or

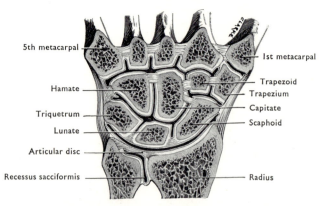

5th metacarpal
1st metacarpal
Trapezoid
Hamate
Trapezium
Capitate
Triquetrum
Scaphoid
Lunate
Articular disc
Recessus sacciformis
Radius

FIG. 89 Coronal section through radiocarpal, intercarpal, carpometacarpal, and intermetacarpal joints to show joint cavities and interosseous ligaments (diagrammatic).

124

with the pisiform joint. With a single cavity these articulations share a synovial membrane which covers all the intra-articular parts not covered with articular cartilage, and a fibrous capsule which surrounds all the bones and holds them together. Thus it is possible to describe **palmar, dorsal, lateral,** and **medial ligaments** of the intercarpal, carpometacarpal and intermetacarpal joints separately, but they are simply parts of the same fibrous capsule and will not be dealt with further, except to note that they are continuous with the capsule of the wrist joint, though there is no continuity with its joint cavity.

Interosseous ligaments are also present which join the three proximal carpal bones and complete the distal articular surface of the wrist joint. Those joining the distal row of carpal bones together are less regular in position, and there are three stout ligaments joining the non-articular parts of the bases of the adjacent metacarpals of the fingers. These limit the distal extent of the corresponding intermetacarpal joints. Interosseous ligaments between the rows of bones are less well developed, but there is an interosseous carpometacarpal ligament joining the adjacent sides of the capitate and hamate bones to the medial side of the base of the third metacrapal. There may also be a ligament joining the capitate and scaphoid bones [FIG. 89].

DISSECTION. Remove the interosseous muscles from the metacarpal bones, and detach the flexor tendons from the fingers, but leave the extensor tendons in position. Define and clean the ligaments which connect the carpus and metacarpus, and those which unite the bases of the medial four metacarpal bones. To display the interosseous carpometacarpal ligament, divide the bands which connect the bases of the third and fourth metacarpal bones, and sever the dorsal ligaments which bind the medial two metacarpal bones to the carpus. Bend the metacarpal bones forcibly forwards, thus exposing the ligament. Display the articular surfaces of the carpometacarpal joints by detaching the metacarpus from the carpus. To see the interosseous ligaments, separate the bones of the distal row of the carpus from one another, and deal similarly with the bases of the metacarpal bones.

Articular Surfaces and Movements [FIGS. 72, 89]

1. **Intercarpal joints.** The bones of the proximal row articulate with one another by flat surfaces, and so do the bones of the distal row, thus allowing a very limited amount of gliding movement which is controlled by interosseous and capsular ligaments. The transverse part of the intercarpal joint, between the proximal and distal rows, is deeply concavo-convex owing to the capitate and hamate bones being inserted into the concavity formed by the triquetrum, lunate and the distal part of the medial surface of the scaphoid; while the convex distal surface of the scaphoid bone fits into the concavity formed by the trapezium and trapezoid bones. Flexion and extension are the main movements at this joint, but there is also some side to side gliding which increases the movements of adduction and abduction at the wrist joint [FIG. 86]. Together these joints supplement the movements of the radiocarpal joint and increase the strength and elasticity of the wrist.

2. **Carpometacarpal** and **intermetacarpal joints.** The metacarpal bone of the thumb articulates with the trapezium by a saddle-shaped joint with a lax capsule; both features which allow a very considerable range of movement which is further increased by the separation of the joint from the other carpometacarpal joints. It should be noted that the movements of the thumb are not in the same plane as the corresponding movements of the fingers, because the thumb lies anterior to the fingers with its flexor surface facing medially and not anteriorly. Thus the metacarpal bone of the thumb can be moved: (1) laterally (extension); (2) medially (flexion); (3) posteriorly towards the palm (adduction); (4) anteriorly (abduction). A combination of these movements, one after the other, constitutes circumduction, but a more important combination is that which produces **opposition**; in this the thumb is first abducted and medially rotated and then flexed, bringing the palmar surface of its terminal segment into contact with that of any of the fingers. This

movement differs from simple flexion with abduction by virtue of the medial rotation of the metacarpal of the thumb, and it is this movement which confers on the thumb its importance in grasping, making it functionally one half of the hand.

The metacarpal of the index finger is fitted around the distal surface of the trapezoid bone. It articulates laterally with the trapezium, and medially with the capitate and the metacarpal of the middle finger, which has a flat joint with the capitate. Movement of both these metacarpals is extremely limited, but the carpometacarpal joints of the ring, and particularly the little finger, allow of some movement. When the hand is clenched the 4th and 5th carpometacarpal joints are flexed, and the presence of an opponens muscle inserted into the 5th metacarpal helps to flex and rotate it slightly laterally, thus assisting in the 'cupping of the hand'.

The nerve supply of the intercarpal, carpometacarpal, and intermetacarpal joints is derived from the anterior and posterior interosseous nerves, and the dorsal and deep branches of the ulnar nerve.

THE METACARPO-PHALANGEAL AND INTERPHALANGEAL JOINTS

The ligaments of the metacarpo-phalangeal joints and interphalangeal joints are alike.

Fibrous Capsules

In each joint the fibrous capsule is thickened in front to form a palmar ligament, and at the sides to form collateral ligaments. On the dorsum of the joint the fibrous capsule is replaced by the extensor tendon, a mechanism which allows the full range of flexion with continuous support for the dorsal surface of the joints.

Collateral Ligaments. The collateral ligaments are strong oblique bands that pass downwards and forwards from the sides of the head of the proximal bone of the joint to the sides of the base of the distal bone [FIG. 67, p. 99].

Palmar Ligament. This is a strong, thick,

fibrous plate. It is attached loosely to the neck of the proximal bone, extends over the palmar surface of the head, and is attached firmly to the base of the distal bone. It forms part of the socket for the head of the proximal bone, whose palmar surface articulates with it when the joint is straight. The margins of each palmar ligament are continuous with the collateral ligaments, and give attachment to the margins of the fibrous flexor sheath ; its palmar surface is covered by the flexor tendon and the synovial sheath.

In a metacarpo-phalangeal joint of a finger, the margins of the palmar ligament give attachment also to the deep transverse metacarpal ligament and partial attachment to the processes of the palmar aponeurosis.

The **nerve supply** of the metacarpo-phalangeal joints and of the interphalangeal joints is derived from the nerves that innervate the skin of the digits to which they belong.

Sesamoid Bones. In the metacarpo-phalangeal joint of the thumb, the palmar ligament is fused with the tendons of the adductor pollicis and flexor pollicis brevis. In the fused ligament and tendons, two little sesamoid bones are developed which articulate with the palmar surface of the head of the first metacarpal bone. Sometimes minute sesamoid bones are found in the palmar ligaments of other metacarpo-phalangeal joints, the joints of the index and the little finger being the most frequent.

DISSECTION. Raise the extensor tendons from the metacarpo-phalangeal joints. If this is done carefully, the dorsal part of the synovial membrane will be left intact.

Movements at the Metacarpo-phalangeal Joints

In each metacarpo-phalangeal joint, the concave surface of the phalanx receives the convex surface of the head of the metacarpal bone. The joints are condyloid ; the movements are therefore : (1) flexion, (2) extension, (3) abduction, (4) adduction, (5) circumduction. There is no provision for active or voluntary rotatory movements at these joints ; but, if a finger is seized by the other hand and twisted, it will be seen that considerable passive rotatory movement is possible.

During flexion of the fingers, the proximal phalanx and the palmar ligament travel forwards upon the head of the metacarpal bone; and the collateral ligaments, owing to the fact that they are attached nearer to the dorsal surface than to the palmar surface of the head, tighten so that lateral movement is restricted. The **interosseous** and **lumbrical** muscles produce this movement, aided by the long and short flexors of the digits.

The proximal phalanges of the fingers, in the movement of extension, can be carried backwards only to a very slight degree beyond the line of the metacarpal bones. The **extensor digitorum** and the **extensores indicis** and **digiti minimi** are the muscles which operate in this movement.

Abduction and adduction are movements of the proximal phalanx away from and towards a line prolonged distally through the middle metacarpal, and are seen when the fingers are spread out and drawn together again. The action of the interosseous muscles in these movements is explained on page 109. It should be noticed that the movements of abduction and adduction are very free in the extended position of the fingers; but, if flexion is induced, the power of separating the fingers becomes more and more restricted, until it becomes lost when the hand is closed.

This is due partly to the arrangement of the collateral ligaments mentioned above but perhaps mainly to the restricting action of the flexors [see p. 109].

Very little abduction or adduction is possible at the metacarpo-phalangeal joint of the thumb. These movements take place at its carpometacarpal joint.

Movements at the Interphalangeal Joints

The interphalangeal joints are hinge joints; therefore the only movements possible are flexion and extension. Flexor digitorum profundus flexes all the joints of the fingers, but flexor superficialis only acts on the proximal interphalangeal and the meta-carpo-phalangeal joints. Extension of the phalanges at the interphalangeal joints is produced not only by the extensors of the digits but also by the interosseous and lumbrical muscles acting through the extensor expansions, into which they are inserted; it is probable that extension of the middle and distal phalanges is brought about chiefly by the interossei and the lumbricals. The interossei and lumbricals, therefore, flex the proximal phalanges at the metacarpo-phalan-geal joints and extend the middle and distal phalanges at the interphalangeal joints.

In the thumb, the flexor pollicis longus and the extensor pollicis longus operate at the interphalangeal joint.

THE LOWER LIMB

INTRODUCTION

The parts of the lower limb are the hip and buttock, the thigh, the leg, and the foot and toes.

The hip and buttock make up what is called the **gluteal region,** which overlies the side and the back of the pelvis, extending from the waist and the small of the back down to the hollow on the side of the hip, and to the fold or groove that limits the buttock below. The hip and the buttock are not sharply distinguished from each other either in anatomical descriptions or in ordinary English usage, but the **hip** (*coxa*) may be taken as the upper part of the region presented in a side view, while the **buttock** (*natis*) is the rounded bulge behind and below. The groove that limits the buttock inferiorly is called the **gluteal fold**. The cleft between the buttocks is called the **natal cleft**, its lower part —*i.e.*, the part in front of the end of the backbone—is included in the perineum.

The skeleton of the hip and buttock is one bone called the **hip bone** ; it is made up of three parts united at the **acetabulum** where the femur articulates with it [FIG. 90]. The **ilium** is the large, upper part, and is felt in the lower margin of the waist. The **ischium** is the lower and hinder part, on which the body rests in the sitting posture. The **pubis** is the anterior part, and is the bone felt at the lower part of the front of the abdomen.

The hip bone forms part of the skeleton of the trunk also. The right and left hip bones, together with the sacrum and the coccyx, make up the skeleton of the pelvis, and the two hip bones together are sometimes called the **pelvic girdle**. At the front the two hip bones articulate with each other to form a joint called the **pubic symphysis** (*symphysis*= union). At the back they articulate with the sides of the sacrum at the **sacro-iliac joints.**

The **thigh** (*femur*) extends from the hip to the knee (*genu*). Its bone is called the **femur.** At its upper end, the femur articulates with the hip bone to form the **hip joint.** At the

knee joint, the femur articulates (1) with the tibia and (2) with the **patella** (knee cap), which lies in the front of the knee joint.

The thigh joins the gluteal region at the hollow on the side of the hip and at the fold of the buttock. Medially, it joins the perineum, which separates it from the other thigh. In front, it extends higher up than it does behind, and joins the front of the abdomen at the groove of the groin or **inguinal region.** The **ham** (*poples*) is the lower part of the back of the thigh and the back of the knee. The hollow of the ham is called the **popliteal fossa.**

The **leg** (*crus*) extends from the knee joint to the ankle joint. Colloquially, the term 'leg' usually means the whole free part of the lower limb, but it never does so in anatomical descriptions. The soft, fleshy part at the back of the leg is the **calf** (*sura*).

The bones of the leg are the **tibia** or shin bone and the **fibula**. They lie side by side— the fibula, which is a very slender bone, lying on the lateral side. At their upper and lower ends, they articulate with each other to form **tibiofibular joints.** Their lower ends articulate also with the talus (*i.e.*, the first bone of the foot) to form the **ankle joint.** The prominent parts of their lower ends, at the sides of the ankle, are called the **lateral malleolus** and the **medial malleolus.** Certain muscles attached to the fibula are called **peroneal** muscles from *peroné*, which is the Greek equivalent of the Latin *fibula* (=a pin or skewer).

The **foot** (*pes*) extends from the point of the heel (*calx*) to the roots of the toes. Its upper surface is usually called the **dorsum** of the foot and its lower surface is the **sole** (*planta*). The foot is divided into the tarsus, the metatarsus and the toes [FIGS. 170, 171].

The **tarsus** is the posterior half. Its bones are called **tarsal bones,** of which there are seven. They are arranged in two rows—a posterior row and an anterior row—with one of the bones set in between the two rows. There are two bones in the first row—set one above the other. The upper bone is the **talus,** which lies below the tibia; the lower bone is the largest bone of the tarsus, and is called the **calcaneus** because it is the skeleton of the heel. There are four bones in the second row. They are placed side by side—the **cuboid bone** most laterally, and then three bones called **cuneiform bones** because they are wedge-shaped (*cuneus* = a wedge). The bone between the rows is called the **navicular bone**; it separates the cuneiform bones from the talus. The tarsal bones articulate with one another forming **intertarsal joints.**

The **metatarsus** has a skeleton of five **metatarsal bones.** They are set side by side behind the toes, and are numbered 1 to 5 beginning with the one behind the big toe. Their posterior ends are called their bases; their anterior ends are called their heads. The bases articulate with one another forming **intermetatarsal joints,** and with the cuboid and cuneiform bones forming **tarsometatarsal joints.**

The **toes** or digits are numbered from medial to lateral side. The first toe is called also the big toe or **hallux,** and the fifth is the little toe, **digitus minimus.** The bones of the toe are called **phalanges.** The big toe has two phalanges. Each of the other toes has three. Each proximal phalanx articulates with the head of a metatarsal bone to form a **metatarsophalangeal joint.** The middle phalanx articulates with the other two to form **interphalangeal joints.** The proximal end of a phalanx is called its base and its distal end is its head.

Bones that are embedded in the substance of tendons are called **sesamoid bones.** The largest is the patella. The others are very small, and some of them are often absent; the two that are always present lie on the plantar surface of the first metatarsophalangeal joint [Fig. 172, 173].

THE FRONT OF THE THIGH

The order of dissection of the Lower Limb depends upon the arrangement that has been made for the general allotment of parts. If, according to a common plan, the limb is to be dissected in continuity with the Pelvis by the same dissectors, it may be advisable to begin with the gluteal region and to dissect the greater part of the thigh before any special dissection of the pelvis from the side is undertaken [see Vol. 2]. If, however, the limb is allotted separately, and the dissection begins at the same time as the dissection of the anterior abdominal wall, then the dissection should begin with the front of the thigh.

Before making the preliminary incisions in the skin, the dissector must study the surface anatomy of the region.

SURFACE ANATOMY

The **pubic symphysis** [p. 129, Fig. 91] is in the median plane, at the lowest part of the front of the abdomen, between the right and left pubic bones. Below and behind the symphysis there is a wide archway, called the **pubic arch,** whose sides are formed by the right and left pubis and ischium. Find the lower part of the symphysis, and press your fingers along one side of the arch. It is at the uppermost part of the medial side of the thigh, in the boundary between the thigh and the perineum. Next, find the upper margin of the symphysis, and draw your finger in a lateral direction. The bone felt is the **pubic crest.** The crest is about 2·5 cm. long, and ends laterally in the **pubic tubercle,** a small, blunt prominence at that distance from the symphysis.

Find the **iliac crest,** which is the bone felt in the lower margin of the waist. Trace it forwards and note that it curves slightly in a medial direction, and slopes markedly downwards. Its anterior end is called the **anterior superior iliac spine,** and in a thin body it can be gripped between finger and thumb. Between this spine and the pubic tubercle there is a shallow, curved groove that separates the front of the thigh from the front of the abdomen. Press your finger along the groove and feel a resilient band: that is the **inguinal ligament,** which stretches between the spine and the tubercle. Run your finger

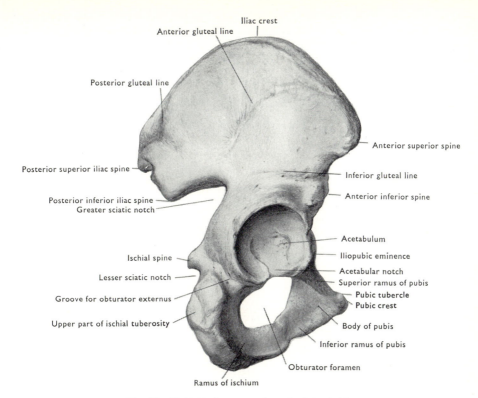

Anterior gluteal line

Iliac crest

Posterior gluteal line

Anterior superior spine

Posterior superior iliac spine

Inferior gluteal line

Posterior inferior iliac spine
Greater sciatic notch

Anterior inferior spine

Acetabulum

Ischial spine

Iliopubic eminence

Lesser sciatic notch

Acetabular notch
Superior ramus of pubis

Groove for obturator externus

Pubic tubercle
Pubic crest

Upper part of ischial tuberosity

Body of pubis

Inferior ramus of pubis

Obturator foramen

Ramus of ischium

FIG. 90   Right hip bone seen from the lateral side.

upwards and backwards from the spine along the outer edge or lip of the iliac crest, until you feel a low prominence called the **tubercle of the iliac crest;** it is at the widest part of the pelvis, and is therefore the highest point of the crest seen from the front, though the actual highest point is further round at the back. A hand's breadth below the tubercle the **greater trochanter** of the femur is near the surface, and forms a wide prominence just in front of the hollow on the side of the hip; the top of the trochanter is about the same level as the pubic crest.

The **head of the femur,** which articulates with the hip bone, is deeply hidden under muscles; but it can be felt. Place your finger on a spot **(mid-inguinal point),** just below the inguinal groove, midway between the anterior

superior iliac spine and the pubic symphysis; press firmly and rotate the limb this way and that; the head of the femur should be felt moving behind the muscle. In the living limb, the pulsations of the **femoral artery** are felt at the same spot.

The **shaft of the femur** is thickly covered with muscles throughout its length.

At the knee, the **patella** is a familiar object. The **ligamentum patellae** stretches downwards from it and leads you to the **tuberosity of the tibia,** which is a blunt prominence on the front of the upper end of the tibia. It is a very strong tendon—5 cm. long and 2·5 cm. wide—that can be gripped between finger and thumb, and is felt best when the knee is half bent. Grasp the patella and try to move it. It is movable when the knee is straight, but

131

not when the knee is bent—for then the ligamentum patellae is put upon the stretch. When the knee is bent, the patella is drawn off the front of the femur on to its lower end, and the **patellar surface** of the femur can be felt (if you press firmly) through the muscles above the patella [FIGS. 155, 161].

The large masses of bone at the sides of the

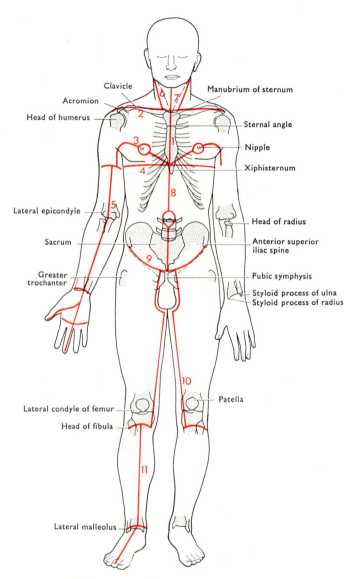

FIG. 91   Landmarks and incisions.   For the bony landmarks of the lower limb, see illustrations of individual bones.

knee are the **lateral** and **medial condyles** of the femur and of the tibia. With the knee bent, feel the sides of the femoral condyles; their most prominent points are called the **lateral** and **medial epicondyles** of the femur, and are nearer the back of the knee than the front.

Straighten the knee, and look at the posterior part of its medial surface. Note a low, longitudinal, fleshy elevation about the width of a finger. It is the lower part of the **sartorius** muscle, which runs downwards from the anterior superior iliac spine obliquely across the thigh, and can be brought into prominence in the living limb by bending it at both knee and hip joints and rotating the thigh outwards. Bend the knee, and note that the muscle slips backwards off the medial condyle of the femur into the medial boundary of the popliteal fossa.

The wide, smooth, fleshy swelling above the medial condyle is the lower part of a large muscle called the **vastus medialis.** When the knee is bent, that swelling is limited posteriorly by a wide, shallow groove. Press your finger into that groove; a tense band is felt in its floor; that is the tendon of a large muscle called the **adductor magnus.** Draw the finger downwards; it will be caught on a small prominence of bone, called the **adductor tubercle,** which projects from the uppermost part of the medial condyle [FIG. 103].

SUPERFICIAL DISSECTION

General instructions for making incisions and for the removal of skin and superficial fascia are given on page 10.

DISSECTION. Reflect the skin by making incisions 9 and 10 [Fig. 91]. Raise carefully the quadrilateral flap of skin thus mapped out from the superficial fascia and turn it laterally, taking particular care in the region of the knee to avoid injury to the patellar plexus of cutaneous nerves.

Superficial Fascia

The superficial fascia of the thigh contains abundant fat, especially on the medial side. The deeper part of the superficial fascia is membranous throughout the region, but especially in the uppermost part it forms a distinct layer, where partially separated from the fatty layer by vessels and lymph nodes [FIG. 100], and the two layers can be identified by a little dissection. Both layers of the superficial fascia are continuous with the corresponding layers on the anterior wall of the abdomen. The membranous layer is loosely attached to the deep fascia of the thigh by areolar tissue except near the inguinal ligament, where there is a linear, fairly firm attachment which begins a little lateral to the pubic tubercle and extends nearly horizontally in a lateral direction for about 8 cm. The medial part of the line of fusion may lie on, or a little below, the inguinal ligament; but, as the lateral part of the ligament passes superiorly, the line deviates further and further away from it.

This connexion is of some practical importance, and, to demonstrate it, the dissectors of

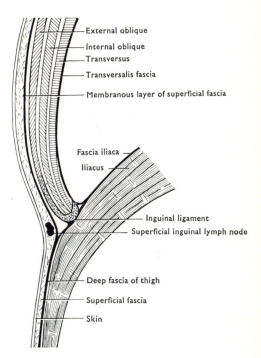

External oblique
Internal oblique
Transversus
Transversalis fascia
Membranous layer of superficial fascia

Fascia iliaca
Iliacus

Inguinal ligament
Superficial inguinal lymph node

Deep fascia of thigh
Superficial fascia
Skin

FIG. 92 Diagram of fasciea and muscles of inguinal and subinguinal regions lateral to femoral sheath. Cf. FIG. 100.

the Lower Limb and the Abdomen must work together.

If urine is effused into the anterior part of the male perineum from a rupture of the urethra, it cannot pass into the medial side of the thigh because of the attachment of the membranous layer of the superficial fascia to the side of the pubic arch and to the front of the pubis, but it can ascend between the membranous layer and the deep fascia to the wall of the abdomen. Having reached the wall of the abdomen, it cannot descend into the front of the thigh because of the connexion between the membranous layer and the deep fascia of the thigh [see Vol. 2].

The dissector will now proceed to display the structures that lie in the superficial fascia and under cover of it.

The edge of fascia now exposed is the lower margin of the **saphenous opening,** an oval

134

gap in the deep fascia, situated just below the medial part of the inguinal ligament. The opening will be exposed later.

The **spermatic cord** is a thick, soft bundle—almost as thick as a little finger—that emerges from the abdomen just above the medial end of the inguinal ligament; it appears through an opening called the **superficial inguinal ring** and descends into the scrotum. It will be cleaned by the dissector of the Abdomen, but the dissector of the Lower Limb will note that it crosses a corner of his territory. In the female, the spermatic cord is replaced by a slender, inconspicuous band, the **round ligament of the uterus,** that emerges through the same point in the abdominal wall and descends into the labium majus.

The removal of the cribriform fascia exposes the greater part of the anterior wall of the **femoral sheath**—that is, the fascial layer that surrounds the uppermost 4 cm. of the femoral artery and vein. The sheath is very liable to be injured as the cribriform fascia is removed. If that has happened, the femoral vessels will be partly exposed. Note that the vein is opposite the opening, while the artery is behind its lateral margin.

DISSECTION. Look for the remaining cutaneous nerves seeking them first, with the help of Figures 93 and 94, at the points where they pierce the deep fascia and trace them downwards. They are named and described on pages 137–9.

The saphenous nerve, the principal distribution of which is in the leg and foot, becomes superficial much lower than the others; it appears behind the vein at the medial side of the knee, and its infrapatellar branch appears in front of the vein above the knee.

Look for a network of slender nerves in front of the patella. It is called the patellar plexus, and is formed by branches of several cutaneous nerves. At the same time, see if there is any evidence of a subcutaneous bursa [p. 140] in front of the patella.

Superficial Inguinal Vessels

Three small arteries—the **external pudendal,** the **superficial epigastric,** and the **superficial circumflex iliac**—pierce the cribriform fascia or the deep fascia of the thigh below the inguinal ligament, and radiate from their origin in the directions that their names imply. They supply the skin of the external genital organs, of the groin and of the lower part of the anterior abdominal wall, and the inguinal lymph nodes [Fig. 93]. They all spring from the femoral artery immediately after it enters the thigh.

The **veins** which accompany these arteries converge towards the saphenous opening and join the great saphenous vein before it pierces the cribriform fascia.

Lymph Nodes and Lymph Vessels

The superficial inguinal lymph nodes are arranged in two main groups: (1) An **upper** group of large nodes spread out immediately below the line where the membranous layer of superficial fascia is fused with the deep fascia of the thigh; one or two small outlying members of this group may be found above the inguinal ligament on the course of the superficial epigastric vessels. (2) A **lower** group

made up of a variable number of large nodes placed along both sides of the upper part of the great saphenous vein [Figs. 93, 136].

In a spare subject the general arrangement of the lymph vessels may also be made out. These groups of lymph nodes receive the superficial vessels of: (1) the lower limb, including the gluteal region, (2) the external genital organs, (3) the perineum, and (4) the lower part of the anterior wall of the abdomen. They receive also some of the lymph vessels from certain organs in the pelvis. Swollen, painful nodes in the groin may therefore signify disease in the superficial parts named above, or they may be a sign of disease in a pelvic organ. Numerous vessels connect the nodes with one another. The efferent vessels pass through the cribriform fascia and the deep fascia around the saphenous opening. They end in the deep inguinal nodes, which lie alongside the upper part of the femoral vessels, and in the external iliac nodes, which lie in the abdomen around the external liac artery [see Vol. 2].

Saphenous Opening

This is an oval aperture in the deep fascia of the thigh. Its position and dimensions should be carefully noted, because through it a femoral hernia makes its way towards the surface. It is about 3 cm. long and 1·5 cm. wide. It is situated just below the inguinal ligament, and its centre is about 3–4 cm. below and lateral to the pubic tubercle. Spread over the opening, there is a thin portion of the deep fascia, the **cribriform fascia,** perforated by certain vessels. (*Cribrum*=a sieve.) These vessels are the great saphenous vein, one or more of the superficial arteries, and some of the lymph vessels that connect the superficial and deep inguinal lymph nodes.

The femoral vein, enclosed with the artery in the femoral sheath, is immediately behind the opening; the artery lies lateral to it.

The upper, lower and lateral margins of the opening form one crescentic, sharp edge of deep fascia called the **falciform margin** of the saphenous opening. The lower margin is better defined than the upper because the

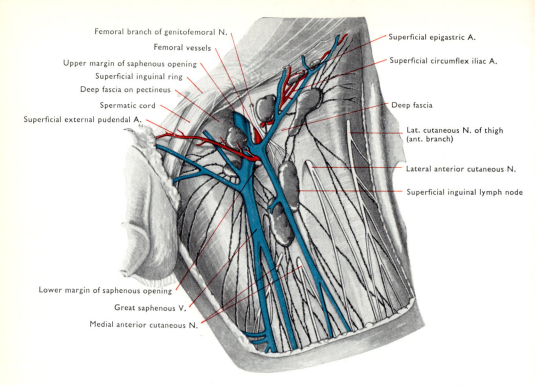

Femoral branch of genitofemoral N.
Femoral vessels
Upper margin of saphenous opening
Superficial inguinal ring
Deep fascia on pectineus
Spermatic cord
Superficial external pudendal A.

Superficial epigastric A.
Superficial circumflex iliac A.
Deep fascia
Lat. cutaneous N. of thigh (ant. branch)
Lateral anterior cutaneous N.
Superficial inguinal lymph node

Lower margin of saphenous opening
Great saphenous V.
Medial anterior cutaneous N.

FIG. 93 Superficial dissection of proximal part of front of thigh. The saphenous opening and the superficial lymph nodes and lymph vessels of the groin are displayed. The lymph vessels may be recognized by their beaded appearance.

great saphenous vein hooks backwards over it to join the femoral vein. On the medial side the deep fascia that covers the pectineus muscle—the **pectineal fascia**—slopes postero-laterally, and disappears behind the femoral sheath [FIG. 99]; the medial margin of the opening is therefore an oblique surface, not a sharp edge.

Great Saphenous Vein

This is the largest superficial vein of the lower limb. In the thigh, it is frequently concealed in the fat, but in the leg it is usually very evident in the living limb—and hence the name (*saphes* = easily seen). In the condition known as 'varicose veins', it is often very conspicuous and tortuous. It begins on the medial side of the dorsum of the foot, crosses anterior to the medial malleolus and, running

obliquely backwards over the medial surface of the distal third of the tibia and along its medial margin, crosses the knee far back on its medial side and inclines anteriorly through the thigh to the saphenous opening. Here it pierces the cribriform fascia and the femoral sheath to enter the femoral vein.

During its ascent through the leg it lies between two membranous layers of fascia and is crossed by a more superficial plexus of veins which tend to join it at the knee. It communicates through the deep fascia with the deep veins, particularly at the ankle and knee, and receives many tributaries, including the superficial veins of the groin which join it near its termination.

There are several valves in its interior which help to divide the column of blood into sections, and so reduce the pressure on the walls of the distal part of the vein.

Superficial Inguinal Ring

This is the aperture in the aponeurosis of the external oblique muscle of the abdominal

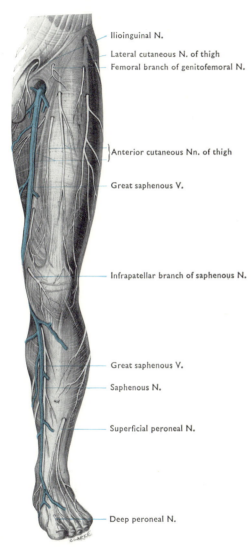

Ilioinguinal N.

Lateral cutaneous N. of thigh

Femoral branch of genitofemoral N.

Anterior cutaneous Nn. of thigh

Great saphenous V.

Infrapatellar branch of saphenous N.

Great saphenous V.

Saphenous N.

Superficial peroneal N.

Deep peroneal N.

FIG. 94 Cutaneous nerves on front of lower limb. See also FIG. 111.

wall through which the spermatic cord (or the round ligament of the uterus) escapes from the abdomen. It has probably been displayed by the dissector of the Abdomen already, and will be studied by him, but the dissector of the Lower Limb will note its position: it is immediately above the pubic tubercle and the medial end of the inguinal ligament.

Cutaneous Nerves

Six cutaneous nerves are met with in the area of the present dissection [FIGS. 94, 95].

From the lumbar plexus in the abdomen.
- Ilio-inguinal nerve.
- Femoral branch of the genitofemoral nerve.
- Lateral cutaneous nerve of thigh.

From the femoral nerve.
- Lateral anterior cutaneous nerve of thigh.
- Medial anterior cutaneous nerve of thigh.
- Saphenous nerve.

They communicate with one another, and the areas of skin supplied by them overlap.

The **ilio-inguinal nerve** (L. 1) escapes through the lateral part of the superficial inguinal ring. Most of its branches go to the scrotum or to the labium majus, according to the sex; but some are distributed to the skin of the adjacent part of the thigh.

The **femoral branch of the genitofemoral nerve** (L. 1, 2) is a slender nerve, not easily found, that pierces the deep fascia about 2 cm. below the inguinal ligament, a little lateral to the saphenous opening. It supplies an area of skin, about the size of the palm of the hand, immediately below the inguinal ligament.

The **lateral cutaneous nerve of the thigh** (L. 2, 3) escapes from the abdomen close to the anterior superior iliac spine, behind the inguinal ligament, and descends over the surface of the sartorius muscle, embedded in a thick ridge of deep fascia which must be slit up to expose the nerve. Five centimetres below the anterior superior spine, the nerve divides into: (1) A **posterior branch** which pierces the deep fascia at once, and runs

137

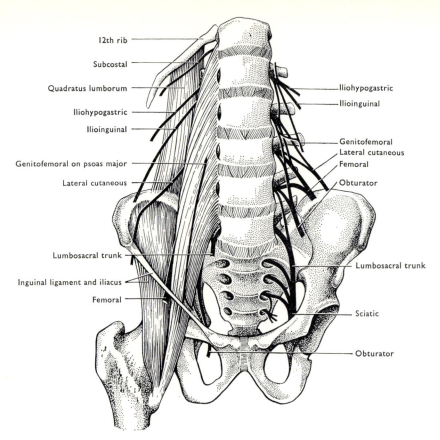

FIG. 95 Lumbar plexus (semi-diagrammatic) in relation to quadratus lumborum and iliopsoas muscles.

backwards and downwards to supply the skin over the greater trochanter and the adjoining part of the gluteal region and thigh. (2) An **anterior branch** which pierces the deep fascia 5 cm. lower down, and descends to the lateral side of the patella, giving branches to the skin of the lateral side and front of the thigh.

The **lateral anterior cutaneous nerve of the thigh** (L. 2, 3) pierces the deep fascia in the middle line of the thigh about the junction of its upper and middle thirds. It appears usually as two branches which perforate the fascia near each other. Both branches extend to the knee.

The **medial anterior cutaneous nerve of the thigh** (L. 2, 3) perforates the deep fascia on the medial side of the thigh as two branches: The **anterior branch** emerges at the junction of the lower and middle thirds of the thigh, in front of the great saphenous vein; it descends to the knee, and its terminal branches turn forwards to reach the front of the patella. The **posterior branch** reaches the surface near the knee, behind the great saphenous vein, and descends to supply the skin on the medial side of the upper part of the leg. The main stem of the medial anterior cutaneous nerve sends a few twigs to the skin of the middle third of the medial side of the thigh, along the line of the great saphenous vein.

138

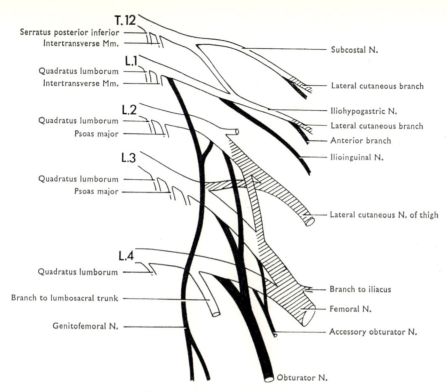

T. 12

Serratus posterior inferior
Intertransverse Mm.

L.1

Quadratus lumborum
Intertransverse Mm.

L.2

Quadratus lumborum
Psoas major

L.3

Quadratus lumborum
Psoas major

L.4

Quadratus lumborum

Branch to lumbosacral trunk

Genitofemoral N.

Subcostal N.

Lateral cutaneous branch

Iliohypogastric N.
Lateral cutaneous branch
Anterior branch

Ilioinguinal N.

Lateral cutaneous N. of thigh

Branch to iliacus

Femoral N.

Accessory obturator N.

Obturator N.

FIG. 96   Diagram of lumbar plexus.
Ventral offsets, black ; dorsal offsets, cross hatched. Cf. the arrangement of the brachial
plexus, FIG. 14. For the sacral part of the lumbosacral plexus, see FIG. 114.

The **saphenous nerve** (L. 3, 4) becomes subcutaneous on the medial side of the knee by perforating the fascia between the sartorius and the tendon of the gracilis muscle, and passes into the leg in front of the great saphenous vein. A small artery—the saphenous branch of the descending genicular artery —is a useful guide to it as it runs downwards along the nerve. Before the saphenous nerve pierces the fascia it gives off the infrapatellar branch which pierces the sartorius muscle and the deep fascia on the medial side of the knee, and curves downwards and forwards to reach the front of the joint below the patella [FIG. 94].

Patellar Plexus. Filaments of four nerves have been traced to the skin of the knee, viz., the saphenous, the lateral anterior cutaneous, and the anterior branches of the lateral cutaneous and the medial anterior cutaneous nerves of the thigh. These filaments interlace with one another and form the patellar plexus, which is situated over the patella, ligamentum patellae, and proximal part of the tibia. As in other peripheral nerve plexuses, the individual nerve fibres do not join.

DISSECTION. Remove the remains of the superficial fascia, in order to expose the deep fascia, but leave the cutaneous nerves and vessels. On the media side of the thigh the deep fascia is very thin and you must take care not to remove it with the superficial fascia. On the front of the knee, look again for evidence of a prepatellar synovial bursa.

Fascia Lata

This is the deep fascia of the thigh.

On the medial side the fascia lata is so delicate and thin that the subjacent muscular fibres shine through it. **On the lateral side** it is very dense and is thickened to form a long, strong, wide band called the **iliotibial tract,** which stretches from the iliac crest to the lateral condyle of the tibia.

Around the root of the limb this sleeve of fascia is attached to the bones of the pelvis and to the inguinal and sacrotuberous ligaments which complete the superficial margin between trunk and lower limb. Thus it is attached : **laterally,** to the iliac crest ; **anteriorly,** to the inguinal ligament ; **medially,** to the pubis and ischium, to the margin of the pubic arch and to the ischial tuberosity ; while **posteriorly** it is continuous with the fascia of the gluteal region, through which it is fixed to the sacrotuberous ligament, the coccyx, the sacrum, and the iliac crest.

Immediately below the inguinal ligament it gives a linear attachment to the membranous layer of the superficial fascia, and it is modified by the formation of the cribriform fascia and the saphenous opening.

On the front and on the sides of the knee it is attached to the capsule of the joint, the medial and lateral margins of the patella, the tuberosity of the tibia, the condyles of the tibia and of the femur, and to the head of the fibula. Posteriorly it forms the strong **popliteal fascia** which roofs over the popliteal fossa and is continuous with the fascia of the back of the leg.

Intermuscular Septa

These are three partitions which pass from the fascia lata to the back of the femur and are called the **lateral, medial** and **posterior intermuscular septa.** They divide the thigh into three compartments for the three great

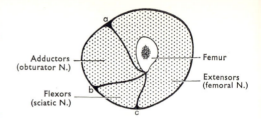

FIG. 97   Diagram to show the arrangement of the three intermuscular septa and the three osteofascial compartments of the thigh seen from above.
a. Medial intermuscular septum
b. Posterior intermuscular septum
c. Lateral intermuscular septum

groups of muscles of the thigh, each associated with its nerve. The **extensor** group on the front, with the **femoral nerve;** the **flexor** group or hamstrings on the back, with the **sciatic nerve ;** and the **adductors** on the medial side, with the **obturator nerve** [FIG. 97].

These three septa will be disclosed in a subsequent dissection. In the meantime, note that the medial and the lateral septa show as white lines on the surface of the fascia in the distal part of the thigh.

The extensor group is composed of four large muscles which collectively are called the **quadriceps femoris,** for they unite together before their insertion into the patella, and therefore resemble four heads of a single muscle. The ligamentum patellae anchors the patella to the tibia, and acts as a continuation of the tendon of the quadriceps. A thin tendinous sheet extends downwards over the front of the patella from the tendon of the quadriceps to the ligamentum patellae ; a synovial bursa may be found on the surface of this sheet.

Patellar Bursae

Because of the need for free movement of the skin on the underlying tissues, *e.g.* in kneeling, and of the deep tissues on each other, there are several synovial bursae in the patellar region. Of these, two may have been found.

A prepatellar bursa lies between the skin and the superficial fascia in front of the lower part of the patella; chronic enlargement of this bursa from friction is known as 'housemaid's knee'.

A **subcutaneous infrapatellar bursa** lies between the skin and the fascia in front of the tuberosity of the tibia and lower half of the ligamentum patellae, and is sometimes divided into upper and lower parts.

Two other constant bursae are found in the deep tissues, and will be seen later:

A **suprapatellar bursa** lies superior to the patella between the tendon of the quadriceps and the front of the femur. It is large and is important in that it nearly always opens into the cavity of the knee joint.

A **deep infrapatellar bursa** is small and lies between the lower end of the ligamentum patellae and the upper end of the tibia.

Inguinal Ligament

The inguinal ligament is the lower border of the aponeurosis of the external oblique muscle of the abdomen thickened and folded backwards upon itself. It presents, therefore, a rounded surface towards the thigh, and a grooved surface towards the abdomen. It extends medially and inferiorly from the anterior superior iliac spine to the pubic tubercle and the adjoining 2–3 cm. of the pecineal line. The fascia lata is attached to it along its whole length, and exercises traction upon it, so that the ligament is convex downwards and loses this curvature when the fascia lata is divided.

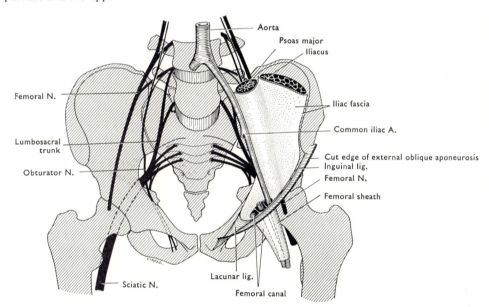

FIG. 98   Diagram to show the routes of entry of nerves and femoral blood vessels into the lower limb, viewed from in front and above. On the right, a portion of the aponeurosis of the external oblique muscle of the abdomen is shown with the inguinal ligament formed from its rolled inferior margin. The lacunar ligament passes posteriorly from this to be attached to the pubis and encircle the medial border of a funnel of fascia, the femoral sheath, which encloses the femoral vessels and femoral canal, and passes into the femoral triangle. The fascia of this sheath is continuous above with the fascia iliaca, which covers the psoas and iliacus muscles on the posterior abdominal wall, and anteriorly with the transversalis fascia, which lines the deep surface of the anterior abdominal wall. Note that the femoral nerve lies posterior to the fascia iliaca and hence is outside the femoral sheath as it enters the thigh. On the left, note how the sciatic and femoral nerves are packed close to the plane of the hip joint, thus minimizing tension on them during movements of the limb.

141

The pectineal part of the inguinal ligament is a thin, triangular, posterior expansion from its medial part, and is called the **lacunar ligament** [FIG. 98]. The apex of the lacunar ligament is at the pubic tubercle; its anterior and posterior margins are attached respectively to the inguinal ligament and the pecten pubis; its base, a free, sharp crescentic margin, abuts on the medial side of the femoral sheath. Its femoral surface faces inferolaterally and gives partial origin to the pectineus muscle.

The point on the inguinal ligament which is equidistant from the pubic symphysis and the anterior superior iliac spine is called the **mid-inguinal point.**

DISSECTION. The femoral sheath was partly exposed when the cribriform fascia was removed [p. 134]. To expose the sheath fully, cut through the fascia lata along the inguinal ligament, and carefully remove the part of it that is lateral to the saphenous opening (including the falciform margin). The removal of the loose fat will then bring the whole sheath into view. With the handle of the knife or a blunt hook, isolate the sheath from the inguinal and lacunar ligaments.

Femoral Sheath

This is a funnel-shaped, fascial tube that surrounds the uppermost 4 cm. of the femoral vessels. The mouth of the funnel opens into the abdomen; the lower part gradually closes upon the vessels, and fuses with their coats about the level of the lower margin of the saphenous opening. The sides of the sheath do not slope equally towards each other. The lateral wall is nearly vertical; the upper part of the medial wall is very oblique.

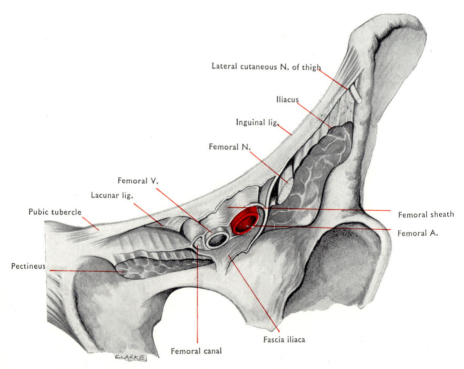

Lateral cutaneous N. of thigh

Iliacus

Inguinal lig.

Femoral N.

Femoral V.

Lacunar lig.

Pubic tubercle

Pectineus

Femoral canal

Fascia iliaca

Femoral sheath

Femoral A.

FIG. 99   Dissection to show emoral sheath and structures which pass between inguinal ligament and hip bone.

Constitution of the Femoral Sheath. The main part of the inguinal ligament is separated from the hip bone by an elongated interval [FIG. 99] filled by structures escaping from the abdomen into the thigh, and the lacunar ligament and pectineus medially. Laterally the interval is filled by the psoas major and iliacus muscles with the femoral nerve between them, and the lateral femoral cutaneous nerve in the latera angle. Lying between and anterior to psoas major and pectineus, and abutting medially on the lacunar ligament, is the femoral sheath and its contents [FIG. 98]. The lower part of the posterior wall of the abdomen, immediately above the thigh, is formed by the iliacus and psoas major muscles. They are covered with that part of the fascial lining of the abdomen which receives the name **fascia iliaca.** The anterior wall of the abdomen, formed internally by the transversus abdominis muscle, is lined, in like manner, with a portion of the general lining termed the **fascia transversalis.** Lateral to the femoral vessels these two fascial layers become continuous with each other and, at the same time, are attached to the back of the inguinal ligament [FIG. 92]. Behind this union the iliacus, the psoas, the femoral nerve, and the lateral cutaneous nerve pass into the thigh. But the external iliac vessels (which become the femoral vessels in the thigh), with the femoral branch of the genitofemoral nerve, lie within the fascial lining of the abdomen; and, as they pass out of the abdomen behind the inguinal ligament, they carry with them a funnel-shaped prolongation of the fascia which is the femoral sheath [FIG. 98].

The dissector will now readily understand that the **anterior wall** of the sheath is formed of **fascia transversalis,** and the **posterior wall**

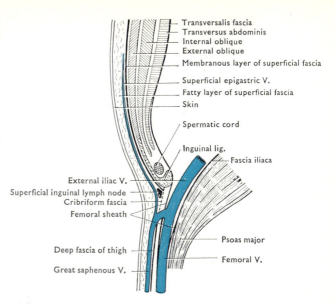

Transversalis fascia
Transversus abdominis
Internal oblique
External oblique
Membranous layer of superficial fascia
Superficial epigastric V.
Fatty layer of superficial fascia
Skin
Spermatic cord
Inguinal lig.
Fascia iliaca
External iliac V.
Superficial inguinal lymph node
Cribriform fascia
Femoral sheath
Psoas major
Deep fascia of thigh
Femoral V.
Great saphenous V.

FIG. 100 Diagram of fasciae and muscles of inguinal and subinguinal regions in the line of the femoral vein. Cf. FIG. 92.

of **fascia iliaca**—each of them being continued into the thigh from the corresponding wall of the abdomen [FIG. 100].

DISSECTION. **Open the femoral sheath by three vertical incisions through the anterior wall—one over the femoral artery, another over the femoral vein in the line of the great saphenous vein, and the third a little medial to the upper part of the vein. The first two should extend downwards for 3–4 cm. from the inguinal ligament, the most medial for only 1 cm.**

Interior of the Femoral Sheath. A little dissection will show that the sheath is divided into three compartments by two antero-posterior septa. The femoral artery and femoral branch of the genitofemoral nerve occupy the **lateral compartment;** the femoral vein fills the **intermediate compartment;** the **medial compartment** lodges a little loose areolar tissue, a small lymph node, and some lymph vessels. This last compartment, from its relation to femoral hernia, has the special name of femoral canal applied to it.

Femoral Canal. The boundaries and extent of the femoral canal are best studied by introducing the little finger into the canal and pushing it gently upwards. The length of the canal is not nearly so great as that of the other two compartments. Indeed, it is not more than 1·5 cm. long. It rapidly diminishes in width from above downwards, and its lower end is closed by the fusion of its walls.

The upper end or mouth of the canal is called the **femoral ring.** It is closed by a plug of fat called the **femoral septum,** and the peritoneum—the innermost, glistening lining of the abdominal walls—overlies the fat, and is slightly dimpled into the ring. It is wide enough to admit the tip of the little finger. With your finger-tip in the ring, feel its boundaries: anteriorly, the inguinal ligament; medially, the lacunar ligament; posteriorly, the pecten of the pubic bone; laterally, the femoral vein.

The canal lies on the pectineus muscle and its fascia; and the upper margin of the saphenous opening crosses its upper part. Lower down, the canal is covered by the cribriform fascia, and is usually crossed by the external pudendal artery.

Femoral Hernia. Femoral hernia is the name applied to the protrusion of some of the contents of the abdominal cavity through the femoral canal into the thigh. The aperture through which vessels, nerves, and muscles pass into the anterior part of the thigh from the abdomen lies posterior to the inguinal ligament, where the anterior and posterior abdominal walls meet inferiorly at an acute angle. The whole weight of the abdominal contents presses downwards against this region, and while the aperture is closed laterally by the fusion of the iliac and transversalis fasciae with each other and with the inguinal ligament, and medially by the lacunar ligament, between these the funnel-shaped extension of the fasciae, the femoral sheath, forms a point of weakness which invites the entry of a loop of intestine. The lateral part of the femoral sheath is filled by the femoral vessels, but the abdominal end of the femoral canal, its widest part (the **femoral ring),** is only covered by a layer of peritoneum and filled with yielding fat (femoral septum). This potential opening is protected anteriorly by the inguinal ligament, but is liable to be enlarged when the ligament is stretched and drawn forwards as the abdominal muscles weaken and the abdomen distends. The opening is larger in the female than the male, because of the wider female pelvis, a feature which accounts for the greater frequency of femoral hernia in the female.

If a loop of intestine or a piece of omentum pushes its way into the femoral canal it carries a sac of peritoneum, the hernial sac, in front of it. This sac comes to lie in the lower part of the canal deep to the cribriform fascia which presents little resistance, so that the sac protrudes anteriorly through it close to the saphenous vein. If the sac and its contents continue to enlarge, it turns superolaterally towards the anterior superior iliac spine, the whole hernia becoming U-shaped. Thus reduction calls for its apex to be drawn down to the saphenous opening before an attempt is made to return it through the distended femoral canal to the abdomen.

The sac may expand in the subcutaneous tissue of the groin, but the femoral ring is relatively unyielding and remains tight round the neck of the sac, the sharp edge of the lacunar ligament effectively preventing enlargement at this level, as the margin of the saphenous opening does at a slightly lower level. This tightness obstructs the gut tube passing through, and may be sufficient so to compress the blood vessels that the intestine in the sac loses its blood supply (strangulation of the hernia) with serious consequences. Surgical interference is directed towards the relief of the tension at the neck, and for this purpose it is usual to divide the lacunar ligament. It should be noted that the small pubic branch of the inferior epigastric artery crosses the abdominal surface of the lacunar ligament and anastomoses with the pubic branch of the obturator artery. In 30 per cent. of cases this anastomosis forms the main obturator artery, which is then called the **abnormal obturator artery,** and as it may

144

cross the lacunar ligament it is liable to injury when this ligament is divided.

The boundaries and contents of the femoral triangle, which occupies the upper third of the front of the thigh, must now be dissected.

DISSECTION. The lateral boundary of the triangle is the sartorius muscle, and the medial boundary is the medial border of the adductor longus [Fig. 101]. Clean these muscles down to the apex of the triangle where they meet, preserving the nerves in relation to the sartorius.

Now place a block under the knee in order to flex the hip joint and relax the boundaries and contents of the triangle.

Raise the femoral nerve from the groove between the psoas and iliacus muscles on a blunt hook and note that it soon ends in a number of muscular and cutaneous branches. Secure the nerve to the pectineus first, and endeavour to trace it medially, behind the femoral

artery, to its muscle. Then clean the other branches of the femoral nerve till they leave the triangle, avoiding injury to the lateral circumflex artery which passes laterally among these nerves near their origin.

Now clean the vessels, retaining the large venous trunks, but removing the venae comitantes of the smaller arteries. Raise the femoral artery, and clean it as far as the apex of the triangle. Secure and clean a small artery called the deep external pudendal. It springs from the upper part of the femoral artery and runs medially. You have probably found the root of the profunda artery already. It is a large artery that springs from the femoral artery about 5 cm. below the inguinal ligament. Follow it downwards amidst the fat behind the femoral vessels till it leaves the triangle. At the same time clean the profunda vein which lies in front of its artery. Two large arteries spring from the profunda near its origin. They are the lateral and medial circumflex arteries. Trace the lateral artery as far as the sartorius. Trace the medial one backwards

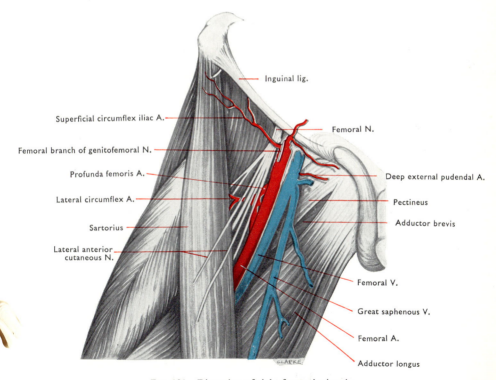

FIG. 101   Dissection of right femoral triangle.

as far as possible into the fat behind the femoral vessels. Preserve the proximal parts of the circumflex veins and note that they end in the femoral vein. Not uncommonly, one or both of the circumflex arteries spring from the femoral artery.

As you clean the femoral vein trace the nerve to the pectineus muscle behind it. Clean the pectineus, and look for the anterior division of the obturator nerve in the interval between it and the adductor longus, as it descends behind them in front of the adductor brevis.

Next clean the surface of the iliacus and psoas major. And, lastly, remove the mass of fat from the angle between the psoas and pectineus—disentangling the medial circumflex artery, which passes backwards between those two muscles.

Femoral Triangle

This is the anterior surface of the hollow that occupies a great part of the upper third of the thigh [FIG. 101]. Its **base** is the inguinal ligament. Its **lateral boundary** is the medial border of the sartorius; its **medial boundary** is the medial border of the adductor longus; and those two muscles meet at the **apex.** The apex is continuous with a narrow intermuscular space, called the **adductor canal,** through which the femoral vessels travel down to the popliteal fossa.

The **roof** is composed of the skin and fasciae. The superficial fascia contains the superficial inguinal lymph nodes with their lymph vessels, the femoral branch of the genitofemoral nerve, branches of the ilioinguinal nerve, the superficial branches of the femoral artery with their companion veins, and the upper part of the great saphenous vein; most of these structures pierce the deep fascia of the roof.

The **floor** is composed of muscles—adductor longus, pectineus, psoas major and iliacus, from medial to lateral side. The adductor brevis may appear in the floor between the pectineus and adductor longus. The floor slopes backwards towards the centre from the lateral and medial boundaries; the space is triangular, therefore, in section as well as in outline. The central hollow is occupied by a mass of fat which contains the profunda and medial circumflex vessels, behind the main femoral vessels.

Contents of the Triangle.

1. The **femoral vessels** traverse the triangle from base to apex; the vein is medial to the artery at the base of the triangle, and behind it at the apex.

2. The **deep external pudendal artery** is a small artery that arises from the medial side of the femoral artery near the base of the triangle. It runs a variable course medially and pierces the deep fascia to be distributed to the scrotum in the male and to the labium majus in the female.

3. The **profunda femoris artery** springs from the lateral side of the femoral, curves downwards behind it and leaves the triangle by passing behind the adductor longus close to the femur. The **profunda vein** is in front of its artery and ends in the femoral vein.

4. The **lateral** and **medial circumflex arteries** spring from the profunda near its origin. The lateral artery runs laterally among the branches of the femoral nerve and leaves the triangle behind the sartorius. The medial artery passes backwards and disappears through the floor of the triangle between the psoas and the pectineus. The **circumflex veins** end in the femoral vein.

5. Three or four **deep inguinal lymph nodes** lie along the medial side of the femoral vein. They receive afferent vessels from the superficial inguinal nodes and from the deep parts of the limb; and they send their efferent vessels to the nodes that lie in the abdomen around the external iliac artery.

6. The **femoral branch of the genitofemoral nerve,** already noticed [p. 137], is distributed to the skin over the femoral triangle.

7. The **lateral cutaneous nerve** of the thigh crosses the lateral angle of the triangle [p. 137].

8. The **femoral nerve.**

Before the contents of the triangle are studied further, another stage of the dissection of the front of the thigh must be carried out.

DISSECTION. Complete the cleaning of the sartorius right down to its insertion into the tibia.

Next make a vertical cut through the deep fascia from the tubercle of the iliac crest to the lateral margin of the patella, and remove the deep fascia between the incision and the sartorius; this will leave the main part of the iliotibial tract in position, but will disclose the tensor fasciae latae, on the lateral side of the upper part of the sartorius, and portions of the four parts of the quadriceps femoris muscle.

Identify (1) the rectus femoris, extending down the middle of the thigh; (2) part of the vastus lateralis, at the lateral side of the rectus; (3) a small part of the vastus intermedius which usually appears to be the lower part of the vastus lateralis; (4) part of the vastus medialis that fills the space between the lower parts of the rectus femoris and sartorius.

Trace the lateral circumflex artery behind the sartorius and the rectus femoris, and follow its three branches; the descending branch follows the anterior border of the vastus lateralis and indicates the line along which the vasti are fused.

Clean the ascending branch of the lateral circumflex artery, and, as you remove the fat, remove also the septum of fascia between the sartorius and the tensor.

Then clean the upper part of the rectus femoris. It arises by two heads which very soon join together. Follow them up to their attachments.

Lift the middle third of sartorius laterally, exposing a narrow strip of fascia joining the vastus medialis to the adductors. This is the roof of the adductor canal which should be divided longitudinally to expose the femoral vessels, saphenous nerve, and the nerve to vastus medialis in the canal [Fig. 102].

Sartorius

This is a long, slender, strap-like muscle with parallel fibres—a characteristic that enables it to be recognized when a portion of it is exposed in the living limb.

It arises from the anterior superior iliac spine, crosses the upper third of the thigh obliquely, and then descends almost vertically to the posterior part of the medial side of the knee; finally, it curves forward to end in a

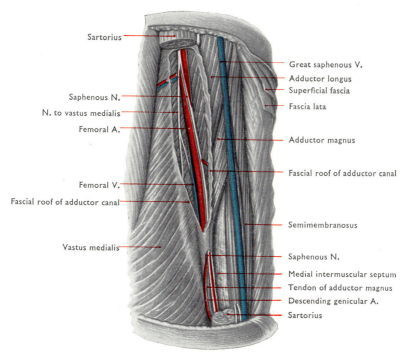

Sartorius
Saphenous N.
N. to vastus medialis
Femoral A.
Femoral V.
Fascial roof of adductor canal
Vastus medialis

Great saphenous V.
Adductor longus
Superficial fascia
Fascia lata
Adductor magnus
Fascial roof of adductor canal
Semimembranosus
Saphenous N.
Medial intermuscular septum
Tendon of adductor magnus
Descending genicular A.
Sartorius

FIG. 102   Dissection of adductor canal in the right thigh.   A portion of the sartorius has been removed.

thin tendon which expands to be inserted into the upper part of the medial surface of the tibia [Fig. 128]. Note that the muscle is fleshy almost to its lower end.

It forms the lateral boundary of the femoral triangle, covers the fibrous roof of the adductor canal and produces a vertical fleshy ridge far back on the medial side of the flexed knee. Thence it curves forwards to its insertion; but when the leg is flexed it slips backwards into the medial boundary of the popliteal fossa, and proceeds straight to its insertion. Its thin, wide tendon is separated by a bursa from the tendons of gracilis and semitendinosus, which lie deep to it and are inserted posterior to it.

Nerve supply: the **femoral nerve.** Action: it flexes both the hip joint and the knee joint, and rotates the thigh laterally to bring the limbs into the position adopted by the cross-legged tailor (*sartor* = a tailor).

Adductor Canal

When the femoral vessels and saphenous nerve leave the femoral triangle, they enter the adductor canal in a deep furrow on the medial side of the thigh bounded anteriorly by the vastus medialis muscle, and posteriorly by the adductor longus and magnus muscles. It is converted into a canal by a strong fibrous membrane which stretches across it, and upon the surface of which the sartorius muscle is placed. When the fibrous membrane which roofs in the canal is traced upwards it is seen to become thin and ill-defined; inferiorly, however, it becomes dense and strong, and at the distal end of the canal it presents a thick, sharply defined margin. The posterior wall of the canal, in its lowest part, presents a deficiency or aperture which leads backwards through adductor magnus into the popliteal fossa, the **tendinous (adductor) opening** through which the femoral vessels leave the canal to become the popliteal vessels.

The saphenous nerve escapes from the canal by passing under cover of the distal margin of the fibrous roof. The nerve to the vastus medialis enters the upper end of the canal, and its branches descend for some distance between the vastus and its fascia before they enter the muscle.

Femoral Artery

The femoral artery is the direct continuation of the external iliac artery of the abdomen, and is the great arterial trunk of the lower limb. It begins behind the inguinal ligament at the mid-inguinal point [p. 142] and is separated from the brim of the pelvis only by psoas major. Here it may be compressed against the bone to control bleeding from a more distal point. Entering the femoral triangle anterior to the head of the femur, it passes towards the apex of the triangle covered only by skin and fasciae and lying on the muscles of the floor. The femoral nerve is lateral to it and the femoral vein moves into a position posterior to it, beginning a slow spiral course round the artery which will bring it to the lateral side at the hiatus in adductor magnus. At the apex of the triangle it enters the adductor canal with the vein, the saphenous nerve, and the nerve to vastus medialis, and lies against the posteromedial aspect of the shaft of the femur. Here it receives a branch from the obturator nerve and is separated from the adductor longus by the femoral vein, while the muscle separates both from the profunda vessels.

The course of the femoral artery may be marked out on the surface by the upper two-thirds of a line drawn from the mid-inguinal point to the adductor tubercle, with the thigh in the position of slight flexion, abduction, and lateral rotation.

Branches. In addition to the three small superficial arteries of the groin and the deep external pudendal, the artery gives off, in the femoral triangle, the profunda femoris which will be traced in a later dissection. The branches which arise in the adductor canal are muscular twigs and the **descending genicular artery,** which springs from the femoral trunk a short distance above the opening in the adductor magnus. It gives branches to muscles and to the knee joint, and one accompanies the saphenous nerve to the medial side of the knee and the leg.

Femoral Vein

This is the direct continuation of the popliteal vein. It begins at the opening in the adductor magnus, traverses the adductor canal and the femoral triangle, and ends behind the inguinal ligament, where it becomes the external iliac vein. It accompanies the femoral artery, but their relations to each other alter at different stages of their course. In the lower part of the adductor canal, the vein is posterolateral to the artery; it inclines medially as it ascends, and, for a considerable distance, is directly behind the artery, but in the upper part of the femoral triangle it is on the medial side of the artery. Slit the femoral vein open with the scissors. Several valves will then be seen. One is almost invariably found immediately above the entrance of the profunda vein.

Tributaries. The veins that join the femoral vein do not correspond strictly to the branches of the artery. The superficial veins of the groin end in the great saphenous vein, which itself joins the femoral; the femoral receives the circumflex veins direct, although the corresponding arteries are usually branches of the profunda.

Femoral Nerve (L. 2, 3, 4)

It arises within the abdomen from the lumbar plexus [Figs. 95, 96], descends in the groove between the iliacus and psoas major, and enters the thigh behind the inguinal ligament and the fascia iliaca. In the thigh it is lateral to the femoral artery, and is separated from it by a small portion of the psoas major muscle and the femoral sheath [Fig. 98].

It ends about 2 cm. below the inguinal ligament by dividing into a number of muscular and cutaneous nerves:

Muscular branches to:
  Pectineus.
  Sartorius.
  Quadriceps femoris.

Cutaneous branches:
  Medial and lateral anterior cutaneous of thigh.
  Saphenous.

The supply to the quadriceps femoris is by separate nerves to its four heads—rectus femoris and the three vasti. The *articular nerves* arise from these four muscular branches. The nerve to the rectus femoris sends a slender branch to the hip joint, and the nerves to the vasti send filaments down through the muscles to the knee joint. Thus the nerves to the heads of the quadriceps that act only on the knee joint send branches to that joint; the nerve to the head that acts also on the hip joint sends a branch to that joint.

The **lateral anterior cutaneous nerve** (L. 2, 3) sometimes pierces the medial border of the sartorius, and is distributed by two branches [p. 138]. The distribution of the lateral cutaneous nerve also should be reviewed [p. 137].

The **medial anterior cutaneous nerve** (L. 2, 3) inclines downwards and medially along the medial margin of the sartorius, crosses in front of the femoral artery at the apex of the femoral triangle, and divides into an anterior and a posterior branch [p. 138].

The **saphenous nerve** (L. 3, 4) is the longest branch of the femoral nerve and the only one that has its main distribution below the knee as far as the medial border of the foot. Note that it accompanies the femoral artery in the adductor canal, emerges from the canal by passing under cover of the lower border of its fibrous roof, and that it appears from under cover of the sartorius at the medial side of the knee.

The **nerve to the pectineus** arises a short distance below the inguinal ligament, and runs medially and downwards behind the femoral vessels to reach its destination.

The **nerves to the sartorius** are two or three in number. As a rule they take origin in common with the lateral anterior cutaneous nerve.

The **nerves to the rectus femoris** (usually two) sink into the deep surface of that muscle. The upper one supplies an articular twig to the hip joint.

The **nerve to the vastus medialis** accompanies the saphenous nerve into the adductor canal and divides into branches which soon sink into the muscle. It sends an articular branch to the knee joint.

The **nerve to the vastus lateralis** passes behind the rectus femoris, and runs downwards with the descending branch of the lateral circumflex artery to enter the anterior border of the muscle. Usually it gives a branch to the knee joint.

The **nerves to the vastus intermedius** are two or three in number, and they sink into its anterior surface. The most medial of them is a long slender nerve which can be traced downwards along the medial edge of the vastus intermedius to the articularis genus muscle. Its terminal filaments are given to the knee joint.

Lateral Circumflex Artery

This is the largest branch of the profunda femoris artery. It arises near the origin of the profunda and runs laterally among the branches of the femoral nerve and then under cover of the sartorius, to the deep surface of the rectus femoris where it ends by dividing into ascending, transverse, and descending branches.

The **ascending branch** reaches the gluteal surface of the ilium by ascending along the intertrochanteric line of the femur under cover of the tensor fasciae latae. It supplies the hip joint and the adjacent muscles. The **transverse branch** is of small size. It sinks backwards through the vastus lateralis, and anastomoses with other arteries at the back of the femur. The **descending branch** runs downwards along the anterior border of the vastus lateralis, gives branches to the quadriceps femoris, and sends a long branch down through the vastus lateralis to the capsule of the knee joint.

Tensor Fasciae Latae

This is a short, thick muscle that lies at the junction of the gluteal region and the upper part of the front of the thigh. It is enclosed between two layers of fascia which are continuous with the iliotibial tract. The muscle arises from the anterior part of the iliac crest, and passes downwards and slightly backwards

to be inserted into the iliotibial tract 3–5 cm. below the level of the greater trochanter. Nerve supply : the **superior gluteal nerve**.

Iliotibial Tract

This thick band of fascia lata on the lateral side of the thigh is attached above to the tubercle of the iliac crest, and below to the lateral condyle of the tibia, the capsule of the knee joint and the patella. From above downwards, it covers part of the gluteus medius, the greater trochanter, the vastus lateralis, part of the vastus intermedius, the lateral condyle of the femur, and the knee joint.

Two muscles are inserted into it : the gluteus maximus behind, at the level of the greater trochanter, and the tensor fasciae in front, below the greater trochanter. The lower part of the tract serves, therefore, as an aponeurotic tendon by means of which those two muscles gain insertion into the anterior surface of the lateral condyle of the tibia ; and the whole tract serves as a powerful brace which, in the erect posture, helps to steady the pelvis and keeps the knee joint firmly extended.

Above the insertion of the gluteus maximus the posterior border of the tract is continuous with the thick fascia on the superficial surface of the gluteus medius, and its anterior border splits to enclose the tensor fasciae latae. Below the gluteus maximus the borders of the tract merge into the rest of the fascia lata ; and its deep surface is connected with the lateral supracondylar ridge and the linea aspera by the lateral intermuscular septum.

DISSECTION. To see the lateral intermuscular septum and the relation of the vastus lateralis to the femur, detach the muscle from the septum and turn it forwards from its bed.

Intermuscular Septa. There are three intermuscular septa of the thigh : lateral, medial, and posterior [p. 140]. The lateral is strong ; the other two are weak and, except in the lower part of the thigh, are represented merely by thin fascial layers on the front and back of the adductor muscles.

The most distinct part of the **medial septum** is in front of the distal part of the adductor magnus; it springs from the fascia lata behind the posterior border of the sartorius and passes to the medial supracondylar ridge. Similarly, the **posterior septum** is the thin layer between the adductor magnus and the semimembranosus, and its lower part is behind the tendon of the adductor magnus.

The **lateral intermuscular septum** is a fibrous partition that separates the vastus lateralis and intermedius from the short head of the biceps

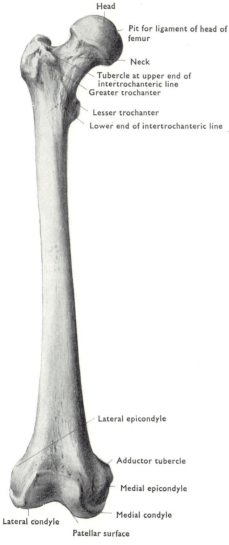

FIG. 103   Right femur (anterior aspect).

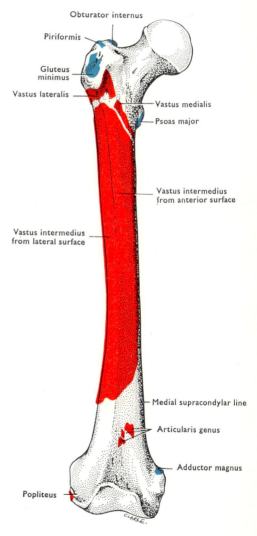

FIG. 104   Right femur (anterior aspect) to show muscle attachments.

151

femoris—one of the muscles of the back of the thigh. The septum springs from the deep surface of the iliotibial tract, and its deep border is attached to the lateral supracondylar ridge and to the linea aspera. Parts of the vastus intermedius and vastus lateralis arise from its anterior surface, and some of the fibres of the short head of the biceps femoris spring from its posterior surface and can be seen shining through it at this stage of the dissection.

Quadriceps Femoris

The quadriceps femoris muscle is composed of the rectus femoris and the three vasti, lateralis, intermedius, and medialis, which clothe the front and sides of the shaft of the femur, and are more or less blended with one another.

Rectus Femoris. The rectus muscle arises by a tendon which splits superiorly to pass (1) to the anterior inferior iliac spine **(straight head,** FIG. 105), and (2) to a long groove immediately above the acetabulum under cover of the gluteus minimus **(reflected head,** FIG. 112). These two tendinous attachments of the muscle take the strain in varying degree according to the extent of flexion or extension at the hip joint.

In the erect posture the two heads of origin of the rectus femoris lie at a right angle to each other and join to form a strong, flattened tendon, which spreads out on the anterior surface of the upper part of the fusiform muscle in the form of an aponeurosis. About 8 cm. above the knee joint, the rectus femoris ends in a strong tendon which begins some distance above on its deep surface in the form of an aponeurosis. The tendon of the rectus femoris joins the other tendons of the quadriceps, and forms with them a common tendon which is inserted into the upper border of the patella.

Vastus Lateralis. This muscle forms the greater part of the fleshy mass on the lateral side of the thigh. Its superficial stratum is a glistening aponeurosis. It overlaps the vastus intermedius, and is partly blended with that muscle. Its anterior border is therefore ill-defined, and the descending branch of the

152

lateral circumflex artery is the best guide to it.

The vastus lateralis has a long, linear origin from the root of the greater trochanter and the linea aspera down to the supracondylar ridge [FIGS. 104, 107]. The fleshy fibres are, for the most part, directed downwards and forwards, the lowest being 3–4 cm. superior to the patella. By means of the common tendon of insertion the muscle gains attachment to the patella, and, at the same time, gives an expansion to the capsule of the knee joint.

DISSECTION. Clean the superior attachments of rectus femoris, then divide it about its middle and pull the lower part forcibly downwards. The narrow interval between the tendons of the vastus intermedius and vastus medialis will then become apparent, and will serve as a guide to the line along which the muscles must be separated. Another guide to the line of separation is a long, slender nerve that descends to supply the articularis genus muscle; it runs along the medial edge of the vastus intermedius. Raise the anterior border of the vastus medialis and divide it transversely about 5 cm. above the patella; pull the muscle medially and examine its origin.

Vastus Medialis. This muscle is intimately related to, but seldom fused with the vastus intermedius.

It has a long linear origin chiefly from the intertrochanteric and spiral lines, the linea aspera and through the medial intermuscular septum to the tendons of adductors longus and magnus. It should be noted that so few muscle bundles arise from the medial surface of the femur that it is almost bare. The fleshy fibres are directed downwards and forwards, and end in the common tendon of the quadriceps muscle, which is inserted into the patella and becomes connected with the capsule of the knee joint. The lowest fibres pass almost horizontally into the medial aspect of the superior half of the patella. These fibres hold the patella medially.

Vastus Intermedius. The vastus intermedius covers and arises from the anterior and lateral surfaces of the shaft of the femur. It is inserted into the patella by means of the common tendon.

Articularis Genus. This muscle consists of a few of the deepest bundles of the vastus intermedius. They spring from the front of the femur and are inserted into the synovial membrane of the knee which bulges upwards between the quadriceps tendon and the femur, *i.e.*, the suprapatellar bursa.

Common Tendon of the Quadriceps. This tendon takes the place of the capsular ligament of the knee joint above the patella. It is inserted into the upper border of that bone; but some fibres are carried downwards, across the front of the patella, into the ligamentum patellae.

Ligamentum Patellae. The patellar ligament is the broad, thick tendon that connects the patella with the tuberosity of the tibia, and through it the quadriceps is attached to the tibia. It is the continuation of the quadriceps tendon.

Actions of Quadriceps. The muscle as a whole is an extensor of the knee, but the rectus femoris can also take part in flexion of the thigh at the hip joint. The articularis genus merely lifts the upper part of the synovial membrane of the knee and prevents it being caught between the patella and femur as the knee joint is extended. Nerve supply: the **femoral nerve.**

THE MEDIAL SIDE OF THE THIGH

If required, the gluteal region and back of thigh may be dissected before the medial side of the thigh.

The group of adductor muscles on the medial side of the thigh is disposed in three strata. The **anterior layer** is composed of the pectineus and the adductor longus, which lie in the same plane. Their adjacent borders touch each other near the pubis, but near the femur they are separated by a small interval. The **middle layer** is the adductor brevis alone and the **posterior layer** is the adductor magnus.

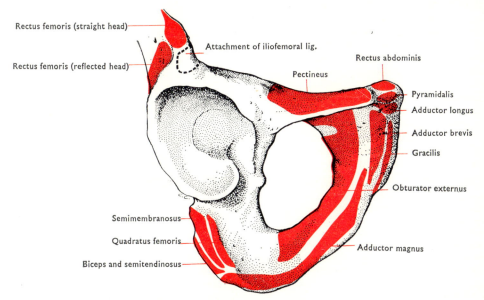

Rectus femoris (straight head)
Rectus femoris (reflected head)
Attachment of iliofemoral lig.
Pectineus
Rectus abdominis
Pyramidalis
Adductor longus
Adductor brevis
Gracilis
Obturator externus
Semimembranosus
Quadratus femoris
Biceps and semitendinosus
Adductor magnus

FIG. 105 Muscle attachments to outer surface of right pubis and ischium. The actual origin of the pectineus is not so extensive as shown; it arises from the upper part of the pectineal surface of the pubis and overlies the remainder.

The gracilis muscle, also an adductor, lies superficially along the medial side of the thigh. It is a long, slender muscle—hence the name gracilis — and is applied against the adductor brevis and adductor magnus.

The two divisions of the **obturator nerve** are interposed between the three muscular layers—the anterior division descending in front of the adductor brevis, and the posterior division behind it. The profunda artery is behind the adductor longus near the femur.

Adductor Longus

This muscle is placed at the medial side of the pectineus. It is triangular in shape, being narrow at its origin and expanded at its insertion. It arises from the front of the body of the pubis immediately below the pubic crest [FIG. 105] by a short, strong, flat band which is so curved upon itself that it is like a round tendon. It is inserted into the linea aspera of the femur by a very thin aponeurosis which lies between the vastus medialis and the other adductors, and is intimately connected with them. Nerve supply: anterior division of the **obturator nerve.** Action: primarily an adductor, it can also act as a lateral rotator and can flex the extended thigh.

DISSECTION. **Divide the adductor longus 2–3 cm. below its origin. Turn the proximal part upwards and note the character of the tendon. Turn the distal portion towards the femur, and secure the nerve of supply. Clean both sides of its aponeurosis as far as possible, separating it from the vastus medialis and the adductor magnus.**

Pectineus

The pectineus is placed between the adductor longus and the psoas major. It is flat, and

154

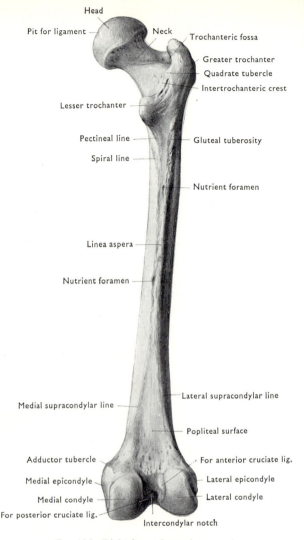

Head
Pit for ligament
Neck
Trochanteric fossa
Greater trochanter
Quadrate tubercle
Intertrochanteric crest
Lesser trochanter
Pectineal line
Gluteal tuberosity
Spiral line
Nutrient foramen
Linea aspera
Nutrient foramen
Lateral supracondylar line
Medial supracondylar line
Popliteal surface
Adductor tubercle
For anterior cruciate lig.
Medial epicondyle
Lateral epicondyle
Medial condyle
Lateral condyle
For posterior cruciate lig.
Intercondylar notch

FIG. 106   Right femur (posterior aspect).

narrows slightly towards its insertion. It has a fleshy origin from the pecten and pectineal surface of the pubis [FIG. 105], and descends laterally and backwards to gain insertion into the upper half of a line that extends from the back of the lesser trochanter to the linea

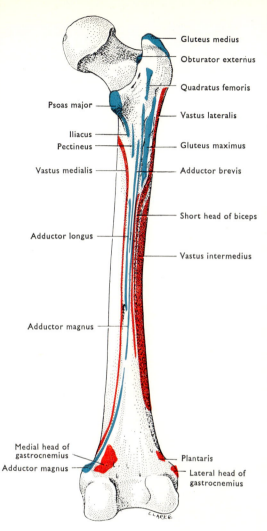

Psoas major

Iliacus
Pectineus

Vastus medialis

Adductor longus

Adductor magnus

Medial head of
gastrocnemius
Adductor magnus

Gluteus medius

Obturator externus

Quadratus femoris

Vastus lateralis

Gluteus maximus

Adductor brevis

Short head of biceps

Vastus intermedius

Plantaris
Lateral head of
gastrocnemius

CLARKE

FIG. 107 Right femur (posterior aspect) to show muscle attachments.

aspera [FIG. 106]. Nerve supply: the **femoral nerve.** Action: it adducts the thigh and assists in flexion.

DISSECTION. Detach the pectineus from its origin and turn it towards its insertion; at its lateral margin, look for an accessory obturator nerve which is occasionally present. Care must be taken not to

injure (1) the anterior division of the obturator nerve, which lies behind the muscle, or (2) the medial circumflex artery which passes backwards between it and the psoas major [Fig. 108]. Trace the medial circumflex artery still further backwards, between the adductor brevis and the obturator externus. The adductor brevis is below the artery; the obturator externus is the fleshy mass above it, closely applied to the front of the pelvis. Clean both these muscles as far as possible.

Accessory Obturator Nerve

This slender nerve, when present, arises either from the lumbar plexus or from the obturator trunk near its origin. It descends across the superior ramus of the pubis along the medial side of the psoas major into the thigh. If small, it ends in the hip joint or in the pectineus; if larger, it usurps the distribution of the obturator nerve to an extent that varies with its size [FIG. 96].

Medial Circumflex Artery

This artery usually springs from the profunda femoris artery at the same level as the lateral circumflex branch, but sometimes it springs directly from the femoral trunk. It passes backwards, out of the femoral triangle, between the psoas and the pectineus, and then between the obturator externus and the adductor brevis, to reach the back of the thigh, where, close to the lesser trochanter, it divides into an ascending and a transverse terminal branch. Before the main trunk divides it gives off: (1) *muscular branches*, and (2) an *articular branch* which enters the hip joint through the acetabular notch.

Adductor Brevis

The adductor brevis is behind the adductor longus and the pectineus, and in front of the adductor magnus. It arises from the front of the os pubis below the origin of the adductor longus [FIG. 105]. As it descends it inclines backwards and laterally and it is inserted into the lower two-thirds of the line which extends from the lesser trochanter to the linea aspera [FIG. 107], and into the

upper part of the linea aspera. Nerve supply:
the **obturator nerve.** Action: like all the other
adductor muscles it is an adductor, and a
lateral rotator of the thigh.

DISSECTION. Divide the adductor brevis close
to its origin and turn it towards its insertion, but do
not injure the anterior division of the obturator nerve
which lies in front of it. When the muscle is reflected
the posterior division of the nerve will be exposed.

Trace it upwards to the obturator externus, and
downwards into the adductor magnus. Clean a further
part of the obturator externus. Define the origin of the
adductor magnus from the side of the pubic arch
and clean its anterior surface as far as possible towards
its insertion, separating it from the adductor brevis.

Obturator Nerve (L. 2, 3, 4)

The obturator nerve arises in the abdomen
proper from the lumbar plexus [FIG. 95,

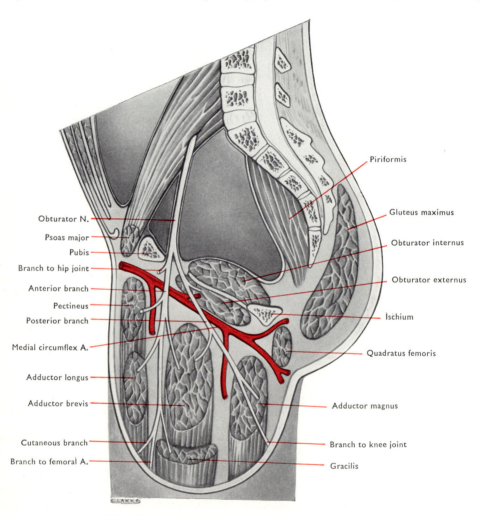

FIG. 108   Scheme of adductor group of muscles and obturator nerve.

p. 138], and descends into the pelvis. It enters the limb with the obturator vessels, through the upper or anterior part of the obturator foramen [FIG. 98]. While still within the foramen it splits into an anterior and a posterior division.

The **anterior division** enters the thigh over the upper border of the obturator externus muscle, and runs downwards on the anterior surface of the adductor brevis, behind the pectineus and adductor longus. It gives branches to the adductor longus, the adductor brevis and the gracilis. In addition, it gives off: (1) an **articular branch** to the hip joint [FIG. 108]; (2) a fine twig which appears at the distal border of the adductor longus, joins the medial anterior cutaneous and saphenous nerves in the subsartorial plexus, and may then become cutaneous to the distal third of the medial side of the thigh; and (3) a terminal twig which goes to the femoral artery [FIG. 108] and breaks up into fine filaments upon its walls.

The **posterior division** of the obturator nerve, as it enters the thigh, pierces the obturator externus near its upper border. It descends between the adductor brevis and the adductor magnus, and is expended chiefly in the supply of the magnus. It gives a branch to the obturator externus, an occasional one to adductor brevis, and an articular branch which pierces the lower part of the adductor magnus and enters the back of the knee joint [p. 177].

Gracilis

This long, slender muscle arises by a thin, wide tendon from the lower half of the body of the pubis, close to the symphysis, and from the upper half of the side of the pubic arch [FIG. 105]. It lies along the medial side of the thigh and knee, and ends in a thin, rounded tendon which inclines forwards, below the knee, and expands to be inserted into the upper part of the medial surface of the tibia [FIG. 128]. Two intercommunicating bursae separate the tendon of the gracilis from the tibial collateral ligament of the knee joint and from the tendon of the sartorius.

Nerve supply: the anterior division of the **obturator nerve.** Action: it adducts the thigh, flexes the knee joint and rotates the flexed leg medially.

Adductor Magnus

The adductor magnus is one of the most powerful muscles of the thigh. It is a thick, flat, fleshy mass which springs from the side of the pubic arch and the lower part of the ischial tuberosity [FIG. 105]. The part from the arch spreads out to be attached to the medial side of the gluteal tuberosity, to the linea aspera, and to the medial supracondylar ridge. The bundles which arise anteriorly pass in a horizontal direction; the more posterior the origin the more oblique the direction taken [FIGS. 107, 121]. Thus the part from the tuberosity descends almost vertically and forms the posteromedial border, which is the thickest part of the muscle. It ends in a strong, rounded tendon which is inserted into the adductor tubercle [FIGS. 106, 117]. The tendon is further attached to the femur by the medial intermuscular septum, which stretches between it and the medial supracondylar ridge and gives origin to lower part of vastus medialis.

At the gluteal tuberosity and the linea aspera the insertion is interrupted by the passage of the perforating vessels. At these spots the muscle fibres are attached to tendinous slips which arch over the vessels. The opening for the femoral vessels is in series with these arches, and is situated at the supracondylar ridge about the junction of the middle and lower thirds of the thigh [FIG. 121].

Nerve supply is double. The part inserted into the adductor tubercle is associated at its origin with the hamstrings and, belonging to the same flexor group, is supplied by the tibial part of the **sciatic nerve ;** the rest of the muscle—the true adductor part—is supplied by the posterior division of the **obturator nerve.**

Action: the adductor portion adducts the thigh, rotates it laterally, and helps to flex the hip joint. The hamstring portion extends the hip joint.

157

DISSECTION. Complete the cleaning of the anterior surface of adductor magnus and obturator externus muscles.

Obturator Externus

This flat, fan-shaped muscle overlies the external surface of the obturator membrane, and arises from its anteromedial half, and also from the medial and lower margins of the obturator foramen [FIG. 105]. It passes backwards and laterally, below the neck of the femur and the capsule of the hip joint, and then curves upwards and laterally on to the back of the neck of the femur, to end in a stout tendon which obtains insertion into the floor of the trochanteric fossa [FIG. 107]. This tendon is examined in the dissection of the gluteal region.

Nerve supply: the posterior division of the **obturator nerve**. Action: it is a flexor and a lateral rotator of the thigh.

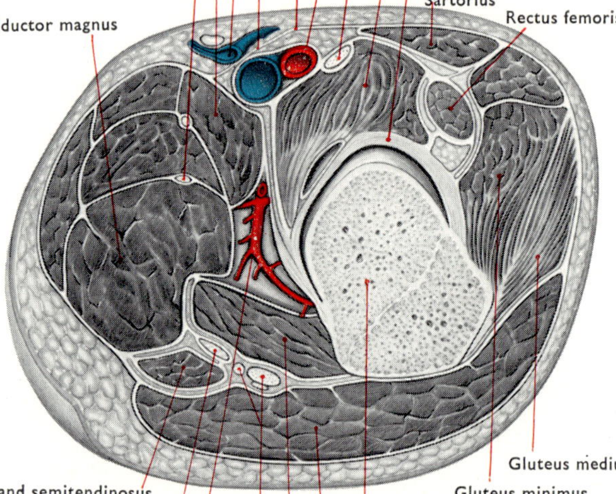

DISSECTION. Detach the obturator externus carefully from its origin in order to expose the obturator artery and its terminal branches. Release the posterior division of the obturator nerve from the substance of the muscle, and avoid injury to its anterior division.

Obturator Artery

The obturator artery arises in the pelvis from the internal iliac, and accompanies the nerve through the obturator foramen. As soon as it enters the thigh, it divides into two terminal branches which diverge from each other and form an arterial circle on the obturator membrane under cover of the obturator externus. Both branches give twigs to the neighbouring muscles, and the **posterior branch** sends an **articular twig**

FIG. 109 Dissection of oblique section through upper part of thigh to show relations of the hip joint. The section is cut transversely to the neck of the femur.

through the acetabular notch into the hip joint. This twig passes along the ligament of the head of the femur and plays a minor part in the supply of that bone; it may be seen in a well injected subject when the joint is opened.

Psoas Major and Iliacus

Both these muscles arise within the abdomen, and enter the thigh behind the inguinal ligament. The tendon of psoas major forms on its lateral side, and is inserted into the lesser trochanter of the femur. The iliacus lies at the lateral side of the psoas and is inserted, by fleshy fibres, into the tendon of the psoas, into the lesser trochanter and the surface of the femur below it. The united iliopsoas first descends over the front of the capsule of the hip joint and then passes backwards inferior to it to reach its insertion. A synovial **bursa** intervenes between it and the front of the capsule, and facilitates the play of the united muscle over the joint. The bursa may communicate with the joint through an aperture in the capsule [FIG. 123]. Nerve supply : ventral rami of L.2 and L.3.

Action : the iliopsoas is the chief flexor of the thigh : conversely, if the lower limbs are fixed, it is a flexor of the trunk as in raising it from the supine position. Flexion of the thigh is accompanied by slight medial rotation owing to the insertion of iliopsoas lateral to the axis of rotation of the femur. But if the

neck of the femur is broken, the iliopsoas rotates the distal fragment laterally.

DISSECTION. Divide the femoral vessels and nerve below the inguinal ligament, and tie them separately to a small piece of wood. Cut through the sartorius and the rectus femoris, about 5 cm. from their origins, and turn them aside. Divide the iliopsoas near its insertion and turn the two parts upwards and downwards. This will expose the psoas bursa and the capsule of the hip joint. Open the bursa, ascertain its extent with the finger, and note whether or not it communicates with the joint.

Turn aside the tensor fasciae latae. Raise the upper part of the rectus femoris and clean its reflected head. Lastly, clean the anterior part of the capsule of the hip joint.

THE GLUTEAL REGION

SURFACE ANATOMY

[FIGS. 110, 112]

In the lower part of the region the **buttock** forms a smooth, rounded elevation which is separated from its fellow by the **natal cleft,** and limited inferiorly by the **gluteal fold.** The groove below the fold is the result of a firm linear attachment of the skin to the deep fascia by fibrous strands that pass through the superficial fascia. The bulging prominence of the buttock is due to a thick layer of fat and the lower part of a large muscle called the **gluteus maximus** that overlie the ischium, which is the skeleton of the buttock. The lower border and **tuberosity** of the ischium [FIG. 90] are roughened by the attachments of muscles. Though the tuberosity is hidden deeply under the fat and gluteus maximus, it can be felt if you place your finger in the medial part of the gluteal fold and press upwards. Note that the gluteal fold does *not* correspond to the lower border of the gluteus maximus, which crosses the fold obliquely along a line from the coccyx to the lateral side of the thigh a hand-breadth below the trochanter.

The terms 'buttock' and 'gluteal region' are not synonymous. The 'region' extends both upwards and forwards for a considerable distance beyond the buttock, and is

limited superiorly by the **iliac crest** [p. 130]. On the side of the trunk, in a muscular man, the outermost muscle of the abdomen **(obliquus externus)** bulges out over the crest so that the crest lies in a groove. Find the highest point of the crest (which is at the level of the fourth lumbar vertebral spine), and note the downward slope of the crest both anteriorly and posteriorly. Its anterior part has been examined already. A line drawn from its anterior superior spine to the front of the greater trochanter marks the anterior limit of the gluteal region and its junction with the upper part of the front of the thigh.

Trace the iliac crest backwards to its posterior end at the **posterior superior iliac spine.** This spine does not form a surface prominence ; on the contrary, it lies in the floor of a dimple of the skin. The dimple is situated a little above the buttock, about three finger-breadths from the median plane, and is at the level of the second spine of the sacrum, opposite the middle of the sacro-iliac joint.

The area between the right and left dimples corresponds to the back of the **sacrum.** The sacrum has usually three tubercles or spines in the median plane, about 2·5 cm. apart. The second spine is midway between the dimples, and is the guide to the other two spines. The natal cleft begins at or near the

159

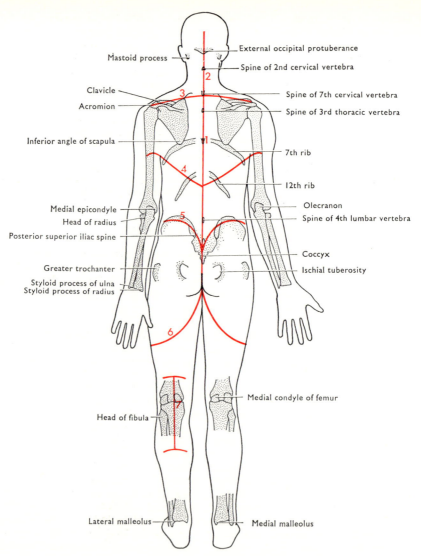

Mastoid process

External occipital protuberance

Spine of 2nd cervical vertebra

Clavicle

Acromion

Spine of 7th cervical vertebra

Spine of 3rd thoracic vertebra

Inferior angle of scapula

7th rib

12th rib

Olecranon

Medial epicondyle

Head of radius

Spine of 4th lumbar vertebra

Posterior superior iliac spine

Coccyx

Greater trochanter

Ischial tuberosity

Styloid process of ulna
Styloid process of radius

Medial condyle of femur

Head of fibula

Lateral malleolus

Medial malleolus

FIG. 110   Landmarks and incisions.   For the bony landmarks of the lower limb, see illustrations of individual bones.

third spine, and deepens as it extends downwards; the lower part of the sacrum and the coccyx lie in its floor. The **coccyx** reaches almost to the anus, and can be distinguished from the sacrum, because it

moves slightly under pressure, except in old people.

Press firmly on the region between the lower part of the sacrum and the ischial tuberosity. The resistance encountered is due to a strong band, called the **sacrotuberous ligament,** which is felt through the fat and the gluteus maximus.

DISSECTION. **Reflexion of Skin. Incisions [Fig. 110 (5 and 6)].** (1) From the posterior superior iliac spine along the iliac crest, as far forwards as the position of the body will permit; (2) from the posterior end of this incision downwards and medially to the median line in the sacral region, and then perpendicularly to the tip of the coccyx; (3) from the tip of the coccyx downwards and laterally over the back of the thigh to the middle of the lateral side of the thigh. Turn this flap of skin laterally.

Superficial Fascia

This has the same general characters as the corresponding layer of fascia in other parts of the body, but is much more heavily laden with fat—more particularly so in the female. It thickens over the upper and lower margins of the gluteus maximus and it is tough and stringy over the ischial tuberosity, where it forms a most efficient cushion upon which the ischium rests while the body is in the sitting posture.

Cutaneous Nerves [FIG. 111]

The cutaneous nerves of the gluteal region are numerous and difficult to find. They converge on the gluteal region from all directions:

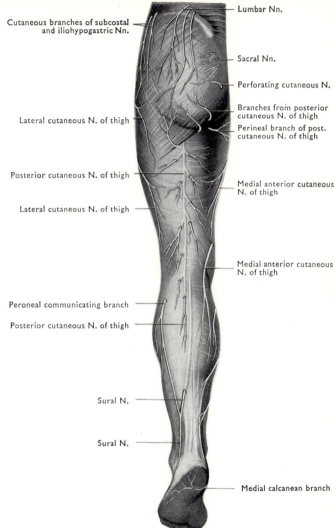

FIG. 111   Cutaneous nerves on back of lower limb.   See also FIG. 94.

1. From above: the lateral cutaneous branches of the **subcostal** (T. 12) and **iliohypogastric** (L. 1) nerves pierce the deep fascia anterior and posterior to the tubercle of the iliac crest, and descend over the lateral surface to the level of the greater trochanter.

2. From in front: branches from the posterior division of the **lateral cutaneous nerve of the thigh** (L. 2, 3) which pierces the deep fascia 5 cm. inferior to the anterior superior iliac spine, supply the antero-inferior region.

3. From below: two or three branches of the **posterior cutaneous nerve of the thigh** curl over the middle third of the lower border of gluteus maximus and supply the postero-inferior part (S. 1, 2, 3).

4. From the medial side: the **dorsal rami** of L. 1–3 and S. 1–3, and inferior to this, the **perforating cutaneous nerve** (S. 2, 3, ventral rami). The lumbar branches are long and pierce the deep fascia above the iliac crest, descending obliquely across it almost to the fold of the buttock. The others are short. The perforating cutaneous pierces the sacrotuberous ligament, gluteus maximus and the deep fascia and appears midway between the coccyx and the ischial tuberosity. These nerves supply the medial and intermediate regions.

DISSECTION. Look first for the branches of the sacral nerves. Reflect the superficial fascia laterally from the median plane between the posterior superior iliac spine and the tip of the coccyx, and secure the nerves as they pierce the deep fascia.

Next identify the branches of the lumbar nerves. Reflect a thin layer of the superficial fascia downwards from the iliac crest and secure twigs of the lumbar nerves as they come up through the deeper layer of the fascia. These twigs will lead to the trunks of the nerves at the iliac crest; the trunks can then be traced and other branches secured. Find the branches of the iliohypogastric and subcostal nerves in the same way.

If the perineum has been dissected, the perforating cutaneous nerve may be found in situ. If not, find it between the coccyx and the ischial tuberosity.

The branches of the posterior cutaneous nerve of the thigh have now to be displayed. Cut through the superficial fascia along the lower border of the gluteus maximus. Do so very carefully for, if you cut the deep fascia also, you are apt to cut the trunk of the posterior cutaneous nerve itself as it escapes from under cover of the gluteus maximus. As soon as the deep fascia is exposed turn the superficial fascia upwards, and look for the branches as they curve upwards round the lower border of the gluteus maximus about its middle third.

After the cutaneous nerves have been demonstrated remove the superficial fascia from the whole of the gluteal region in order that the deep fascia may be examined.

Deep Fascia

The deep fascia now exposed differs in character in its anterior and posterior parts.

In front of the gluteus maximus, where the fascia lies over the anterior part of the gluteus medius, it is dense, opaque, and pearly white in colour—in marked contrast with the deep fascia over the gluteus maximus itself, which is thin and transparent. When the dense portion reaches the anterior border of the gluteus maximus it splits into two lamellae which enclose the muscle between them. Both lamellae give origin to some of its fibres, and they send their septa into the muscle to divide it into coarse bundles.

DISSECTION. Follow the branches of the posterior cutaneous nerve of the thigh to the trunk of that nerve at the lower border of the gluteus maximus. When the trunk of the nerve is secured, proceed to clean the gluteus maximus—a difficult process, owing to the septa of deep fascia.

Do not remove the thick, opaque fascia which covers the insertion of the muscle.

As the upper border of the muscle is defined, note the connexion of the fascia with the layer on the deep surface of the muscle and with the fascia on the gluteus medius.

Gluteus Maximus

The gluteus maximus is a powerful muscle which arises from: (1) the rough, upper part of the area of the ilium behind the posterior gluteal line; (2) the back of the sacrum and coccyx; and (3) the sacrotuberous ligament.

From this extensive origin, the fasciculi of the muscle proceed obliquely downwards and forwards towards the upper part of the shaft of the femur, but only a portion of the muscle is inserted into the bone. Three-quarters of it is inserted into the iliotibial tract; only the lower deep quarter is inserted into the gluteal tuberosity. As the upper part approaches its insertion it becomes aponeurotic; and this sudden thinning of the muscle accounts for the hollow of the hip behind the greater trochanter. It has been noted already that the lower border of the muscle does not correspond to the fold of the buttock but crosses it obliquely.

Three **synovial bursae** underlie the muscle: (1) A multilocular bursa separates its lower edge from the tendons that arise from the ischial tuberosity, *i.e.*, the origin of the ham-

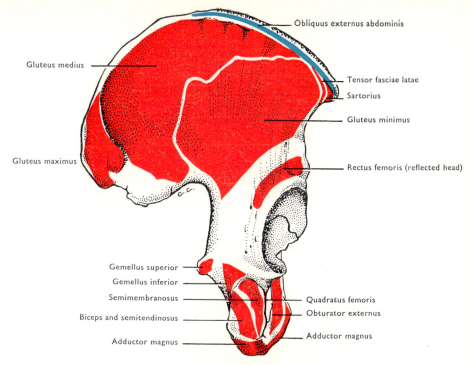

Gluteus medius

Gluteus maximus

Obliquus externus abdominis

Tensor fasciae latae

Sartorius

Gluteus minimus

Rectus femoris (reflected head)

Gemellus superior

Gemellus inferior

Semimembranosus

Biceps and semitendinosus

Adductor magnus

Quadratus femoris

Obturator externus

Adductor magnus

FIG. 112   Muscle attachments to outer surface of right hip bone.

strings; it is usually difficult to define it, owing to the small size of its loculi and the stringiness of the fibrous tissue between them. (2) A large bursa separates the aponeurotic part from the greater trochanter. (3) Another large bursa separates the aponeurotic part from the upper part of the vastus lateralis.

Nerve supply: **inferior gluteal nerve.** Action: it is the chief extensor of the thigh at the hip joint, and comes powerfully into action to straighten the lower limb on the trunk, or the trunk on the lower limb, in the act of rising from the stooping and squatting positions, and in running and climbing.

DISSECTION.   As the gluteus maximus is reflected be careful not to injure the structures which lie closely subjacent to it. The nerves most liable to injury are the posterior cutaneous nerve of the thigh and the perforating cutaneous nerve, which is very liable to injury when

the fibres of the gluteus maximus are being raised from the sacrotuberous ligament.   That ligament itself is liable to be cut if it is not identified before the medial part of the muscle is reflected.

Cut through the muscle from (1) its upper border, two finger-breadths above the greater trochanter, to (2) the lower border 2–3 cm. medial to its insertion into the femur.

To facilitate this procedure pass two fingers deep to the muscle (from upper or lower border, whichever is the more convenient) separating it from subjacent structures as the cut is made.

When the muscle is divided reflect the lateral part to its insertion, open the two bursae deep to the aponeurosis and explore their extent with the finger tip. The upper of the two is a large loose sac between the aponeurosis and the greater trochanter of the femur; the other lies below it and in front of the part of the muscle inserted into the gluteal tuberosity of the femur. A slight touch of the knife is sufficient to open it, and the glistening tendon of the vastus lateralis comes into view.

Then reflect the medial part of the muscle towards its origin, working close to the deep surface of the muscle to avoid injuring the posterior cutaneous nerve of the thigh. As soon as the vessels and nerves which enter the muscle appear, clean and turn them medially with the muscle (removing the veins, if necessary). These vessels and nerves are: (1) the superficial branch of the superior gluteal artery, encountered as the upper part of the muscle is followed towards the ilium; and (2) the inferior gluteal nerve and artery, encountered as the lower part is turned towards the ischial tuberosity. Look for the synovial bursa on the tuberosity.

Identify the sacrotuberous ligament again. The gluteus maximus arises from it and conceals it; but it can be felt through the muscle as a firm resisting band that stretches upwards and medially from the ischial tuberosity. Detach the gluteus maximus carefully from the ligament. As you do so, secure the perforating cutaneous nerve and divide the coccygeal branches of the inferior gluteal artery which pierce the ligament to enter the muscle.

Bony Landmarks under Gluteus Maximus

The **greater trochanter** is situated in the lower and lateral part of the area exposed. The **gluteal tuberosity** is inferior to it, and receives the lower deep fibres of the gluteus maximus. The **ischial tuberosity** is about 8 cm. medial to the distal part of the greater trochanter, and gives origin to the hamstring muscles. Rotate the thigh laterally (*i.e.*, move it so that its anterior surface is turned away from the median plane); the trochanter is then approximated to the

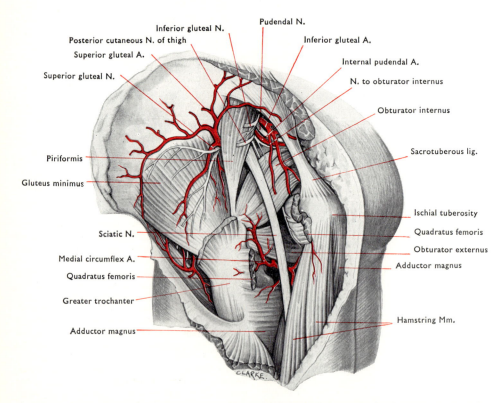

FIG. 113 Dissection of left gluteal region. Gluteus maximus and gluteus medius have been removed, and quadratus femoris has been reflected. In the specimen, the inferior gluteal artery was medial to the internal pudendal instead of lateral to it.

tuberosity, and it recedes from the tuberosity when the thigh is rotated medially.

Sacrotuberous Ligament

This is a long, strong band that extends upwards and medially from the tuberosity of the ischium to the margins of the sacrum and coccyx, and to the posterior iliac spines, inferior and superior. It holds down the posterior part of the sacrum and thus prevents the weight of the body depressing its anterior part. The inferior or medial border of the ligament forms the posterior boundary of the perineum. Its upper or lateral margin forms the posterior boundary of two openings called the greater and lesser sciatic foramina, which are separated from each other by the sacrospinous ligament.

Sacrospinous Ligament

The sacrospinous ligament is a short, thick triangular band that extends medially from the spine of the ischium to the last piece of the sacrum and the first piece of the coccyx. Its medial part is hidden under cover of the sacrotuberous ligament, but its lateral part can be felt by the finger tip placed about 2–3 cm. above the upper border of the tuberosity of the ischium. It is the posterior, ligamentous part of the muscle **coccygeus.**

With the help of a pelvis with the ligaments *in situ*, note the connexions of the sacrotuberous and sacrospinous ligaments, and the position of the sciatic foramina.

Sciatic Foramina

The **greater sciatic foramen** is the upper of the two. It is bounded by the greater sciatic notch of the hip bone and by both the ligaments. It transmits the piriformis muscle with the superior gluteal nerve and vessels **above** it, and the inferior gluteal nerve and vessels, the sciatic nerve and other nerves and vessels **below** it.

The **lesser sciatic foramen** is bounded by the lesser sciatic notch of the hip bone and by both the ligaments. It transmits the tendon of the obturator internus muscle, and the nerve to obturator internus, the pudendal nerve and the internal pudendal vessels which emerge

through the greater sciatic foramen below the piriformis and disappear immediately into the lesser foramen.

DISSECTION. Begin with the superficial branches of the superior gluteal artery. They enter the upper part of the gluteus maximus; follow them to the point where they emerge through the cleft between the gluteus medius and the upper border of the piriformis muscle. Clean the piriformis from the greater sciatic foramen to the greater trochanter. Then clean the posterior cutaneous nerve of the thigh, following it upwards to the lower border of the piriformis. Secure its perineal branch, which passes below the ischial tuberosity towards the perineum.

Follow the inferior gluteal vessels and nerve upwards to the lower border of the piriformis.

Flex the knee, and keep it flexed by supporting the leg on a large block. That relaxes the hamstring muscles and the sciatic nerve, which is the next structure to be cleaned. It is the thick, firm, white cord that emerges below the piriformis. Cut its fascial covering at the level of the top of the greater trochanter. Insert the handle of the knife and run it upwards, along the lateral border of the nerve to the lower border of the piriformis, and downwards as far as possible. Clean the fascia from the back of the nerve, and secure the branches to the hamstring muscles that spring from its medial border about the level of the ischial tuberosity. They will be followed to the muscles later; meanwhile note and preserve the branches of the medial circumflex femoral artery which pass to these muscles with their nerves.

Next pull the upper part of the sciatic nerve laterally, exposing the bony dorsum of the acetabulum and the slender nerve to the quadratus femoris, and trace it downwards until it disappears in front of a slip of muscle called the superior gemellus. About a finger-breadth medial to the sciatic nerve look for the nerve to the obturator internus, the internal pudendal vessels and the pudendal nerve lying on the spine of the ischium and the sacrospinous ligament. Clean and preserve the artery and the nerves, but remove the veins.

Now proceed to clean and examine the muscles that are anterior to (i.e., deep to) the sciatic nerve. First, the tendon of the obturator internus passing from the lesser sciatic foramen to the greater trochanter, with a fleshy slip along each border—the superior and inferior gemellus. Below that, the quadrilateral sheet—quadratus femoris—extending from the ischial tuberosity to the back of the greater trochanter; and, below the quadratus, the upper border of the adductor magnus. Clean the transverse branch of the medial circumflex artery, which emerges between the quadratus and adductor magnus, and look for a small artery, called the first perforating, as it pierces the adductor magnus at the medial border of the gluteal tuberosity.

After the muscles are cleaned, divide the tendon of the obturator internus about a finger-breadth from the lesser sciatic notch. Raise the medial part of the tendon, turn it backwards to find the bursa between it and the floor of the notch; note the grooved character of the deep surface of the tendon.

Turn next to the hamstring muscles which spring from the tuberosity of the ischium; separate the common tendon of the biceps femoris and the semitendinosus from the flattened tendon of the semimembranosus, which lies immediately subjacent. Then pull the hamstrings laterally and display the origin of the adductor magnus from the tuberosity.

STRUCTURES UNDER COVER OF
THE GLUTEUS MAXIMUS

For the bursae, see page 162.

Inferior Gluteal Nerve

The **inferior gluteal nerve** (L. 5; S. 1, 2), springs from the sacral plexus, enters the gluteal region through the lower part of the greater sciatic foramen, and supplies gluteus maximus. It divides into two or three branches which break up into numerous twigs, entering the deep surface of gluteus maximus in an irregular line between the upper two-thirds and lower third of the muscle. As it emerges from the pelvis it is accompanied by the **posterior cutaneous nerve of the thigh,** which descends to the thigh on the back of the sciatic nerve.

Inferior Gluteal Artery

This branch of the internal iliac artery, issues from the pelvis below piriformis, descends with the sciatic nerve, and is continued with the posterior cutaneous nerve to the back of the thigh as a fine cutaneous artery. It supplies large muscular branches to the gluteus maximus, cutaneous branches to the buttock and the back of the thigh, and the **companion artery of the sciatic nerve**—a very slender artery that accompanies the nerve for some distance, and then sinks into its substance. It anastomoses with the circumflex femoral arteries.

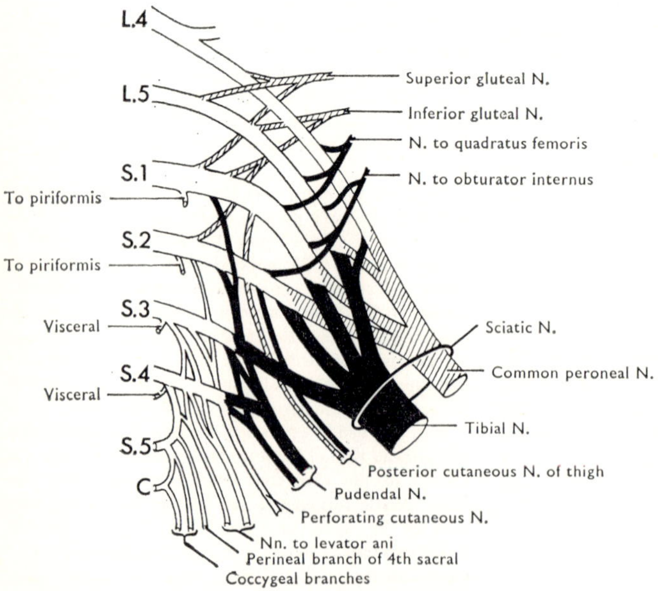

Sciatic Nerve (L. 4, 5; S. 1, 2, 3)

This, the thickest nerve in the body, is a terminal branch of the sacral plexus, and enters the gluteal region through the lower part of the greater sciatic foramen. At first it has the form of a flattened band, but soon it becomes oval or round.

The sciatic nerve traverses the gluteal region in the interval between the greater trochanter of the femur and the tuberosity of the ischium, enclosed in a sheath of fascia; it usually ends half-way down the back of the thigh by dividing into two large branches.

FIG. 114   Diagram of sacral plexus.
Ventral offsets, black; dorsal offsets, cross hatched. Cf. arrangement of the brachial plexus, FIG. 14. For the lumbar part of the lumbosacral plexus, see FIG. 96.

166

These divisions of the sciatic nerve are known as the **common peroneal** (fibular) and the **tibial nerves** from their distribution in the leg and their relation to its bones.

In the gluteal region the sciatic nerve is under cover of the gluteus maximus, and lies, from above downwards, on: (1) the ischium and the nerve to the quadratus femoris; (2) the tendon of the obturator internus with the two gemelli muscles; (3) the quadratus femoris. As it enters the thigh it lies on the adductor magnus. The nerves to one or more of the hamstring muscles issue from the medial side of the main trunk at the level of the ischial tuberosity, or a little lower down.

The level of division of the sciatic nerve is variable and it sometimes splits into the common peroneal and tibial nerves before it leaves the pelvis; the tibial nerve then emerges from the pelvis below the piriformis, but the common peroneal nerve pierces the muscle.

Internal Pudendal Artery, Pudendal Nerve and Nerve to Obturator Internus [FIG. 113]

These structures run only a very small part of their course in the medial part of the gluteal region. They emerge from the pelvis through the greater sciatic foramen and cross the spine of the ischium and the sacrospinous ligament; they then enter the lesser sciatic foramen and pass out of view. The nerve to the obturator internus lies on the base of the ischial spine, and furnishes a twig to the superior gemellus. The internal pudendal artery, with a companion vein on each side, crosses the tip of the spine. The pudendal nerve lies on the sacrospinous ligament, close to the ischial spine.

Small Lateral Rotator Muscles of Thigh

These are the piriformis, the obturator internus and the two gemelli, the quadratus femoris, and the obturator externus. They are not all completely exposed by reflexion of the gluteus maximus. The piriformis and obturator internus emerge from the pelvis, and only part of the obturator externus, which lies anterior to the quadratus femoris, is seen

from behind when that muscle has been reflected. But they are all inserted into the greater trochanter, and they are related to the back of the hip joint.

Piriformis. The piriformis muscle arises within the pelvis chiefly from the middle three pieces of the sacrum. After it has passed through the greater sciatic foramen its fleshy belly rapidly tapers to a rounded tendon which passes superficial to the tendon of the obturator internus, and is inserted into the upper border of the greater trochanter [FIG. 104]. It is closely adherent to the subjacent obturator tendon for some distance. Nerve supply: branches in the pelvis from the **first** and **second sacral nerves.**

Obturator Internus. [FIG. 113]. This muscle has a large, fan-shaped, fleshy belly which arises, within the pelvis, from the side and front walls of the pelvic cavity. Its fibres converge on the tendon, which issues through the lesser sciatic foramen, bends at a right angle, and runs laterally across the back of the hip joint to be inserted into the medial surface of the greater trochanter [FIG. 104]. The deep surface of the tendon is divided into four or five portions by longitudinal grooves, and is separated by a *bursa* from the lesser sciatic notch.

Gemelli. The gemellus superior arises from the upper margin of the lesser sciatic notch. Its fibres run along the upper border of the tendon of the obturator internus, and are inserted obliquely into it. The gemellus inferior arises from the lower margin of the lesser sciatic notch, and is inserted into the lower border of the obturator tendon in a similar manner.

Close to their origins the gemelli meet under cover of the obturator tendon, and form a fleshy bed on which the tendon lies; near the trochanter their fibres overlap the obturator tendon, and tend to cover its superficial surface.

Quadratus Femoris. The quadratus femoris lies between the gemellus inferior and the adductor magnus. It arises from the lateral border of the ischial tuberosity, and proceeds horizontally to **gain** insertion into the back of the greater trochanter and the adjoining part of the shaft of the femur [FIG. 107].

The **nerve to quadratus femoris** arises from the sacral plexus, escapes from the pelvis through the lower part of the greater sciatic foramen, and descends over the ischium and the capsule of the hip joint, under cover of the sciatic nerve, the obturator internus and the gemelli. It gives a twig to the hip joint, supplies the inferior gemellus, and sinks into the deep surface of the quadratus femoris.

Obturator Externus. This muscle arises from the front of the pelvis [FIG. 105] and winds backwards below the hip joint. Its tendon is seen here passing obliquely upwards and laterally on the back of the neck of the femur to be inserted into the trochanteric fossa.

Medial Circumflex Artery

This artery arises from the profunda in the femoral triangle. It passes backwards among the muscles of the medial side of the thigh, and ends near the upper border of the adductor magnus by dividing into ascending and transverse branches.

The **ascending branch** runs obliquely upwards and laterally towards the trochanteric fossa, giving off muscular twigs. The **transverse branch** passes backwards, and then, curving downwards, it breaks up into branches which enter the hamstring muscles. It anastomoses with the terminal twig of the transverse branch of the lateral circumflex artery, which, in a well-injected subject, will be noticed

appearing from amidst the fibres of the upper part of the vastus lateralis. An arterial circle is thus formed around the upper part of the femur; it communicates proximally with the inferior gluteal artery and distally with the first perforating artery. This series of inosculations is sometimes spoken of as the **cruciate anastomosis** of the thigh.

The **structures superior to piriformis** lie close to the ilium, and are the gluteus medius and minimus, and the tensor fasciae latae, together with the superior gluteal vessels and nerve which supply them.

The posterior part of the gluteus medius was covered by the gluteus maximus; its anterior border is overlapped by the tensor fasciae latae; the rest of it is invested by the dense fascial layer already referred to, and is the fleshy substance felt through the skin and fasciae below the iliac crest on the side of the hip in the living body.

Gluteus Medius

This wide, thick muscle arises from the large area between the anterior gluteal line and the iliac crest [FIGS. 112, 107]. The fibres converge to form a flattened band, partly fleshy and partly tendinous, which is inserted into the posterosuperior angle of the greater trochanter and the oblique ridge on its lateral surface. A small *bursa* separates the tendon from the anterior part of the lateral surface of the trochanter.

Nerve supply: **superior gluteal nerve.** Action: as a whole the muscle is an abductor of the thigh. It is mainly concerned with preventing the pelvis from tilting to the opposite side when that foot is raised from the ground; its anterior fibres can rotate the thigh medially.

and reflect the two parts. As the lower part of the muscle is reflected look for the small bursa that lies between it and the trochanter. When the upper part of the muscle is raised, the branches of the superior gluteal vessels and nerve will be exposed; clean and preserve them, except the twigs which enter the gluteus medius and interfere with its reflexion. Follow the branches of the artery and nerve to tensor fasciae latae and clean the surface of the gluteus minimus.

Superior Gluteal Nerve

This nerve (L. 4, 5 ; S. 1) arises from the sacral plexus, and escapes from the pelvis through the upper part of the greater sciatic foramen. It then turns forward, between the gluteus medius and minimus, and immediately divides into two or more branches. The upper branch or branches sink into the gluteus medius. The lowest branch crosses the middle of the gluteus minimus, and giving branches to both the gluteus medius and minimus, it passes between their anterior borders and ends in the deep surface of tensor fasciae latae.

Superior Gluteal Artery [Fig. 113]

This is a large vessel which springs from the internal iliac artery and escapes from the pelvis with the nerve and the vein. Immediately after its exit it divides into a superficial and a deep division.

The **superficial division** has been seen during the reflexion of the gluteus maximus. Its branches are distributed to the deep surface of that muscle.

The **deep division** bifurcates, close to its origin, into a superior and an inferior branch. The inferior branch accompanies the lowest branch of the nerve. The superior branch follows the upper border of the gluteus minimus close to the anterior gluteal line of the ilium.

Gluteus Minimus

This is also a thick, wide muscle. It arises from the broad area of the ilium between the anterior and inferior gluteal lines [Fig. 112, p. 163]. The muscular fibres pass gradually into an aponeurotic tendon which covers the superficial surface of the distal part of the muscle and narrows to be inserted into the lower and lateral part of the front of the greater trochanter [Fig. 104]. It is intimately connected, near its insertion, with the capsule of the hip joint, and it is separated from the upper and anterior part of the trochanter by a small bursa.

Nerve supply : **superior gluteal nerve.** Action : the same as gluteus medius.

DISSECTION. Detach the gluteus minimus from its origin and turn it downwards, separating it from the capsule of the hip joint. Open the bursa, and examine its extent.

Structures under Cover of the Gluteus Minimus

The upper and posterior parts of the **capsule of the hip joint** are now exposed. Note that the capsule is loosely attached to the back and upper part of the neck of the femur, about a finger-breadth medial to the trochanter, but firmly attached to the acetabular rim. Many of the fibres of the posterior part of the capsule run circularly around the neck of the femur and are named the **zona orbicularis** [see. p. 181].

The **reflected tendon of the rectus femoris** is attached to the floor of a groove situated immediately above the margin of the acetabulum, and is there embedded under the superficial fibres of the capsule [p. 152]. To expose it, cut through these fibres parallel with the direction of the tendon.

THE POPLITEAL FOSSA

The dissection of the popliteal fossa should be carried out before the back of the thigh is disturbed, in order that its contents may be examined before the medial and lateral boundaries of its upper portion are displaced.

The popliteal fossa lies behind the knee, opposite the lower third of the femur, the knee joint and the upper part of the tibia. It appears as a hollow when the knee joint is flexed because the tendons which form its superior boundaries stand out from the femur on their way to the leg bones, but it bulges slightly when the joint is fully extended and the tendons lie close to the femur.

Palpate the bony points and tendons in your own limb as they are difficult to feel in the fixed cadaver. With the knee flexed, identify the **condyles** of the tibia and femur on the lateral and medial sides of the knee. The condyles of the tibia and femur are easily differentiated anteriorly because of the wide gap between them. Follow the lateral condyle of the tibia posteriorly, and note a pronounced bony protuberance immediately below its posterolateral aspect, the **head of the fibula.** Behind the lateral side of the knee identify a thick round cord descending to the head of the fibula, the tendon of insertion of **biceps femoris.** Keeping your fingers on this tendon, flex and extend the knee and note how the tendon passes on to the posterolateral aspect of the femoral condyle in extension, but still

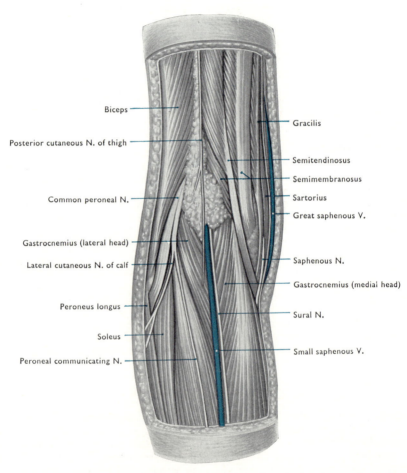

Fig. 115 Left popliteal region after removal of the deep fascia—the muscles and fat being left undisturbed.

produces a slight longitudinal ridge. Slip your finger to the medial side of this ridge and press deeply: the bone which can be felt is the lateral condyle of the femur. If the finger is moved from side to side, a round cord can be felt immediately medial to the tendon of biceps; this is the **common peroneal nerve.** Now move your finger round the lateral side of the tendon of biceps into the groove which lies anterior to it and separates it from a broad firm area, the **iliotibial tract,** which can be traced inferiorly to a tubercle on the anterolateral surface of the lateral condyle of the tibia. With the knee fully extended, the anterior margin of the iliotibial tract can be felt about 2·5 cm. posterolateral to the lateral margin of the patella. With the knee flexed, press your finger into the interval between the head of the fibula and the femoral condyle; the **fibular collateral ligament** of the **knee joint** is felt there as a rounded cord. Then place your finger on the back of the head of the fibula, push the soft parts medially and move the finger sideways to feel the common peroneal nerve again.

Place your fingers under the medial side of the popliteal fossa, and with your foot on the floor, attempt to flex the knee. The slender tendon which stands out is the semitendinosus, and immediately medial to it and on a slightly deeper plane is the larger tendon of semimembranosus. Anteromedial to this is the tendon of gracilis, which is often obscured by the muscle fibres of the posterior part of sartorius.

In the upper part of the popliteal region the muscles of the two sides are fairly close together; the distal part of the belly of the semimembranosus is thick, and it bulges near the mid line of the limb as the muscle contracts on walking. In the middle of the fossa the pulsations of the **popliteal artery** are felt when deep pressure is made. In the lower part the two heads of the **gastrocnemius** muscle form two rounded cushions that merge inferiorly into the calf.

Above the popliteal region the back of the thigh is smooth and rounded; but, in a thin person, the outlines of the bellies of the hamstring muscles may be seen faintly.

DISSECTION. Reflexion of the Skin. Place a block under the knee to support the limb and to make the bounderies of the popliteal fossa tense. Make incision 7 [Fig. 110, p. 160]. Separate the two flaps of skin from the superficial fascia and turn them aside.

Superficial Fascia

The superficial fascia of the popliteal region presents no peculiar features and, as a rule, it contains only a moderate amount of fat, the small saphenous vein and three cutaneous nerves.

DISSECTION. Look first for the small saphenous vein ascending from the calf and piercing the deep fascia over the distal part of the fossa. As the upper part of the vein is being cleaned, secure the terminal part of the posterior cutaneous nerve of the thigh, which runs alongside the vein. At a higher level, in the midline of the popliteal area, one or more twigs from the posterior cutaneous nerve may be found piercing the deep fascia.

The posterior branch of the medial anterior cutaneous nerve of the thigh has been found already on the medial side of the thigh [Fig. 94]. Follow it now, as it descends to the back of the calf. The peroneal communicating nerve (a branch of the common peroneal) may be found at the lower and lateral part of the popliteal area as it pierces the deep fascia [Fig. 111]. Sometimes, however, the nerve pierces the deep fascia much lower down and will not be found until the back of the leg is dissected. After the structures mentioned have been secured and cleaned, remove the remains of the superficial fascia, but avoid injury to the deep fascia.

Deep Fascia

The popliteal fascia is thin, but it possesses considerable strength owing to the transverse fibres which are interwoven amidst its longitudinal fibres. It is firmly attached, on each side, to the tendons of the muscles which bound the popliteal fossa.

BOUNDARIES OF THE POPLITEAL FOSSA

The fossa is bounded above and laterally by the biceps femoris muscle; above and medially by the semitendinosus and the semimembranosus muscles, supplemented by the

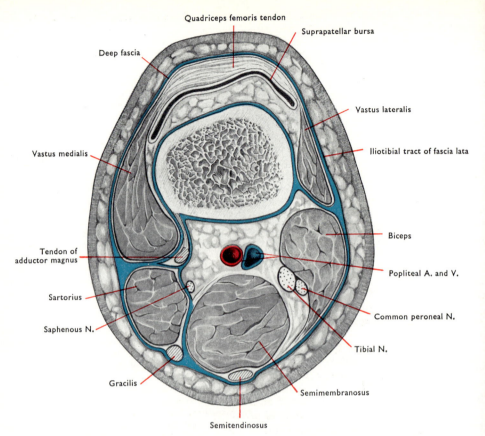

Quadriceps femoris tendon

Suprapatellar bursa

Deep fascia

Vastus lateralis

Vastus medialis

Iliotibial tract of fascia lata

Tendon of
adductor magnus

Biceps

Popliteal A. and V.

Sartorius

Saphenous N.

Common peroneal N.

Tibial N.

Gracilis

Semimembranosus

Semitendinosus

FIG. 116 Transverse section though proximal part of popliteal region of thigh.

gracilis, the sartorius and the tendon of the adductor magnus—the semitendinosus lying on the back of the semimembranosus, while the other muscles lie anteriorly. The lower part of the fossa is bounded by the two heads of the gastrocnemius as they converge [FIG. 115], and the lateral head is supplemented by a small muscle called the plantaris, which lies along its medial border.

When the popliteal fossa is opened up by dissection it has the appearance of a diamond-shaped space of considerable size; but it should be appreciated that the muscles are tightly packed together when the fascia is in position, and that the fossa is merely a small

intermuscular interval between the distal ends of the hamstring muscles [FIGS. 115, 116]. Thus in life the fossa is less than 2·5 cm. wide at its broadest part, and only a small portion of the popliteal artery, just above the knee joint, is not covered by muscles.

DISSECTION. Make an incision through the deep fascia along the medial margin of the upper lateral boundary; turn the fascia laterally and expose the biceps femoris. Clean the muscle and its tendon. Make an incision through the deep fascia along the lateral margin of the upper medial border, and reflect the fascia towards the medial side to expose the semitendinosus tendon and semimembranosus muscle. Follow the tendon of the semitendinosus to the level

172

of the medial condyle of the tibia; then pull it aside and clean the distal part of the semimembranosus and its tendon. Pull the part of that muscle which lies at the level of the medial condyle of the femur towards the medial side of the knee and display the semimembranosus bursa, which lies between the semimembranosus and the medial head of the gastrocnemius. Open the bursa and find whether it communicates with the bursa in front of the gastrocnemius, and whether that bursa communicates with the cavity of the knee joint. Now pull the semitendinosus and semimembranosus laterally, and clean the gracilis. The saphenous nerve emerges between the gracilis and the sartorius, accompanied by an artery; secure the artery and nerve and follow them downwards with the great saphenous vein.

Lastly pull the gracilis medially and clean the distal part of the adductor magnus.

CONTENTS OF THE POPLITEAL FOSSA
[FIGS. 117, 118]

The principal objects in the fossa are the **tibial** and **common peroneal nerves** and the **popliteal artery** and **vein,** with their branches and tributaries; but the most superficial structure in the upper part of the space is the **posterior cutaneous nerve of the thigh.** This nerve runs along the middle line, immediately subjacent to the popliteal fascia,

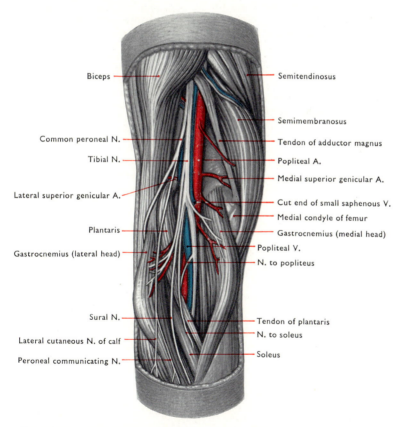

Biceps — — — Semitendinosus

— — Semimembranosus

Common peroneal N. — — Tendon of adductor magnus

Tibial N. — — Popliteal A.

— Medial superior genicular A.

Lateral superior genicular A. — — Cut end of small saphenous V.

— Medial condyle of femur

Plantaris — — Gastrocnemius (medial head)

— Popliteal V.

Gastrocnemius (lateral head) — — N. to popliteus

Sural N. — — Tendon of plantaris

— N. to soleus

Lateral cutaneous N. of calf — — Soleus

Peroneal communicating N. —

FIG. 117 Dissection of left popliteal fossa. The upper boundaries have been pulled apart and the aponeurosis to which the two heads of the gastrocnemius are attached has been split and the heads separated. For deeper dissection see FIG. 118.

until it pierces that fascia in the lower part of the space. It sends one or two branches through the fascia to the skin.

The tibial nerve is separated from the posterior cutaneous nerve of the thigh by a thin layer of fat, and lies superficial to the popliteal vessels, which are situated in a much deeper plane, in close contact with each other. The common peroneal nerve lies along the upper lateral boundary of the fossa. Both these nerves give off branches, most of which are easily found, but their articular branches are delicate and are easily destroyed by the dissector who does not exercise care. One of the articular nerves is derived from the posterior division of the obturator nerve. It is a slender filament that descends in close apposition to the popliteal artery.

Other important contents of the fossa are **lymph nodes,** some of which lie relatively superficial, near the point where the small saphenous vein pierces the popliteal fascia, but the majority are deeply placed alongside the popliteal vessels.

DISSECTION. Secure the posterior cutaneous nerve of the thigh at the point where it pierces the popliteal fascia, and follow it to the upper angle of the fossa; then remove the remains of the popliteal fascia from the upper part of the popliteal area.

Now pull the posterior cutaneous nerve aside with a hook, and cut through the fat in the upper angle of the fossa till a large nerve—the tibial—is exposed. Follow the nerve downwards and secure its cutaneous, muscular and articular branches. Its cutaneous branch—the sural nerve—descends between the two heads of the gastrocnemius. Follow that branch to the distal angle of the fossa. The articular branches are three in number—superior medial genicular, inferior medial genicular and middle genicular. The superior branch arises at or above the upper angle of the fossa, and the other two at lower levels. Follow them as far as possible. The muscular branches arise about the middle of the fossa and pass to the two heads of the gastrocnemius, the plantaris, the soleus and the popliteus. Separate the heads of the gastrocnemius and trace these branches to the muscles—except the nerve to the popliteus, which lies deeply and will be followed in a subsequent dissection.

Return to the upper angle of the fossa and secure the

common peroneal nerve. Follow it to the lateral angle and thence to the back of the head of the fibula, avoiding injury to its branches. Look for its genicular branches. They arise high up in the fossa or above the fossa; the upper one passes out of the fossa above the lateral femoral condyle; the lower one accompanies the nerve trunk out of the fossa. Secure the peroneal communicating branch and the lateral cutaneous nerve of the calf. They arise from the common peroneal near the lateral angle of the fossa (sometimes by a common stem). Follow them downwards.

Next clean the plantaris and the two heads of the gastrocnemius, dividing the muscular arteries if they are in the way. Separate the plantaris from the lateral head, avoiding injury to the nerve to the soleus which passes between them.

Now clean the popliteal vessels and their branches and tributaries. Begin by pulling the tibial nerve laterally and clearing away the fat that lies superficial to the vessels. The popliteal vein is encountered first. Look in the groove between the upper part of the artery and the vein for the genicular branch of the obturator nerve. It is a mere filament, and easily escapes notice. If you find it, trace it downwards to the back of the knee joint, and upwards into the substance of the adductor magnus.

Then clean the popliteal vein. Not uncommonly, there are accessory venous channels that communicate with the main vein and anastomose with one another around the artery. If they are present, remove them, but be careful of the branches of the artery, and preserve the small saphenous vein.

Next clean the popliteal artery and its branches. The muscular branches are met with first. Clean them and divide them, noting particularly the large size of the branches that enter each head of the gastrocnemius with its nerve at a well-defined neurovascular hilum. Now scrape the fatty tissue from the popliteal surface of the femur with the handle of the knife, but take care of the articular vessels and nerves. The articular or genicular arteries spring from the popliteal artery; they lie close to the floor of the fossa and are joined by the genicular nerves. They were seen, therefore, when the nerves were traced. Follow the two superior and inferior pairs out of the fossa, and the single, middle artery to the middle of the posterior capsule of the knee joint.

FLOOR OF THE POPLITEAL FOSSA

The floor is formed from above downwards by: (1) the popliteal surface of the femur; (2) the capsule of the knee joint; and (3) a strong fascia which covers the popliteus muscle.

Tibial Nerve

This nerve (L. 4, 5 ; S. 1, 2, 3) is the larger of the two terminal branches of the sciatic nerve and begins about the middle of the back of the thigh. It enters the fossa at its upper angle emerging from under cover of the biceps femoris, and bisects the fossa. It lies superficially in the fossa and crosses the vessels from lateral to medial as it descends [Fig. 117]. Thus the branches which it gives to the lateral head of gastrocnemius, plantaris, and soleus in the lower part of the fossa, cross superficial to the vessels to reach these muscles.

Branches. The **sural nerve** is the cutaneous branch. It arises about the middle of the fossa, and runs downwards in the furrow between the two heads of the gastrocnemius into the back of the leg, and thence, along the lateral side of the foot, to the little toe [Fig. 111].

Muscular branches supply both heads of the gastrocnemius, the plantaris, the soleus and the popliteus : they come off in the distal part of the fossa. The branch to the soleus passes between the plantaris and the lateral head of the gastrocnemius, and enters the superficial surface of the soleus near its upper end. (The soleus receives another motor nerve on its deep surface.) The branch to the popliteus arises lower down than the others, and having crossed behind the popliteal artery, descends over the popliteus muscle.

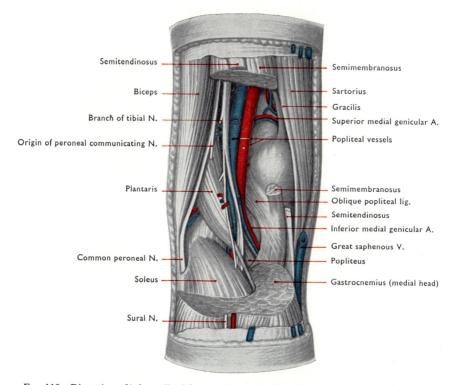

Fig. 118   Dissection of left popliteal fossa. The two heads of the gastrocnemius and portions of the semimembranosus and semitendinosus have been removed. For more superficial dissections, see Figs. 115, 117.

and gains the anterior surface of the muscle by winding round its distal border. It will be seen better when the popliteus muscle is dissected. This little nerve gives branches also to the interosseous membrane and the superior tibiofibular joint.

Articular branches are given off in the upper part of the fossa—sometimes even above the fossa. They accompany the corresponding genicular arteries, and supply the ligaments and synovial membrane of the knee joint. The **superior medial genicular nerve** runs medially, above the medial condyle of the femur, deep to the muscles. The **middle genicular nerve** pierces the oblique popliteal ligament of the knee joint to supply the cruciate ligaments in the interior.

The **inferior medial genicular nerve** is larger than the other two, and more easily found. It runs downwards and medially along the upper border of the popliteus muscle, and then curves forwards below the medial condyle of the tibia, under cover of the tibial collateral ligament of the knee.

Common Peroneal Nerve

This nerve (L. 4, 5; S. 1, 2) is the smaller of the two terminal divisions of the sciatic nerve. It arises about the middle of the thigh, runs downwards and laterally along the medial border of the biceps femoris, and leaves the popliteal fossa at its lateral angle. Here it crosses the plantaris and the lateral head of the gastrocnemius, passes behind the head of the fibula, and turning forwards ends between the lateral side of the neck of the fibula and the peroneus longus by dividing into two branches named the **superficial peroneal nerve** and the **deep peroneal nerve**. In the fossa it is covered only by skin and fasciae and, in the living limb, it can easily be rolled under the finger where it lies on the fibula.

Cutaneous Branches. The **peroneal communicating nerve** arises in the upper part of the popliteal fossa, and runs downwards into the calf to join the sural nerve at a varying level. It frequently takes origin by a common stem with the following branch.

The **lateral cutaneous nerve of the calf** arises

from the common peroneal on the lateral head of the gastrocnemius. It pierces the deep fascia almost at once, and descends to supply the skin of the lateral and anterior surfaces of the upper part of the leg.

Articular Branches. The **superior** and **inferior lateral genicular** nerves accompany the lateral genicular arteries. They are of small size, and it is difficult to find them.

The **recurrent genicular nerve** springs from the termination of the common peroneal nerve. It runs upwards to the front of the knee, and will be dissected at a later stage.

Popliteal Artery [FIGS. 118, 119]

The popliteal artery is the continuation of the femoral artery. It begins behind the femur at the tendinous opening in the adductor magnus, and it terminates at the distal

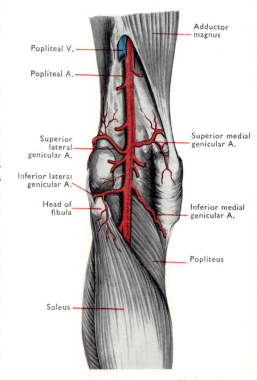

FIG. 119   Left popliteal artery and its branches.

border of the popliteus muscle by dividing into the anterior and posterior tibial arteries. The division is hidden from view at present by the upper border of the soleus muscle; but it will be exposed when the leg is dissected.

The artery lies deep on the floor of the fossa in contact with the femur, the capsule of the knee joint, and the fascia covering popliteus. It is covered by semimembranosus above, by the heads of gastrocnemius and the soleus below, and is crossed posteriorly by the vein and the tibial nerve.

Branches. Muscular branches are distributed to the hamstring muscles and to the muscles of the calf of the leg.

Cutaneous branches are irregular twigs that arise from the muscular branches; the most constant of them accompanies the upper part of the sural nerve.

Articular branches lie on the floor of the fossa and accompany the genicular nerves.

Two **superior genicular arteries** spring from the main trunk in the interval between the upper parts of the condyles of the femur. Two **inferior genicular arteries** arise opposite the knee joint. Their course around the knee joint is shown in FIGURES 119 and 144.

The **middle genicular artery** springs from the

popliteal as it lies on the oblique popliteal ligament of the knee joint. It pierces that ligament to reach the synovial membrane and the cruciate ligaments in the interior of the joint.

Genicular Branch of the Obturator Nerve. This slender filament is the continuation of the posterior division of the obturator nerve. It enters the popliteal fossa by piercing the distal part of the adductor magnus close to the linea aspera, then lies on the posterior surface of the popliteal artery, and enters the knee joint after passing through the oblique popliteal ligament.

Popliteal Vein

This vessel is formed by the junction of the venae comitantes of the anterior and posterior tibial arteries near the distal border of popliteus. It lies in the same fibrous sheath as the popliteal artery and crosses it superficially from medial to posterolateral as it ascends. It receives tributaries corresponding to the branches of the artery, and the small saphenous vein. By slitting it open with the scissors the dissector will see that it has three (sometimes four) valves in its interior.

THE BACK OF THE THIGH

DISSECTION. Reflexion of Skin. Make a vertical incision through the middle of the belt of skin which still covers the region [Fig. 110], and reflect the two flaps.

Look for the branches of the posterior cutaneous nerve of the thigh along the middle of the back of the thigh; they vary in number, and position [Fig. 111, p. 161]. To facilitate the search for them, find the trunk of the nerve in the gluteal region, and pull gently on it.

Follow the branches of the lateral cutaneous and the medial anterior cutaneous nerves from the portions of those nerves which were displayed when the front of the thigh was dissected.

Remove the remains of the superficial fascia to display the deep fascia.

Divide the deep fascia by a longitudinal incision, taking care not to injure the posterior cutaneous nerve of the thigh which lies immediately under cover of the

fascia. Turn the two flaps of deep fascia aside, and clean the posterior cutaneous nerve.

Then clean the posterior surfaces of the hamstring muscles. Having done so, follow the sciatic nerve from the buttock downwards, and trace its branches into the hamstring muscles and adductor magnus; special care should be taken to identify the nerve of supply to the short head of the biceps which, unlike the others, arises from the lateral side of the main nerve. At the same time, note the muscular arteries that run with or near the nerves; they come from the perforating branches of the profunda artery.

Now clean the semitendinosus and both heads of the biceps thoroughly from end to end (retaining their nerves), and dissect their attachments carefully. Pull the semitendinosus and the long head of the biceps laterally, and deal in like manner with the semimembranosus.

Posterior Cutaneous Nerve of Thigh [S. 1, 2, 3]

This long slender nerve arises in the pelvis from the sacral plexus. It escapes from the pelvis through the lower part of the greater sciatic foramen in close company with the inferior gluteal nerve and vessels, and descends in the gluteal region, under cover of the gluteus maximus, over the back of the sciatic nerve or along its medial border. Leaving the gluteal region, and entering the back of the thigh, the sciatic nerve disappears under cover of the long head of the biceps, while the posterior cutaneous nerve runs straight down the middle of the back of the thigh immediately under cover of the deep fascia. It pierces the deep fascia at the back of the knee, and its terminal part descends in the superficial fascia as far as half-way down the calf of the leg.

Branches. All are cutaneous [FIG. 111].

(1) Two or three **gluteal branches** arise in the gluteal region, and wind round the lower border of the gluteus maximus to supply a limited area of skin in the lower part of the buttock. (2) A **perineal branch** arises in the gluteal region and turns medially below the ischial tuberosity across the back of the hamstring muscles to reach the perineum; it gives off a few fine branches to the skin of the uppermost part of the medial side of the thigh, and its terminal branches help to supply the skin of the external genital organs. (3) Several small **branches to the thigh** pierce the deep fascia and supply skin of the medial side and the back of the thigh. (4) The terminal branch ramifies to supply the skin of the upper half of the calf of the leg.

FLEXOR MUSCLES

Their fleshy bellies make up the muscular mass on the back of the thigh; and their tendons in the ham or popliteal region give them the colloquial name of the **hamstrings.**

Biceps Femoris

The **long head** arises, by a tendon common to it and the semitendinosus [FIG. 112, p. 163], from the upper medial part of the ischial tuberosity. Some fibres from the sacrotuber-

ous ligament are continued into it. The **short head** arises from the linea aspera and the upper half of the lateral supracondylar ridge. The tendon of insertion descends across the posterolateral surface of the knee joint to reach its insertion into the head of the fibula. Near the insertion, the tendon overlies the fibular collateral ligament of the knee, which first grooves the tendon deeply and then splits its lower end into two unequal parts [FIG. 128].

Nerve supply: that to the long head is derived from the **tibial part** of the **sciatic nerve,** and that to the short head from the **common peroneal part;** in a wound, one head may therefore be paralysed without the other head being affected. Action: it flexes the knee joint and rotates the flexed leg laterally. The long head is also an extensor of the hip joint.

Semitendinosus

This muscle arises—in common with the long head of the biceps—from the tuberosity of the ischium [FIGS. 112, 128]. The muscular belly ends, in the distal third of the thigh, in a long, cylindrical tendon which passes downwards on the semimembranosus muscle. At the medial side of the knee, the tendon bends forwards, and spreads out to be inserted chiefly into the upper part of the medial surface of the tibia with the tendon of the gracilis. The **subtendinous bursa** of the **sartorius** separates these tendons from the tendon of that muscle, and another bursa separates the semitendinosus from the tibial collateral ligament of the knee; the two bursae communicate so freely that they are, in fact, one bilocular bursa.

Nerve supply: it has an incomplete tendinous intersection on its posterior surface and therefore receives two branches from the **tibial part** of the **sciatic nerve,** one above and one below it. Action: it is a flexor of the knee, a medial rotator of the flexed leg, and an extensor of the hip joint.

Semimembranosus

The semimembranosus arises by a broad tendon from the upper lateral part of the tuberosity of the ischium [FIGS. 112, 141].

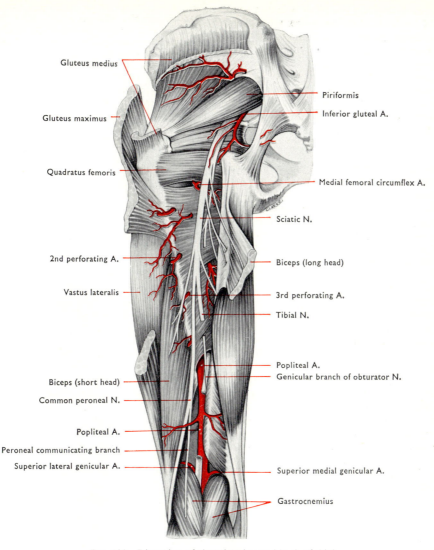

Gluteus medius

Gluteus maximus

Quadratus femoris

2nd perforating A.

Vastus lateralis

Biceps (short head)

Common peroneal N.

Popliteal A.

Peroneal communicating branch

Superior lateral genicular A.

Piriformis

Inferior gluteal A.

Medial femoral circumflex A.

Sciatic N.

Biceps (long head)

3rd perforating A.

Tibial N.

Popliteal A.

Genicular branch of obturator N.

Superior medial genicular A.

Gastrocnemius

FIG. 120   Dissection of gluteal region and back of thigh.

The tendon of origin passes downwards and medially in front of the biceps femoris and the semitendinosus, and is folded in such a manner as to form a groove in which the semitendinosus lies. The fleshy belly arises from this tendon and, at the back of the knee, it becomes a thick, flattened tendon which is inserted chiefly into the floor of the groove on the back of the medial condyle of the tibia. It sends extensions which form: (1) the oblique popliteal ligament of the knee joint, and (2) the fascia of the popliteus, through

179

which it obtains an insertion into the soleal line of the tibia. The **semimembranosus bursa** lies between the tendon and the medial head of the gastrocnemius, and often curves round the medial side of the gastrocnemius to communicate with a bursa which lies between that head and the back of the knee joint.

Nerve supply: the **tibial part** of the **sciatic nerve.** Action: its actions are the same as those of the semitendinosus.

SCIATIC NERVE

The sciatic nerve emerges from the pelvis through the greater sciatic foramen, descends through the gluteal region [p. 166] and the back of the thigh under cover of the long head of the biceps on the posterior surface of the adductor magnus. It ends, at a variable point above the popliteal fossa, by dividing into the common peroneal and tibial nerves.

In the thigh it is close to the back of the femur, and its compression against the femur gives rise to a 'sleeping foot'.

Branches. The branches that spring from the trunk of the sciatic nerve supply the hamstrings and the ischial part of the adductor magnus. Separate branches arise for the two heads of the biceps; the branch to the short head comes from the common peroneal part of the nerve, and the branch to the long head from the tibial part. Two branches pass to the semitendinosus, and those for the semimembranosus and the adductor magnus often arise by a common stem. The portion of the adductor magnus supplied by the sciatic nerve belongs to the flexor group and is essentially a part of the hamstrings.

ADDUCTOR MUSCLES AND PROFUNDA FEMORIS ARTERY

DISSECTION. To bring the adductor magnus more fully into view, detach the hamstring muscles from their origins and turn them aside. First, detach the common tendon of the biceps and semitendinosus. Examine the origin of the semimembranosus again and then detach it also. The posterior surface of the adductor magnus, now fully exposed, should be cleaned, taking care to preserve the branch from the sciatic nerve that runs across it to enter the muscle near its medial border. Define the extensive insertion of the muscle into the

back of the femur. At the same time secure the perforating arteries. They are a series of four arteries which perforate the adductor magnus at its insertion. Trace them laterally through the gluteus maximus and the short head of the biceps into the vastus lateralis.

Define again the attachments of the pectineus and the adductors longus and brevis to the femur. The adductor longus requires most care becasue of its extreme thinness as it approaches the bone. The profunda vessels lie behind the longus, close to the femur—the vein in front of the artery. Clean the profunda vein and preserve it, but remove its tributaries. Then clean the artery. Divide the branches which it gives to muscles in this situation, but clean and preserve those of its branches which cling to the femur: they are the perforating arteries.

Profunda Femoris Artery

This large vessel is the chief artery of supply to the muscles of the thigh. It arises, in the

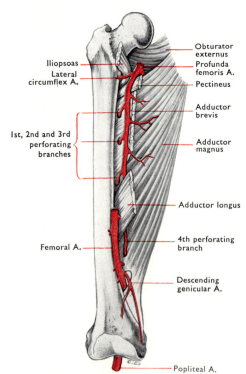

FIG. 121 Profunda femoris artery and its branches. The upper part of adductor longus has been removed to expose the artery.

Obturator externus
Iliopsoas
Lateral circumflex A.
Profunda femoris A.
Pectineus
Adductor brevis
1st, 2nd and 3rd perforating branches
Adductor magnus
Adductor longus
4th perforating branch
Femoral A.
Descending genicular A.
Popliteal A.

femoral triangle, from the posterolateral side of the femoral artery, about 4–5 cm. below the inguinal ligament. It descends curving medially behind the femoral vessels, leaves the femoral triangle by passing posteriorly between the pectineus and the adductor longus, and then descends behind the adductor longus, close to the femur. It gives off the **lateral** and **medial circumflex** arteries, a number of muscular branches, and the first three **perforating arteries,** and ends a little below the middle of the thigh as a fine terminal vessel, called the **fourth perforating artery,** which passes backwards through the adductor magnus.

The **circumflex arteries** have been studied already [pp. 150, 168]. The **muscular branches** are inconsistent; they supply the adductor muscles, and some of them pierce the adductor magnus to reach the hamstring muscles.

Perforating Arteries. These four arteries arise in series from the profunda—the first, where it slips behind the adductor longus, and the fourth as its terminal branch. They wind round the back of the femur, sometimes grooving the bone, and they all end in the vastus lateralis. As they pierce the muscles attached to the back of the femur they are protected by fibrous arches. On their way they give branches to the adductors and the hamstrings; the second or the third sends a **nutrient artery** into the femur, and another nutrient artery may arise from the fourth.

Arterial Anastomoses. In the back of the thigh there is a longitudinal anastomosis between the branches of the internal iliac, the femoral, and the popliteal arteries. Thus the gluteal arteries anastomose with each other and with the circumflex femoral arteries; the latter link up with the perforating arteries which anastomose among themselves, and with the branches of the popliteal artery to the hamstrings. Thus an alternative arterial supply to the limb exists by this route.

THE HIP JOINT

The hip joint is the most perfect example in the body of a ball-and-socket joint. It does not allow so free a range of movement as that which takes place at the shoulder joint, but what it loses in this respect it gains in strength and stability. Its great strength and security depend: (1) upon the depth of the acetabulum and upon the fact that its mouth is reduced in width by a circular band called the labrum acetabulare, which is attached to its lips; (2) upon the tension and strength of the ligaments; (3) upon the length and oblique direction of the neck of the femur; (4) upon the strength of the surrounding muscles; and (5) upon atmospheric pressure.

LIGAMENTS OF THE HIP JOINT

Articular Capsule

The fibrous capsule is exceedingly strong, and surrounds the joint on all sides. **Proximally,** it is attached around the acetabulum. **Distally,** it clasps the neck of the femur: the anterior part of this attachment is to the whole length of the intertrochanteric line and to the root of the greater trochanter, and it is very firm and strong. Posteriorly, it falls short of the intertrochanteric crest by about a finger-breadth, and its attachment to the neck of the femur is weak.

When the capsule of the hip joint has been carefully cleaned, it will be seen that the fibres which compose it run in two different directions. The majority pass obliquely from the hip bone to the femur. There are, however, other fibres which encircle the capsule more or less parallel to the margin of the acetabulum. They constitute the **zona orbicularis** and are seen to advantage in the posterior and inferior parts of the capsule, where they were noted during the dissection of the gluteal region [p. 169]. The oblique fibres are most massed on the front of the joint.

There are three thickened portions of the capsule.

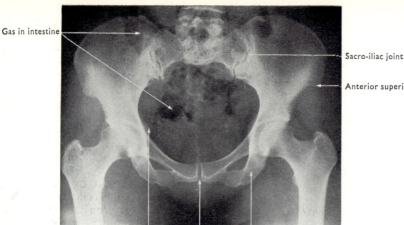

Gas in intestine

Sacro-iliac joint

Anterior superior iliac spine

Ischial spine Pubic Ischial
symphysis tuberosity

FIG. 122 Radiograph of female pelvis. This has been taken with the pelvis slightly tilted so that the coccyx and ischial spines lie at a higher level than normal. Note how the inferior margins of the neck of the femur and the superior ramus of the pubis lie in a continuous arched line.

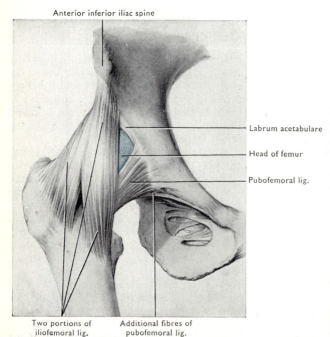

Anterior inferior iliac spine

Labrum acetabulare

Head of femur

Pubofemoral lig.

Two portions of Additional fibres of
iliofemoral lig, pubofemoral lig.

FIG. 123 Dissection of hip joint from the front.

Iliofemoral Ligament. The iliofemoral ligament is placed over the front of the joint, and is the thickest and most powerful part of the capsule. Proximally, it is attached to the inferior half of the anterior inferior iliac spine and to the depressed surface immediately lateral to that spine. Distally, it widens to be attached to the intertrochanteric line of the femur. It is thicker at the sides than in the middle, and these thickenings give the ligament the appearance of an inverted Y [FIG. 123].

The iliofemoral ligament is more than 0·5 cm. thick, and is one of the strongest ligaments in the body—its only rival being the interosseous sacro-iliac ligament. A strain varying from 250 lbs to 750 lbs is required for its rupture. It is rarely torn asunder in dislocation of the hip joint, and, consequently, the surgeon is able in most cases to overcome the displacement by manipulation.

Pubofemoral Ligament. The pubofemoral ligament is the name applied to fasciculi which spring from the pubic bone and the obturator membrane, and join the lower and anterior part of the capsule. When the bursa of the iliopsoas is continuous with the cavity of the joint the aperture of communication is placed between this band and the iliofemoral ligament.

Ischiofemoral Ligament. The ischiofemoral ligament is a comparatively weak band which springs from the ischium below the acetabulum, and passes upwards and laterally to blend with the posterior part of the capsule.

Movements Permitted at the Hip Joint

Test the range of movement of your own joint. **Flexion,** or forward movement, is very free and is only checked by the thigh coming into contact with the abdominal wall. **Extension,** or backward movement, is very restricted by the iliofemoral ligament; the ability to carry the limb posteriorly to the horizontal plane is achieved by flexing the trunk on the opposite limb, i.e., tilting the pelvis forwards on that joint. In the erect posture the line of gravity falls slightly behind the line joining the central points of the two hip joints, but the taut iliofemoral ligaments prevent extension of the joints and materially assist in the maintenance of this posture. **Abduction,** or lateral movement of the limb, is checked by the pubofemoral ligament. **Adduction,** or medial movement (e.g., as in crossing one thigh over the other), is limited by the lateral portion of the iliofemoral ligament and the upper part of the capsule. **Rotation medially** tightens the ischiofemoral ligament, and is therefore, in a measure, restrained by it. **Rotation laterally** is limited by the lateral portion of the iliofemoral ligament. In **circumduction,** which is produced by combination of the movements of flexion, abduction, extension, and adduction, different parts of the fibrous capsule are tightened at different stages of the movement.

DISSECTION. The hip joint should now be opened. Isolate the iliofemoral ligament by incisions along its borders, and then remove all other parts of the capsule. The object of this dissection is to enable the dissector to appreciate the thickness and great strength of the iliofemoral ligament.

Transverse Ligament of Acetabulum

This is a strong band of fibres that bridges across the acetabular notch, and is attached to the margins of the notch. It completes the rim of the acetabulum, and converts the notch into a foramen through which vessels and nerves enter the joint.

Labrum Acetabulare

The acetabular lip is a firm fibrocartilaginous ring which is fixed to the rim of the acetabulum. It deepens the cavity of the acetabulum, and at the same time narrows its mouth to a slight extent. The labrum fits closely upon the head of the femur, and, acting like a sucker, exercises an important influence in retaining it in place. Both surfaces of the labrum are covered with synovial membrane; its free margin is thin, but it is much thicker at its attachment to the acetabular rim.

Ligament of the Head of Femur

This band is flat and fan-shaped. Its narrow end is implanted into the pit on the head of the femur; its flattened end is bifid, and is fixed to the margins of the acetabular notch, and also to the transverse ligament. This attachment can be defined by the removal of the synovial membrane and some areolar tissue. The ligament is surrounded by a prolongation of the synovial membrane; and a small artery runs along it to the head of the femur.

It is doubtful if it plays any part in the mechanism of the hip joint, as it is often a very weak structure. It becomes very tense when the thigh is slightly flexed and then adducted—which, however, is an attitude seldom taken up.

Synovial Membrane and Interior of the Joint

A mass of soft fat occupies the non-articular fossa of the acetabulum. Upon this the ligament of the head of the femur is placed and articular twigs from the obturator vessels and

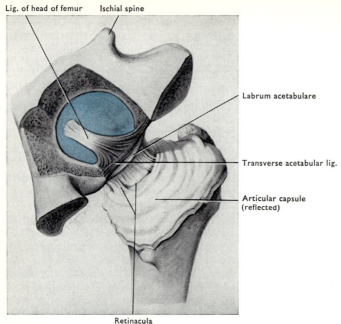

Lig. of head of femur   Ischial spine

Labrum acetabulare

Transverse acetabular lig.

Articular capsule
(reflected)

Retinacula

FIG. 124   Dissection of right hip joint from pelvic side. The floor of the acetabulum has been removed, and the articular capsule of the joint thrown laterally towards the trochanters.

nerve enter it by passing through the acetabular notch.

The **synovial membrane** lines the inner surface of the fibrous capsule; it is reflected from it on to the neck of the femur, and it clothes the bone as far as the margin of the articular cartilage of the head. Along the line of reflexion some fibres of the fibrous capsule run upwards on the neck of the femur and raise up ridges of the synovial membrane. These fibres are termed the **retinacula** of the neck of the femur.

In intracapsular fracture of the neck of the emur the retinacula may escape rupt ure,

and they may then, to some extent, hold the fragments in apposition—hence the name retinacula. Like the ligament of the head, they serve as pathways for small arteries of supply to the head of the femur, so that their rupture in a fracture of the neck may imperil the blood supply to the head.

At the acetabular attachment of the capsule the synovial membrane is reflected on to the labrum acetabulare and invests both its surfaces. It covers also the articular surface of the transverse ligament and the cushion of fat which occupies the acetabular fossa. Lastly it gives a tubular investment to the ligament of the head of the femur.

Blood Vessels and Nerves

The **arteries** that supply the hip joint are derived from the gluteal, circumflex and obturator arteries. The **nerves** come from: (1) the nerve to quadratus femoris, (2) the femoral, through the nerve to rectus femoris, (3) the anterior division of the obturator nerve, and (4), occasionally, the accessory obturator.

REMOVAL OF THE LOWER LIMB. If the dissection of other parts necessitates the removal of the lower limb, this can be done by dividing the ligament of the head of the femur and the iliofemoral ligament, otherwise the limb may be left attached to the hip bone.

THE LEG AND THE FOOT

SURFACE ANATOMY

The head of the fibula, the condyles and tubercle of the tibia have been examined already. Identify them again.

The malleoli are the prominences at the sides of the ankle, which grip the talus between them. The **medial malleolus** is a thick, downward projection from the lower end of the tibia; the **lateral malleolus** is the lower end of the fibula. Their posterior surfaces are in the same coronal plane. The lateral malleolus is the narrower and therefore does not extend forwards so far as the medial one does, but it juts downwards further and articulates, therefore, with a larger area of the talus.

The **neck of the fibula** and the greater part of its **shaft** are buried among muscles, but can be felt through them. The lower, anterolateral part of the shaft is subcutaneous, and is the bone felt above the lateral malleolus.

The shin is the **anterior border of the shaft of the tibia.** It is inconspicuous but it is subcutaneous, and is readily felt if the finger is passed along it. It runs slightly sinuously from the tuberosity of the tibia to the anterior margin of the medial malleolus; it is a sharp edge except towards its lower end. The **medial surface of the tibia,** wide and flat, is easily felt from end to end. Its uppermost part is covered by the tendons of the sartorius, gracilis and semitendinosus; the rest is subcutaneous. The **medial border** of the tibia also is easily felt from end to end; the saphenous nerve and the great saphenous vein run along it [FIG. 94].

On the back of the leg the fleshy prominence of the calf is due to the gastrocnemius and the underlying soleus. These two muscles are thrown into contraction when the heel is raised, *e.g.,* in standing on the toes. The outlines of the two heads of the gastrocnemius are then clearly seen if the limb is thin; it is obvious also that the soleus reaches further down, and that, at the middle of the calf, it is wider than the gastrocnemius. The muscles taper inferiorly to become continuous with the **tendo calcaneus,** which is the strong, thick tendon above the heel. Grasp the tendo calcaneus between finger and thumb. Note that it is nearly 2·5 cm. behind the bones of the leg, the interval being filled with fat and fibrous tissue. Press the fingers on the anterior wall of the hollows at the sides of the tendo calcaneus: the backs of the malleoli can be felt, though tendons cover them and, on the medial side, the pulse of the **posterior tibial artery** may be felt in the living limb [FIG. 142].

The bone of the heel is the calcaneus. Grip its posterior part (tuber) between finger and thumb. The **lateral** and **medial processes** of its lower surface make low, blunt prominences on the sides near the sole. Its **lateral surface** is nearly all subcutaneous, and is easily felt below the lateral malleolus as a wide surface that extends forwards from the back of the heel for 5 cm. or more. The **peroneal trochlea** (when present) is felt as a little prominence about a finger-breadth below the lateral malleolus. On the medial side, the **sustentaculum tali** provides the bony resistance felt a thumb-breadth below the medial malleolus.

The **talus** rests on the upper surface of the calcaneus. Its **body** is hidden below the tibia, between the malleoli; but when the foot is plantar flexed (*i.e.,* when the toes are pointed) the anterior part of the body protrudes from below the tibia. Invert the foot (*i.e.,* twist it so that the sole faces medially). The **head** of the talus then makes a rounded prominence about 2·5 cm. in front of the lateral malleolus and, lateral to the head of the talus, the anterior end of the calcaneus makes an uneven projection.

On the medial side of the foot the landmark most often referred to is the **tuberosity of the navicular bone.** It makes a prominence, blunt and indistinct but easily felt, 2·5–3·5 cm. below and in front of the medial malleolus, about midway between the back of the heel and the root of the big toe, at the level of the lip of the shoe. The bones felt in front of the tuberosity are first the **medial cuneiform bone** and then the **first metatarsal bone.**

On the lateral side the **tuberosity of the fifth metatarsal bone** is a prominent landmark, midway between the point of the heel and the root of the little toe. The **cuboid bone** lies hidden in the side of the foot between that tuberosity and the calcaneus. The **head of the fifth metatarsal bone** is at the root of the little toe, at the widest part of the foot, and forms a rounded bulge. Note that it is much further back than the root of the big toe, and that, when the foot is shod, it is so far from the toe of the shoe that it may be mistaken for the base of the fifth metatarsal bone.

On the dorsum of the foot the metatarsus and the anterior part of the tarsus are under the extensor tendons and the extensor digitorum brevis muscle but the **metatarsal bones** can be felt individually through them. The **extensor digitorum brevis** forms the soft, fleshy pad in front of the lateral malleolus. When the foot and toes are raised, the tendons spring up, and can be individually recognized by the student after he has dissected the region. Unlike the joints of the fingers, the joints of the toes do not have landmarks to indicate their position; their position is ascertained by manipulation.

The sole of the foot has the shape of a half-dome, the ball and lateral margin of the foot and the pad of the heel forming a curved line of contact with the ground. Inside this curve, the sole is concave and slopes upwards to the highest part of the arch on the medial margin of the foot midway between the pad of the heel and the ball of the great toe. It is this dome that is flattened in the condition known as flat foot. The ball of the foot lies under the metatarsophalangeal joints, and that of the great toe is large because of the size of the bones, and the two sesamoid bones on its plantar surface.

The smaller toes are usually flexed so permanently that the only parts seen in the sole are the pads that cover the terminal phalanges; the other phalanges are hidden in a narrow groove. But the groove widens medially so that the skin over the other phalanges of the second and big toes can be seen.

THE FRONT OF THE LEG AND DORSUM OF FOOT

It is convenient to dissect the dorsum of the foot at the same time as the front of the leg, so that the structures that pass over the ankle may be studied in their continuity.

DISSECTION. Raise the knee on a block; bend the foot down, i.e. plantar flex the ankle joint, and fasten it to the table with hooks. Reflect the skin from the lateral and medial sides of the leg as well as from the front by making incision 11 [Fig. 91, p. 132].

Raise the four flaps of skin thus mapped out from the subjacent fatty tissue, and dissect out the superficial veins and nerves.

The lateral cutaneous nerve of the calf was found in the dissection of the popliteal fossa. Trace it now to its termination on the anterolateral aspect of the leg.

Dissect the cutaneous veins next, for, on the dorsum of the foot, they are more superficial than the nerves, and in other situations they serve as guides to the nerves. Begin with the dorsal venous arch. It lies across the anterior part of the metatarsus. Follow it to the medial border of the foot, where it joins the commencement of the great saphenous vein. Next follow that vein upwards to the medial border of the tibia. Do not follow it further at present, but secure the saphenous nerve, which lies close to it, and follow the nerve into the foot.

Now follow the dorsal venous arch to the lateral margin of the foot, where it joins the commencement of the small saphenous vein. Follow the small saphenous vein backwards below the lateral malleolus, and there secure the sural nerve, which lies adjacent to the vein. Follow the sural nerve to the little toe, and, about the middle of the lateral border of the foot, secure the communicating twig which it gives to the lateral branch of the superficial peroneal nerve.

Come back to the dorsal venous arch. Find the dorsal digital veins and trace them on to the toes.

Now cut down through the fat, at the junction of the middle and distal thirds of the leg, about 2–3 cm. to the medial side of the fibula, and secure the trunk of the superficial peroneal nerve as it pierces the deep fascia. Follow it downwards to its division into medial and lateral branches, and then trace them and their subdivisions to their terminations on the toes.

Lastly dissect in the fascia between the first two metatarsal bones and find the cutaneous branch of the deep peroneal nerve as it pierces the deep fascia; trace it and its branches to the adjacent sides of the first and second toes.

CUTANEOUS VEINS

There are two **dorsal digital veins** in each toe. Those along adjacent sides of two toes unite to form a common stem which ends in the dorsal venous arch; those from the medial side of the big toe and lateral side of the little toe join the ends of the arch.

The **dorsal venous arch** lies in the superficial fascia on the anterior parts of the shafts of the metatarsal bones, superficial to the terminal branches of the superficial peroneal nerve, and receives the veins of the dorsum of the foot and toes. Its medial end joins the medial dorsal digital vein of the big toe to form the great saphenous vein and its lateral end unites with the lateral dorsal digital vein of the little toe to form the small saphenous vein.

The **small saphenous vein** runs backwards below the lateral malleolus, and then upwards behind it into the leg.

The **great saphenous vein** passes backwards along the medial side of the foot, and ascends in front of the medial malleolus into the leg, where it passes obliquely across the distal third of the tibia to reach its medial border, along which it ascends. In the lower part of the leg, the great saphenous vein and the saphenous nerve are very liable to injury, for they lie quite superficially between the skin and the bone.

Most of the superficial veins of the medial side of the foot and of the front of the leg end in the great saphenous vein; some of them form communications with the deep veins of the sole and the anterior tibial vein.

CUTANEOUS NERVES

The front of the leg, the dorsum of the foot, and the greater part of the dorsal surfaces of the toes are each supplied by three nerves, of which only the superficial peroneal is common to all three areas [FIG. 94].

The front of the leg is supplied on the medial side and in the infrapatellar region by the **saphenous nerve** (L. 3, 4), the remainder of the upper two-thirds by the **lateral cutaneous nerve of the calf,** and the lower third by the **superficial peroneal.**

The dorsum of the foot is supplied by the saphenous nerve on the medial side, by the **sural** nerve on the lateral side, and by the **superficial** peroneal nerve in the intermediate region.

The adjacent sides of the first and second toes are supplied by the **medial division** of the **deep peroneal nerve,** the lateral side of the little toe by the **sural nerve,** and all the remaining parts by branches of the **superficial peroneal nerve.**

The skin on the dorsal surfaces of the terminal phalanges is supplied by the plantar nerves, the lateral plantar supplying the fifth and lateral side of the fourth toes, the medial plantar supplying the remainder.

Superficial Peroneal Nerve (L. 4, 5; S. 1)

This is one of the two terminal branches of the common peroneal nerve. It begins on the lateral side of the neck of the fibula, descends between the muscles on the lateral side of the leg, and becomes cutaneous by piercing the deep fascia at the junction of the middle and distal thirds of the leg. It divides, either at once or shortly afterwards, into a medial and a lateral branch.

The **medial branch** supplies the medial part of the dorsum of the foot and divides into two branches; one is distributed to the medial side of the big toe, the other to the adjacent sides of the second and third toes. It also gives a communicating twig to the deep peroneal nerve [FIG. 94]. The **lateral branch** supplies the intermediate part of the dorsum of the foot, and also divides into two branches, of which one supplies the adjacent sides of the third and fourth toes, and the other, after receiving a twig from the sural nerve, supplies the adjacent sides of the fourth and fifth toes [FIG. 94]. The branches of both divisions lie deep to the dorsal venous arch.

Sural Nerve (S. 1, 2)

This nerve arises from the tibial nerve, descends over the gastrocnemius, pierces the deep fascia about half-way down the back of the leg, and is joined shortly afterwards by the peroneal communicating branch (L. 5; S. 1, 2) of the common peroneal nerve [FIG. 111]. It descends behind the lateral malleolus, and then, curving forwards below the malleolus, it runs along the lateral border of the foot to the little toe, giving branches on its way to the lateral part of the dorsum of the foot, and communicating with the superficial peroneal nerve. After it pierces the deep fascia it lies alongside the small saphenous vein.

DISSECTION. Remove the remains of the superficial fascia to display the deep fascia.

DEEP FASCIA

The deep fascia does not form a complete investment for the leg. It is absent over the subcutaneous part of the medial surface of the tibia, and is attached to the anterior and medial borders of that bone. It is absent over the triangular subcutaneous surface of the fibula also, being attached to the borders of that area. It is very thick in the proximal part of the front of the leg where it gives origin to the subjacent muscles. It becomes thinner towards the distal part of the leg, but thickened bands (**retinacula**) are formed in it at the ankle, and these act as slings around the tendons, holding them in position when the muscles of the leg contract. It becomes exceedingly thin and fine on the dorsum of the foot.

Retinacula

The **superior extensor retinaculum** is a strong, broad band which stretches across the front of the leg from tibia to fibula, immediately above the ankle joint.

The **inferior extensor retinaculum** is distal to the ankle joint. Laterally, it is fixed firmly to the anterior part of the calcaneus. Medially, it divides into two diverging bands. The upper band is attached to the medial malleolus; the lower band passes to the medial side of the foot, and merges into the deep fascia of the sole. The tendons that are strapped down by the extensor retinacula can be seen through the deep fascia as they emerge from under cover of the inferior retinaculum. From medial to lateral side they are : tibialis anterior, extensor hallucis longus, extensor digitorum longus and peroneus tertius [FIGS. 126, 131].

The two muscles on the lateral side of the leg are the **peroneus longus** and **peroneus brevis.** Their tendons descend over the back of the lateral malleolus, and then curve forwards below the malleolus. A thickened portion of the deep fascia straps them down on the back of the lateral malleolus, and is called the **superior peroneal retinaculum.** Another band—the **inferior peroneal retinaculum**—straps them down on the lateral surface of the calcaneus [FIG. 132]. Postero-inferior to the medial malleolus is the **flexor retinaculum.**

Intermuscular Septa [FIG. 125]

The deep fascia of the front and the lateral side of the leg sends in septa between the

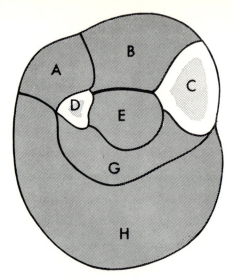

FIG. 125 Diagram of osteofascial compartments of leg. The interosseus membrane lies between B and E.

A. Peroneal muscles   Superficial peroneal N.
B. Extensors   Deep peroneal N.
C. Tibia
D. Fibula
E. Tibialis posterior
G. Long flexors of toes } Tibial N.
H. Superficial muscles of calf

muscles. These septa give partial origin to the muscles ; they are seen as white lines in the partially dissected limb, and their positions are indicated by narrow grooves in a thin, living limb when the muscles are thrown into contraction.

Two of the septa are longer and stronger than the others, and are called the anterior and posterior intermuscular septa of the leg. The **anterior septum** separates the extensors on the front of the leg from the two peroneal muscles, and it is attached to the anterior border of the fibula. The **posterior septum** is interposed between the peroneal muscles and the muscles on the back of the leg, and is attached to the posterior border of the fibula. The leg is thus subdivided into three main osteofascial compartments—anterior (B), lateral (A) and posterior (E, G, H) in FIGURE 125.

DISSECTION. Remove the deep fascia from the front of the leg, but retain the extensor retinacula by separating them artificially with the knife from the deep fascia with which they are continuous. While thus defining their margins and while removing the deep fascia, take great care not to injure the synovial sheaths of the tendons that lie under cover of them. In the proximal part of the leg, leave the deep fascia in position, for it is impossible to raise it from the muscles without lacerating their surfaces. At a lower level it can readily be separated. Divide it in a longitudinal direction midway between the tibia and fibula. Turn aside the medial piece until its attachment to the tibia is demonstrated; then turn aside the lateral piece until its continuity with the anterior intermuscular septum is displayed.

Examine the three tendon sheaths which lie deep to the extensor retinaculum [see below and Fig. 126]. Make a small incision through the deep fascia into each sheath in turn, either at the lower border of the inferior retinaculum or between its two bands, and insert a blow-pipe or the needle of the syringe. If injection fails, examine the extent of the sheaths with a blunt probe.

Synovial Sheaths on Dorsum of Foot

There are three synovial sheaths in front of the ankle and on the dorsum of the foot—one around the tendon of the tibialis anterior, the second around the tendon of the extensor hallucis longus, and the third encloses the tendons of the extensor digitorum longus and peroneus tertius.

The first extends from the upper border of the superior retinaculum to within a short distance of the insertion of the tibialis anterior into the medial cuneiform bone. The second begins between the retinacula, and extends to the first phalanx of the big toe. The third extends from the lower border of the superior retinaculum to the middle of the dorsum of the foot. The sheaths facilitate the movements of the tendons when the muscles are in action, and they are of surgical importance because they are liable to become inflamed.

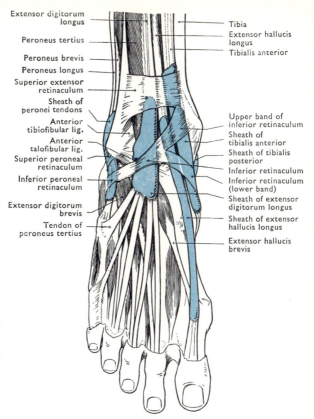

FIG. 126 Synovial sheaths of dorsum of foot.

CONTENTS OF THE ANTERIOR COMPARTMENT OF LEG

Four muscles are brought into view when the deep fascia of the front of the leg has been removed, viz., the tibialis anterior on the tibia, the extensor digitorum longus, the extensor hallucis longus, and the peroneus tertius all on the fibula. These muscles arise partly from the bones of the leg, but to a large extent they take origin also from the deep fascia, the fascial septa, and the interosseous membrane.

The **anterior tibial vessels** and the **deep peroneal nerve** descend in this compartment. At first they are deeply placed, but as they

189

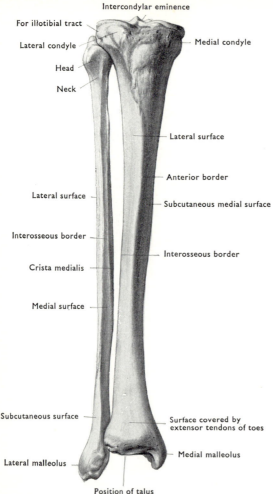

Intercondylar eminence

For iliotibial tract

Lateral condyle

Head

Neck

Medial condyle

Lateral surface

Anterior border

Lateral surface

Subcutaneous medial surface

Interosseous border

Interosseous border

Crista medialis

Medial surface

Subcutaneous surface

Surface covered by
extensor tendons of toes

Lateral malleolus

Medial malleolus

Position of talus

FIG. 127   Right tibia and fibula (anterior aspect).

of the peroneal artery as it pierces the interosseous membrane and descends into the foot [Fig. 129].

As you clean each structure follow it into the dorsum of the foot and onwards to its termination, clearing away the deep fascia. The dorsalis pedis is the continuation of the anterior tibial artery into the foot. Clean it and its branches [Fig. 131].

The small muscle on the dorsum of the foot is the extensor digitorum brevis. Clean it and follow its tendons to the toes.

On the second or the third toe clean the extensor expansion formed over the proximal phalanx by the long and short extensor tendons; trace the middle part of the expansion to the base of the middle phalanx and the two outlying parts to the base of the distal phalanx. Define the margins of the expansion and find slender tendons that join the margins; they come from the small lumbrical and interosseous muscles in the sole.

Tibialis Anterior

This powerful muscle lies along the lateral side of the shin and takes origin chiefly from the upper half of the lateral surface of the tibia, and from the interosseous membrane [FIG. 130]. A strong tendon issues from its fleshy belly in the distal third of the leg, and reaches the dorsum of the foot by passing through both the extensor retinacula. On the foot it inclines medially, turns round the medial margin, and gains insertion into the medial side of the medial cuneiform bone near the sole, and into the adjoining part of the base of the first metatarsal bone.

Nerve supply: the **deep peroneal nerve** and the **recurrent genicular nerve.** Action: it is a dorsiflexor and an invertor of the foot, *i.e.,* it swings the rest of the foot on the talus so as to make the sole face medially.

Extensor Digitorum Longus

The extensor digitorum longus is a long, thin sheet of muscle which arises, for the most part, from the upper three-fourths of the anterior surface of the fibula [FIGS. 129,

approach the ankle they come nearer to the surface.

DISSECTION. To expose the anterior tibial vessels and deep peroneal nerve in their entire course, separate the tibialis anterior and the extensor digitorum longus from each other by carrying the knife upwards along the septum between them. Draw the peroneus tertius muscle aside, and find the perforating branch

190

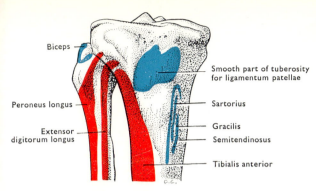

Biceps

Peroneus longus

Extensor
digitorum longus

Smooth part of tuberosity
for ligamentum patellae

Sartorius

Gracilis

Semitendinosus

Tibialis anterior

FIG. 128   Front of upper part of bones of leg with attachments
of muscles mapped out.

Nerve supply of extensor digitorum longus: the **deep peroneal nerve.** Action: it extends the interphalangeal and metatarsophalangeal joints of the lateral four toes, and dorsiflexes the foot.

Peroneus Tertius

This is a small muscle, not always present; it is continuous at its origin with the extensor digitorum longus, of which it appears to be a separated part. It arises from the distal fourth of the anterior surface of the fibula and from the interosseous membrane, and it ends in a slender tendon which expands to be inserted into the dorsal surface of the base of the fifth metatarsal bone. Nerve supply: the **deep peroneal nerve**. Action: it dorsiflexes the ankle and everts the foot, *i.e.*, swings the rest of the foot round the talus so as to make the sole face laterally.

Extensor Hallucis Longus

The long extensor of the big toe is a thin muscle hidden between the tibialis anterior and the extensor digitorum longus, but it comes to the surface near the ankle. It arises from the middle two-fourths of the anterior surface of the fibula, and also from the interosseous membrane. Its tendon passes deep to the superior retinaculum, crosses in front of the distal part of the anterior tibial artery, and descends in front of the ankle joint into the dorsum of the foot. It then passes through the inferior retinaculum [FIG. 131], to be inserted into the base of the distal phalanx of the big toe, occasionally giving a slip to the base of the proximal phalanx also. Nerve supply: the **deep peroneal nerve.** Action: it extends the phalanges of the big toe and dorsiflexes the foot.

Deep Peroneal Nerve

This is one of the two terminal branches of the common peroneal nerve. It arises on the lateral side of the neck of the fibula, under

130]. Its tendon descends behind the superior and inferior extensor retinacula and in front of the ankle joint, and divides into four slips which diverge to reach the lateral four toes, where they are inserted into the middle and distal phalanges. On the dorsum of the first phalanx of the **second, third** and **fourth** toes each slip is joined, on its lateral side, by a tendon from the extensor digitorum brevis.

On each of those three toes the two tendons unite and form an expansion on the dorsum of the first phalanx. Each expansion divides into a middle part and two collateral parts. The middle part, slender and very short, is inserted into the base of the middle phalanx; the collateral parts are stronger, and unite together to be inserted into the base of the terminal phalanx. Each expansion is joined by thin extensions of the slender tendons that pass obliquely upwards across the metatarsophalangeal joints from one lumbrical and two interossei to each expansion. Thus five tendons gain insertion into the second and third phalanges of those three toes. The lumbrical and interosseous muscles flex the metatarsophalangeal joint, and may aid the extensors in extending the interphalangeal joints.

The little toe has only one extensor tendon, but it expands, divides, and is inserted in the same way; it is joined by the tendons of one lumbrical and one interosseous muscle.

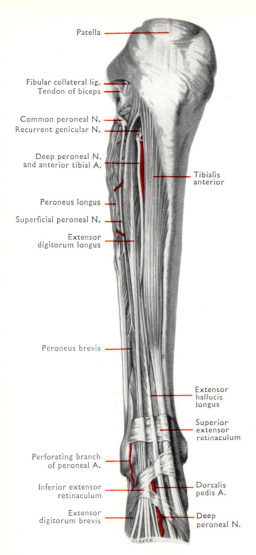

Patella

Fibular collateral lig.
Tendon of biceps

Common peroneal N.
Recurrent genicular N.

Deep peroneal N.
and anterior tibial A.

Tibialis
anterior

Peroneus longus

Superficial peroneal N.

Extensor
digitorum longus

Peroneus brevis

Extensor
hallucis
longus

Superior
extensor
retinaculum

Perforating branch
of peroneal A.

Inferior extensor
retinaculum

Dorsalis
pedis A.

Extensor
digitorum brevis

Deep
peroneal N.

Fig. 129   Dissection of front and lateral side of
leg.

cover of the peroneus longus muscle, and
pierces the anterior intermuscular septum and
the extensor digitorum longus to enter the
anterior compartment of the leg. In that
compartment it runs downwards to the ankle
joint, deeply placed between the tibialis

192

anterior and the long extensors and accompanied by the anterior tibial vessels on the
interosseous membrane. Near the ankle it is
crossed by the extensor hallucis, and running
over the front of the tibia, passes on to the
talus midway between the malleoli. It ends on
the dorsum of the foot, close to the ankle
joint, and between the tendons of extensor
digitorum longus and extensor hallucis
longus, by dividing into lateral and medial
branches.

Branches. In the leg the deep peroneal
nerve gives **muscular branches** to the four
muscles of the anterior compartment, and a
fine **articular twig** to the ankle joint.

The **medial terminal branch** is continued
forwards on the dorsum of the foot, under
cover of the deep fascia, and crossed by
the tendon of the extensor hallucis brevis.
The dorsalis pedis and first dorsal metatarsal
artery are usually between it and extensor
hallucis, but may be [as in Fig. 131] on the
lateral side of the nerve.

At a variable point in the first interosseous
space it pierces the deep fascia, and divides to
supply the contiguous margins of the big toe
and the second toe [p. 187]. Before it reaches
the surface it furnishes **articular twigs** to
the tarsometatarsal and metatarsophalangeal
joints of the big toe, and frequently also a fine
muscular twig to the first dorsal interosseous
muscle.

The **lateral terminal branch** of the deep
peroneal nerve turns abruptly laterally, under
cover of the extensor digitorum brevis, and
ends on the dorsum of the tarsus in a gangli-
form enlargement. Branches proceed from the
enlargment to supply the extensor digitorum
brevis and the numerous joints in the neigh-
bourhood. One fine filament can, in some
bodies, be traced to the second dorsal interosseous muscle.

Anterior Tibial Artery

This, the smaller of the two terminal
branches of the popliteal artery, takes origin
in the back of the leg, at the distal border of
the popliteus muscle, opposite the tuberosity
of the tibia [see Fig. 119]. It enters the front

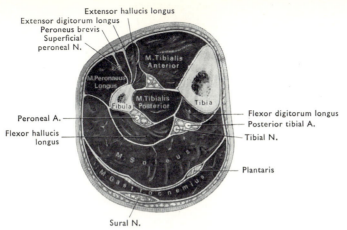

Extensor hallucis longus
Extensor digitorum longus
Peroneus brevis
Superficial
peroneal N.

M.Tibialis Anterior

M.Peronaeus Longus

Fibula

M.Tibialis Posterior

Tibia

Peroneal A.

Flexor hallucis longus

Flexor digitorum longus
Posterior tibial A.

Tibial N.

M. Soleus

M. Gastrocnemius

Plantaris

Sural N.

Fig. 130   Transverse section through middle of leg seen from above.

of the leg by passing forwards through an opening in the upper part of the interosseous membrane. As it passes forwards it lies close to the medial side of the neck of the fibula, and is found there in the present dissection. In the front of the leg it takes a straight course to the front of the ankle joint, midway between the malleoli, where it ends by becoming the **dorsalis pedis artery.**

It is closely accompanied by two **venae comitantes,** and running with the deep peroneal nerve, has the same relations.

Branches. Muscular branches come off at irregular points along the whole length of the artery. Other small branches are the **anterior recurrent artery** which runs upwards through the tibialis anterior muscle, and **malleolar** branches that ramify over the malleoli. The lateral one is the larger of the two malleolar arteries, and it anastomoses with the **perforating branch** of the **peroneal artery,** which appears from the back of the leg by piercing the interosseous membrane above the lateral malleolus.

Dorsalis Pedis Artery

The continuation of the anterior tibial, it begins on the front of the ankle joint and runs forwards on the dorsum of the foot, alongside the deep peroneal nerve and its medial terminal branch, as far as the proximal part of the first interosseous space. There it leaves

the dorsum of the foot by dipping plantarwards, between the two heads of the first dorsal interosseous muscle, to end in the sole of the foot by uniting with the lateral plantar artery in the formation of the plantar arch [Figs. 151, 152].

It is crossed, as it enters the dorsum of the foot, by the inferior extensor retinaculum and, as it leaves the dorsum, by the extensor hallucis brevis.

Branches. On the dorsum of the foot it gives off: (1) small tarsal arteries, (2) the arcuate artery and (3) the first dorsal metatarsal artery. Its termination in the sole will be examined later.

The **arcuate artery** arises opposite the bases of the metatarsal bones and runs laterally across them, under cover of the extensor tendons. It sends forwards three **dorsal metatarsal arteries** over the lateral three intermetatarsal spaces, each of which divides into two **dorsal digital arteries** for contiguous sides of the toes; the lateral one sends a twig to the lateral side of the little toe.

The **first dorsal metatarsal artery** arises at the point where the dorsalis pedis dips towards the sole. It runs forwards over the first dorsal interosseous muscle, and divides into **dorsal digital branches** for the medial side of the big toe and the adjacent sides of the big toe and second toe.

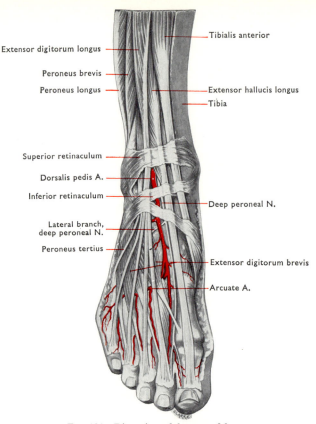

Extensor digitorum longus

Peroneus brevis

Peroneus longus

Tibialis anterior

Extensor hallucis longus

Tibia

Superior retinaculum

Dorsalis pedis A.

Inferior retinaculum

Lateral branch,
deep peroneal N.

Peroneus tertius

Deep peroneal N.

Extensor digitorum brevis

Arcuate A.

FIG. 131   Dissection of dorsum of foot.

Extensor Digitorum Brevis

This muscle arises from the anterior part of the superior surface of the calcaneus, and also from the stem of the inferior extensor retinaculum. It forms a fleshy cushion on the lateral part of the dorsum of the foot and breaks up into four segments.

The most medial of the four is called the **extensor hallucis brevis.** It ends in a tendon which crosses the distal part of the dorsalis pedis artery, and is inserted into the base of the proximal phalanx of the big toe. It is an extensor of the first metatarsophalangeal joint.

The remaining three segments end in tendons which join the long extensor tendons for the second, third and fourth toes and, by

means of the extensor expansions [see p. 191], they gain insertion into the middle and terminal phalanges of those toes. Nerve supply: lateral terminal branch of the **deep peroneal nerve.** Action: Extension of the interphalangeal and metatarsophalangeal joints.

Extensor Retinacula

There are two thickenings of the deep fascia which strap down the tendons of the tibialis anterior, the peroneus tertius and the long extensors, and prevent them from springing forwards when the muscles contract. They are distinguishable from the adjoining deep fascia only by their greater thickness, and have to be artificially separated from it by dissection [FIGS. 126, 131, 132].

194

The **superior extensor retinaculum** is a strong band, 2·5 cm. or more in width from above downwards, situated immediately above the ankle joint. Its ends are firmly attached to the anterior borders of the tibia and the fibula. The long extensors, the peroneus tertius, the anterior tibial vessels and the deep peroneal nerve pass behind it; but its medial part splits to enclose the tendon of the tibialis anterior and its synovial sheath, forming a kind of sling for that tendon. To make certain of these points, divide the fibular attachment of the retinaculum and pull it towards the tibial side.

The **inferior extensor retinaculum** is the more important of the two. It is shaped like the letter Y placed on its side, and lies across the dorsum of the foot close to the ankle joint. The stem of the Y is lateral and is firmly attached to the anterior part of the upper surface of the calcaneus. Its deep surface gives partial origin to the extensor digitorum brevis, and is connected with the interosseous ligament that binds the calcaneus and the talus together. Traced medially the stem divides, one band inclining upwards to be attached to the anterior margin of the medial malleolus, while the other band, passing horizontally to the medial side of the foot, blends with the deep fascia of the sole of the foot.

The deep surface of the retinaculum is adherent to the tarsal bones and ligaments, except where the dorsalis pedis vessels and deep peroneal nerve pass under cover of it. In three places it is split into two layers for the passage of tendons and their synovial sheaths: (1) in the medial part of the stem, for the extensor digitorum longus and the peroneus tertius; (2) in both arms of the Y, for the extensor hallucis longus; and (3) more medially in both arms, for the tibialis anterior; the layer that overlies the tibialis anterior is sometimes very thin.

THE LATERAL SIDE OF THE LEG

The **peroneal tendons** descend behind the lateral malleolus—the longus lying superficial to the brevis—and are bound down by the thickened portion of the deep fascia called the superior peroneal retinaculum. They then curve forwards, below the malleolus, over the lateral surface of the calcaneus and are held in contact with it by the inferior peroneal retinaculum. In the living limb these tendons are less obvious than those of the anterior compartment because they hug the posterior aspect of the lower end of the fibula. The tendon of peroneus brevis is, however, clearly visible on the lateral aspect of the calcaneus when the foot is everted.

The **synovial sheath** begins about 5 cm. above the tip of the lateral malleolus, and is at first a single sheath that envelops both tendons; but on the lateral surface of the calcaneus it divides into two sheaths. The sheath of the peroneus brevis envelops it almost to its insertion. The sheath of the longus follows it across the sole to its insertion, but is often interrupted at the lateral side of the foot.

DISSECTION. Identify the upper margin of the superior retinaculum. Remove the deep fascia immediately above it very carefully, and expose the synovial sheath. Pinch up the sheath and either inflate it or inject it in the way described on page 189. If that fails, expose the peroneal tendons between the two retinacula, and examine the extent and subdivisions of the sheath with a blunt probe. Then clean the retinacula, and define their borders and connexions.

Peroneal Retinacula [FIG. 132].

These are the thickened bands of the deep fascia that prevent displacement of the peroneal tendons. They are not so sharply marked off from the adjacent fascia as the extensor retinacula are, and require more careful dissection for their definition.

The **superior peroneal retinaculum** bridges over the peroneal tendons as they lie on the back of the lateral malleolus. It is attached to the back of the lateral malleolus and to the lateral surface of the calcaneus, and it is connected also with the layer of fascia that lies deeply in the back of the leg. It is lined with the common synovial sheath of the peronei.

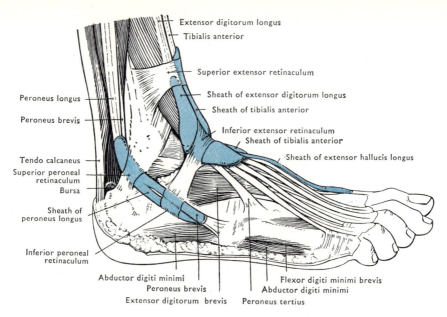

Extensor digitorum longus
Tibialis anterior
Superior extensor retinaculum
Sheath of extensor digitorum longus
Sheath of tibialis anterior
Peroneus longus
Peroneus brevis
Inferior extensor retinaculum
Sheath of tibialis anterior
Sheath of extensor hallucis longus
Tendo calcaneus
Superior peroneal retinaculum
Bursa
Sheath of peroneus longus
Inferior peroneal retinaculum
Abductor digiti minimi
Peroneus brevis
Extensor digitorum brevis
Flexor digiti minimi brevis
Abductor digiti minimi
Peroneus tertius

FIG. 132   Dissection showing synovial sheaths of tendons of lateral aspect of foot.

The **inferior peroneal retinaculum** lies across the peroneal tendons when they reach the lateral surface of the calcaneus. Superiorly it is attached to the anterior part of the upper surface of the calcaneus, and is continuous there with the stem of the inferior extensor retinaculum. Inferiorly it is attached to the lateral surface of the calcaneus below and between the peroneal tendons. Each tendon, therefore, lies in a separate tunnel, which is lined with the branch of the synovial sheath that envelops the tendon.

DISSECTION. Open up the lateral compartment of the leg to display its contents. Divide the deep fascia over the peroneal muscles by a longitudinal incision, and turn the flaps aside until their continuity with the intermuscular septa is demonstrated, but do not injure the peroneal retinacula.

Next separate the two peroneal muscles from each other; clean them, and secure their nerves of supply. Then cut through the upper part of the peroneus longus in order to find the terminal part of the common peroneal nerve; trace its recurrent genicular branch upwards, and the superficial peroneal nerve downwards.

PERONEAL MUSCLES

The peroneus longus and brevis are separated from the extensors by the anterior intermuscular septum and from the muscles of the calf by the posterior septum. They arise partly from the fibula, but most of their fibres spring from the intermuscular septa and the deep fascia that covers them. Nerve supply: the **superficial peroneal nerve.** Action: they are evertors of the foot, and to some extent, plantar flexors.

Peroneus Longus

The peroneus longus muscle arises from the upper two-thirds of the lateral surface of the fibula. Its tendon begins a short distance above the ankle, descends behind the lateral malleolus, and curves forwards below it. The tendon then runs over the lateral surface of the calcaneus to the lateral border of the foot behind the base of the fifth metatarsal bone. Here it enters the groove on the plantar surface of the cuboid bone and runs obliquely across the sole of the foot to be inserted into the base of the first metatarsal bone and into the adjoining part of the medial cuneiform bone. Its position in the sole will be examined later.

Peroneus Brevis

This muscle arises from the lower two-thirds of the lateral surface of the shaft of the fibula, overlapping the peroneus longus in the middle third. Its tendon descends over the back of the lateral malleolus, under cover of the peroneus longus, and then turns forwards, on the lateral surface of the calcaneus, above the longus, to gain insertion into the tuberosity on the base of the fifth metatarsal bone. Occasionally it sends forwards a slender slip to join the extensor tendon of the little toe.

The **peroneus tertius** [p. 191], which acts with the other peroneal muscles in eversion of the foot, is a separated slip of the extensor digitorum longus and is supplied by the **deep peroneal nerve.**

Terminal Branches of the Common Peroneal Nerve

This nerve has been traced as far as the neck of the fibula. At that point it disappears by passing forwards through the deepest fibres of the peroneus longus muscle close to the bone. As it lies between them, it gives off a small **recurrent genicular branch** to the knee joint, and then divides into the **deep** and the **superficial peroneal nerves.**

The recurrent branch pierces the extensor digitorum longus, and then accompanies the anterior tibial recurrent artery through the upper part of the tibialis anterior (which it supplies) to reach the capsule of the knee joint; it gives a branch also to the superior tibio-fibular joint.

The **deep peroneal nerve** pierces the extensor digitorum longus to reach the anterior compartment of the leg, where it has already been dissected.

The Superficial Peroneal Nerve

The superficial peroneal nerve descends in the substance of the peroneus longus till it reaches the peroneus brevis, and, for a short

distance, lies between these two muscles; it then passes obliquely over the anterior border of the brevis and descends, under cover of the deep fascia, in the groove between the peroneus brevis and the extensor digitorum longus. In the distal third of the leg it pierces the deep fascia, and divides into a medial and a lateral branch, which descend into the foot [p. 187].

It supplies the peroneal muscles, the skin of the lower part of the front of the leg, nearly the whole of the dorsum of the foot, and most of the toes.

THE MEDIAL SIDE OF THE LEG

This region corresponds to the medial surface of the tibia, most of which is covered only with the skin and the superficial fascia, for the deep fascia blends with the periosteum at the borders of the bone—except in the upper part, where a thin layer of deep fascia covers the expanded tendons of sartorius, gracilis and semitendinosus that overlie the bone.

DISSECTION. The distal parts of the great saphenous vein and the saphenous nerve have already been cleaned. Now trace them to the knee. Clean the tendons of sartorius, gracilis and semitendinosus, examine their attachments and turn them forwards; examine the bursae between them and under cover of them. The deeper bursa overlies the tibial collateral ligament of the knee; and, as the bursa has probably been opened, the surface of the ligament is smooth and glistening. Clean the ligament from end to end; define its borders, and clean the articular vessels and nerve that pass under cover of it.

The tibial collateral ligament of the knee partly covers the insertion of the semi-membranosus into the tibial condyle, and is covered by the tendons of sartorius, gracilis, and semitendinosus, and the complex bursa between them.

THE BACK OF THE LEG

This is an extensive dissection that includes the superficial muscles of the calf, inserted into the bone of the heel by the tendo calcaneus, and the deep flexor muscles whose tendons pass into the sole of the foot on the medial side of the ankle with the tibial nerve and posterior tibial vessels.

DISSECTION. Make a transverse incision across the distal part of the heel and carry the extremities of the incision forwards along the medial and lateral borders of the foot; then remove the skin from the whole of the back of the leg, avoiding injury to the superficial veins and nerves.

Complete the cleaning of the great saphenous vein and the saphenous nerve on the medial side of the knee, if that has not been done already.

Trace the posterior branch of the medial anterior cutaneous nerve of the thigh downwards over the medial part of the calf [Fig. 135], and the posterior cutaneous nerve of the thigh downwards over the middle of the calf.

The upper part of the small saphenous vein has been found in the popliteal fossa, and its lower part on the lateral border of the foot; now clean the intervening part.

Find the sural nerve again where it lies alongside the lower part of the small saphenous vein. Follow it upwards to the point where it pierces the deep fascia; then trace it upwards to its origin from the tibial nerve, incising the deep fascia to expose it. Five to seven centimetres above the heel it is joined by the peroneal communicating nerve. Follow that nerve upwards to the point where it pierces the deep fascia, and then onwards to its origin from the common peroneal nerve.

Look for the medial calcanean nerves in the fascia at the medial side of the heel. They are small and difficult to find. The small arteries, if injected, are guides to them.

At this stage the dissector should revise the saphenous veins and the cutaneous nerves which have been seen in previous dissections,

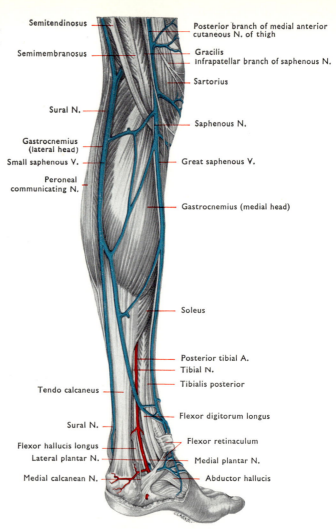

FIG. 133   Superficial dissection of leg viewed from posteromedial side, showing veins and nerves.

Note the numerous anastomoses between the great and the small saphenous veins.

but are now, for the first time, displayed from beginning to end [FIGS. 94, 133–135].

Great Saphenous Vein

This is the longest vein in the body. It begins at the medial border of the foot by the

198

union of the dorsal venous arch with the medial digital vein of the big toe. It ascends in front of the medial malleolus, passes obliquely upwards and backwards across the medial surface of the distal third of the tibia, and then vertically upwards, along the medial border of the tibia, to the posterior part of the medial side of the knee. In this part of its course it is enclosed in a membranous sleeve of fascia which separates it from a more superficial venous plexus at least in the lower two-thirds of the leg. Thence, it passes obliquely upwards, forwards and laterally, through the superficial fascia of the front of the thigh, to the saphenous opening, where it pierces the cribriform fascia and the femoral sheath and terminates in the femoral vein [Figs. 93, 94, 100].

In addition to the veins of origin and the three veins which join it just before it pierces the cribriform fascia, it receives numerous unnamed tributaries, and communicates with the deep veins of the limb by means of anastomosing channels which pierce the deep fascia.

The great saphenous vein contains a number of valves; they divide the long column of blood into a series of segments, and so diminish the pressure on the walls of the more distal parts of the vein. But the superficial veins of the leg are often dilated and tortuous (varicose), and in that condition the valves are incompetent.

Small Saphenous Vein

The small saphenous vein

is formed, in the lateral border of the foot, by the union of the lateral dorsal digital vein of the little toe with the lateral end of the dorsal venous arch. From its point of commencement it runs backwards below the lateral malleolus, and then upwards behind it

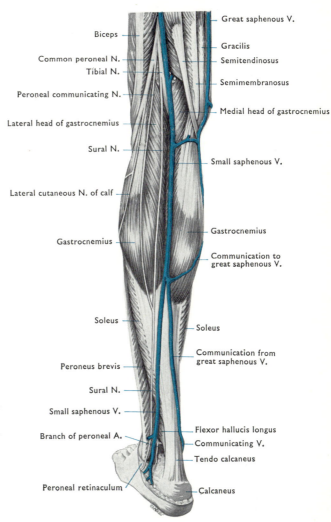

Biceps

Common peroneal N.

Tibial N.

Peroneal communicating N.

Lateral head of gastrocnemius

Sural N.

Lateral cutaneous N. of calf

Gastrocnemius

Soleus

Peroneus brevis

Sural N.

Small saphenous V.

Branch of peroneal A.

Peroneal retinaculum

Great saphenous V.

Gracilis

Semitendinosus

Semimembranosus

Medial head of gastrocnemius

Small saphenous V.

Gastrocnemius

Communication to great saphenous V.

Soleus

Communication from great saphenous V.

Flexor hallucis longus

Communicating V.

Tendo calcaneus

Calcaneus

FIG. 134 Superficial dissection of leg viewed from posterolateral side, showing veins and nerves.

In the specimen there were numerous large anastomosing channels between the small and the great saphenous veins.

into the leg. There it ascends a little lateral to the tendo calcaneus at first, and then along the middle line of the calf to the lower part of the popliteal region, where it pierces the popliteal fascia and terminates in the popliteal vein.

The small saphenous vein receives tributaries from the lateral border of the foot, the heel and the back of the leg.

The two saphenous veins are connected together by a fairly large vein which springs from the small saphenous vein immediately before it pierces the deep fascia, and terminates in the great saphenous vein above the middle of the thigh. This vein sometimes forms the direct continuation of the small saphenous vein which has then either a very small or no connexion with the popliteal vein.

Saphenous Nerve

The saphenous nerve (L. 3, 4) is the longest branch of the femoral nerve. It arises about 2 cm. below the inguinal ligament, and descends through the femoral triangle and the adductor canal with the femoral artery. It leaves the canal by passing behind the lower edge of its fibrous roof, and lies directly under cover of the sartorius. It becomes superficial by curving around the posterior border of the sartorius—between it and the tendon of the gracilis—a little above the knee. It then descends posteromedial to the knee, pierces the deep fascia and enters the leg. In the leg it accompanies the great saphenous vein first along the

medial border of the tibia, and then obliquely forwards across the distal third of the tibia. It enters the foot by passing downwards in front of the medial malleolus—still in company with the vein—and it ends in the skin at the middle of the medial border of the

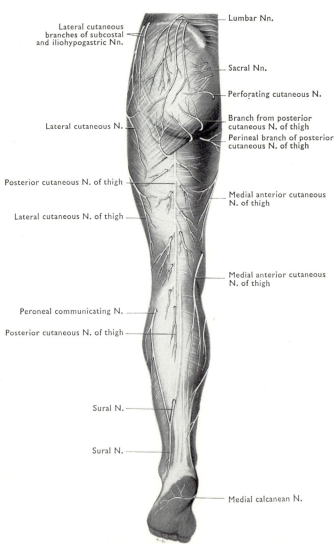

FIG. 135   Cutaneous nerves on back of lower limb.   See also FIG. 94.

200

foot. After it leaves the adductor canal, and before it emerges between the sartorius and gracilis, it gives off an **infrapatellar branch** [FIG. 94, p. 137], which pierces the sartorius on its way to the patellar plexus. Beyond the knee its branches are distributed to the skin of the medial side of the leg and foot.

Sural Nerve

This nerve (S. 1, 2) arises in the popliteal fossa from the tibial nerve, descends in the groove between the two deep heads of the gastrocnemius, pierces the deep fascia of the leg about midway between the knee and the ankle, and accompanies the small saphenous vein into the lateral border of the foot and little toe.

Shortly after it pierces the deep fascia, it is joined by the peroneal communicating nerve. On the side of the foot it communicates with the branch of the superficial peroneal nerve passing to the contiguous sides of the fourth and fifth toes. It supplies the skin of the lower, lateral part of the back of the leg, the lateral border of the foot and adjoining part of the dorsum, and the lateral side of the little toe.

Peroneal Communicating Nerve (L. 5; S. 1, 2). This nerve arises in the popliteal fossa from the common peroneal nerve, frequently in common with the lateral cutaneous nerve of the calf [p. 176]. It crosses superficial to the lateral head of the gastrocnemius, pierces the deep fascia, and passes downwards and medially to join the sural nerve at the upper part of the lateral border of the tendo calcaneus. It supplies skin in the proximal two-thirds of the back of the leg.

Medial Anterior Cutaneous Nerve of Thigh (L. 2, 3; pp. 138, 149). Its **posterior branch** pierces the deep fascia a little above the knee, behind the sartorius and the great saphenous vein, and descends to supply the skin of the upper part of the medial side of the leg [FIG. 135].

The posterior cutaneous nerve of the thigh and the lateral cutaneous nerve of the calf are described on pages 176, 178, 187.

LYMPH VESSELS AND LYMPH NODES OF THE LOWER LIMB
[FIGS. 136, 137]

The dissectors will have seen the inguinal lymph nodes, and may have found one or two of the popliteal group, but they will not have been able to trace the lymph vessels except for a short distance from the nodes in the groin.

As in other parts of the body there are superficial and deep groups of both nodes and vessels.

The **superficial lymph nodes** are the superficial inguinal nodes, and they are in two groups—upper and lower [p. 135].

The **deep lymph nodes** are related to the main blood vessels. They are: the deep inguinal nodes [p. 146], the popliteal nodes [p. 174], and a single anterior tibial node which lies close to the anterior tibial artery in the upper part of the front of the leg.

The **deep lymph vessels** are much less numerous than the superficial vessels, though they drain all the structures that lie deep to the deep fascia. They run along the principal blood vessels, and most of them end in the deep inguinal nodes—the exception being those from the deep parts of the gluteal region and upper part of back of thigh, which accompany the gluteal vessels into the pelvis and end in the internal iliac nodes. Those from the leg are interrupted in the popliteal nodes; the anterior tibial node is placed in the path of those that run along the anterior tibial vessels.

The **superficial lymph vessels** collect the lymph from the skin and the subcutaneous tissues.

In the sole of the foot, as in the palm of the hand, there is a dense cutaneous plexus of lymph capillaries, and the origin of the lymph vessels from the plexus resembles that of the hand [p. 47]; but the great projection of the heel causes a slightly different orientation of the vessels as they leave the foot. The vessels from the lateral border of the foot, from the back of the heel, and from part of the back of the leg [FIG. 137] accompany the small saphenous vein to the popliteal nodes. The vessels from the distal parts of the plantar

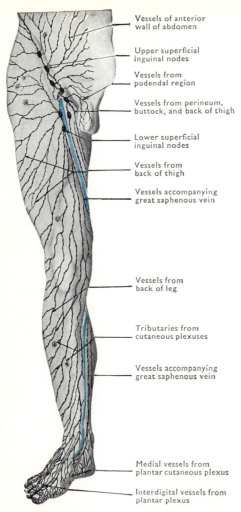

Vessels of anterior
wall of abdomen

Upper superficial
inguinal nodes

Vessels from
pudendal region

Vessels from perineum,
buttock, and back of thigh

Lower superficial
inguinal nodes

Vessels from
back of thigh

Vessels accompanying
great saphenous vein

Vessels from
back of leg

Tributaries from
cutaneous plexuses

Vessels accompanying
great saphenous vein

Medial vessels from
plantar cutaneous plexus

Interdigital vessels from
plantar plexus

'Lymphshed' of
gluteal region

Vessels from buttock
and back of thigh passing,
by lateral route, to
superficial inguinal nodes

Vessels passing by
medial route

'Lymphshed' of
back of thigh

Popliteal node
(deep to fascia)

Vessels accompanying
small saphenous vein

Tributary from
cutaneous plexus

Vessels of calf passing
to front of leg

Vessels of heel passing to
popliteal nodes by small
saphenous route

Lateral vessels from
plantar plexus

FIG. 136 Superficial lymph vessels of anterior
surface of lower limb.

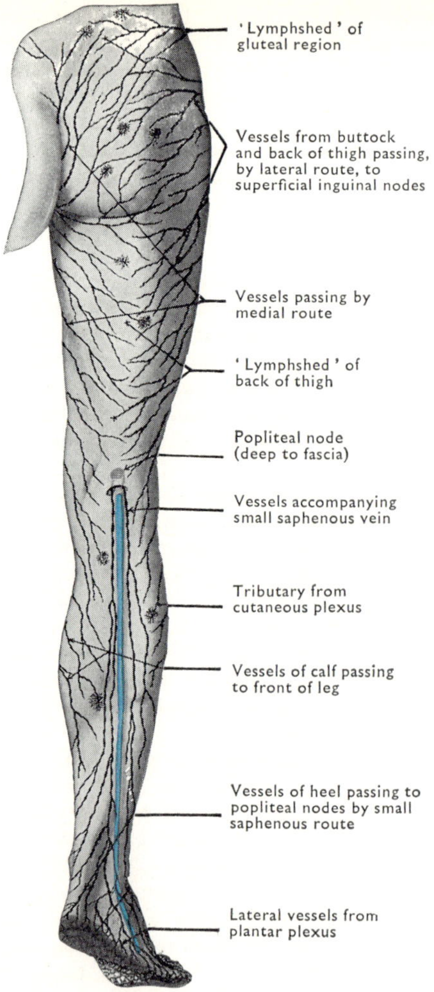

FIG. 137 Superficial lymph vessels of posterior
surface of lower limb.

surfaces of the toes pass to the dorsum of the
foot at the interdigital clefts. Then, together
with vessels that arise from the plantar
capillary plexus, and from the dorsum and
medial border of the foot, they ascend across
the front of the ankle and the medial malleolus,
and constitute the main stream along the line
of the great saphenous vein. They are joined

by vessels from the front and medial side of
the leg, and from the medial side and greater
part of the front of the thigh ; all these vessels
end in the lower group of superficial inguinal
nodes. The vessels from the upper part of
the front of the thigh, the back of the thigh,
and the gluteal region converge upon the
upper group of superficial inguinal nodes, to

which vessels proceed also from the perineum and the lower part of the anterior wall of the abdomen. The efferents from these nodes pass to the deep inguinal nodes.

Thus all the lymph of the lower limb passes through the deep inguinal nodes except the lymph from the deep parts of the gluteal region and back of the thigh. The efferent vessels from these nodes pass behind the inguinal ligament to the external iliac nodes, whence the lymph is carried onwards, through the common iliac nodes and the lumbar nodes, to the lumbar lymph trunks on the posterior abdominal wall.

The student should compare the arrangement of the lymph vessels of the Lower and Upper Limbs [pp. 47–49]. He should note, in particular, the manner in which the superficial lymph vessels of each limb converge upon the important groups of lymph nodes at the roots of the limbs (armpit and groin), and that these groups receive also the superficial vessels of the trunk, and thus share a very wide territory between them.

The lymph vessels begin in a similar manner in the hand and in the foot; in each limb chief and subsidiary streams are formed, each associated with a vein. The chief stream in the lower limb follows the great saphenous vein to the nodes in the groin, which correspond to the nodes in the axilla. The subsidiary stream in the lower limb follows the small saphenous vein to the nodes in the popliteal fossa. These popliteal nodes correspond to the nodes at the bifurcation of the brachial artery *plus* the superficial cubital nodes; the lymph vessels that follow the small saphenous vein correspond, therefore, to those of the upper limb that pierce the deep fascia with the basilic vein.

DISSECTION. Remove the remains of the superficial fascia from the back of the leg, and clean the deep fascia.

DEEP FASCIA

The proximal part in the calf is continuous with the popliteal fascia; it is thin and transparent, but thickens considerably as the heel is approached. On the lateral side of the ankle it forms the **superior peroneal retinaculum** [p. 195]. On the medial side it is greatly strengthened to form a broad band which bridges across the interval between the calcaneus and the medial malleolus; this **flexor retinaculum** straps down the tendons of the long flexors of the toes and the tibialis posterior and retains them in place as they pass from the back of the leg into the foot.

THE POSTERIOR OSTEOFASCIAL COMPARTMENT OF THE LEG

This compartment is bounded posteriorly and at the sides by the deep fascia which extends from the medial border of the tibia to the posterior intermuscular septum, and anteriorly by the tibia, the interosseous membrane, the fibula and the posterior intermuscular septum [FIG. 125, p. 188]. The compartment is subdivided into three by two strong fascial septa.

The **first septum** extends from the medial border of the tibia to the posterior border of the fibula; it covers the long flexors of the toes and enclosing the posterior tibial vessels, separates them from the superficial muscles of the calf [FIG. 130].

Inferiorly it underlies the tendo calcaneus, helps the investing fascia to form the superior peroneal retinaculum, and is continued into the flexor retinaculum where it forms the greater part of its thickness.

Superiorly it is attached to the soleal line of the tibia and to the back of the fibula below the origin of the soleus muscle. Between those attachments it surrounds the popliteal vessels, being continuous with the fascia on the popliteus muscle anteriorly, and posteriorly forming a tendinous arch from which the soleus muscle takes origin.

The **second septum** covers the tibialis posterior. It is attached medially to the proximal part of the soleal line of the tibia and to the vertical ridge on the posterior surface of the tibia, and laterally to the medial crest of the fibula. Above it blends with the interosseous membrane; inferiorly it fuses with the deep surface of the first septum in the distal part of the leg.

203

DISSECTION. First clean the flexor retinaculum carefully, and secure the medial calcanean arteries and nerves, which pierce it. Note that it is continuous proximally with the deep fascia of the back of the leg, and that distally it gives attachment to a muscle called the abductor hallucis. Then make a longitudinal incision through the deep fascia, down the middle of the back of the leg, from the popliteal region to the calcaneus. Turn the two flaps to the sides, detaching their distal parts from the retinacula.

Next clean the gastrocnemius and the tendo calcaneus and remove the pad of fat that separates the tendon from the first fascial septum.

If the medial head of the gastrocnemius was not divided when the popliteal fossa was dissected, divide it now at the level of the knee joint, and turn it laterally; then clean the lower muscular branches of the popliteal artery and the nerves which supply the gastrocnemius, noting the large size of the arteries that enter with them.

Raise the proximal part of the divided head, and note the bursa which intervenes between it and the semimembranosus.

Next follow the nerve to the soleus, which was found when the popliteal fossa was dissected [see p. 175]. Lastly clean the plantaris, and follow its slender tendon to its insertion.

SUPERFICIAL MUSCLES

The superficial muscles of the calf of the leg are the gastrocnemius, the plantaris and the soleus, from superficial to deep. The tendons of the gastrocnemius and soleus unite to form the tendo calcaneus.

Gastrocnemius

The gastrocnemius arises from the distal end of the femur by two heads, which bound the distal part of the popliteal fossa. The **lateral head** springs from an impression on the lateral surface of the lateral condyle of the femur. The **medial head** takes origin from a rough, raised area on the popliteal surface of the femur above the medial condyle.

Each head arises from the bone mainly by a tendon which spreads out over its superficial surface and gives origin to the short fibres of the muscle belly. The two fleshy bellies thus swell out as they descend, and near the middle of the leg they end in a thin, aponeurotic tendon, which runs up on the deep surface

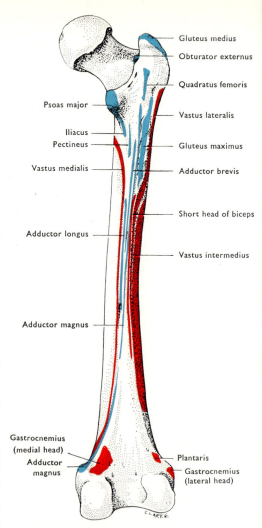

FIG. 138   Right femur to show muscles attached to posterior aspect.

of each. They do not blend with each other, but are separated by a furrow in which the sural nerve and the small saphenous vein lie. The medial belly is slightly larger and extends a little lower than the lateral belly [FIGS. 115, 134]—a feature that is sometimes conspicuous in the well-developed calf of a living limb.

The medial head is separated from the back of the capsule of the knee joint by a **bursa** which may communicate with the cavity of the joint and with the semimembranosus bursa. The lateral head often contains a small sesamoid bone (the 'fabella') opposite the lateral condyle; occasionally it is separated by a bursa from the capsule of the knee joint. The common tendon of the two heads joins the tendon of the soleus to form the tendo calcaneus a short distance below the middle of the leg.

Nerve supply: the **tibial nerve,** each head having a well-marked neurovascular hilum [p. 8]. Action: it is a powerful plantar flexor of the ankle that comes into action in maintaining the standing position and in providing the necessary impetus for walking. The origins from the femur imply that it may act also as a flexor of the knee, and it does so act to assist the hamstrings against resistance; but the two actions cannot be carried out efficiently at the same time. After supracondylar fracture of the femur the gastrocnemius rotates the distal fragment backwards, and treatment is therefore carried out with the knee bent to relax the muscle.

Plantaris

The plantaris has a small, fleshy belly (not more than 8–10 cm. long) which lies partly hidden by the medial side of the lateral head of the gastrocnemius. It arises from the popliteal surface of the femur and ends in a very long, slender tendon which passes between the gastrocnemius and soleus, to run along the medial side of the tendo calcaneus and gain insertion into the calcaneus. It may be closely connected or blended with the tendo calcaneus, or with the fascia of the leg. Like the palmaris longus in the forearm, the muscle is occasionally absent. Nerve supply: the **tibial nerve.** Action: It acts with the gastrocnemius.

DISSECTION. Divide the lateral head of the gastrocnemius at the level of the knee joint. Turn the proximal part upwards, and examine it to see if it contains a sesamoid bone; then look for a bursa which is occasionally present between it and the capsule

of the knee joint. Turn the distal part downwards and note the manner in which the two heads join their common aponeurotic tendon, and the union of that tendon with the tendon of the soleus.

Now clean the posterior surface of the soleus, and define its origin. Note that some of its fibres pass directly to the deep surface of the tendo calcaneus.

Soleus

The soleus is a flat, thick and powerful muscle which arises from the back of the head and the upper third of the posterior surface of the shaft of the **fibula,** from the soleal line and the middle third of the medial border of the tibia [FIG. 141], and from the tendinous arch joining these across the popliteal vessels. The soleus ends in a strong, stout tendon which joins with the tendon of the gastrocnemius to form the tendo calcaneus. Nerve supply: branches of the **tibial nerve** enter the superficial and deep surfaces. Action: it stabilizes the ankle joint in standing, and plantar flexes it when walking, running or standing on the toes.

Tendo Calcaneus

This is the most powerful tendon in the body. It narrows as it descends, but expands slightly to be inserted into the smooth middle portion of the posterior surface of the calcaneus. The fleshy fibres of the soleus are continued downwards on its deep surface almost to the heel. A small **bursa** separates the tendon from the upper part of the posterior surface of the calcaneus.

DISSECTION. Separate the soleus muscle from the tibia and the tendinous arch over the vessels. Turn it laterally; sever the arteries which enter it, but preserve its nerves.

The first fascial septum is now fully exposed. Note its connexions [see p. 203]. Separate it from the flexor and peroneal retinacula; then divide it longitudinally along the middle line of the leg, and turn the two pieces to the sides.

This opens the middle section of the back of the leg and exposes the neurovascular bundle, the flexor hallucis longus laterally, and the flexor digitorum longus medially, with the tendon of tibialis posterior emerging from beneath it in the distal part of the leg.

DISSECTION. Clean the tibial nerve and secure its muscular branches; they arise as a rule in the upper part of the leg. Next clean the terminal part of the popliteal artery and the first part of the anterior tibial artery and its branches; then the posterior tibial vessels and their branches and tributaries. The peroneal artery arises from the posterior tibial about 2–3 cm. below the commencement of the parent trunk. It soon disappears under cover of the flexor hallucis longus; do not trace it further at present.

Clean the flexors of the toes. Then separate the two muscles and push the flexor hallucis longus laterally, separating its deep surface from the second fascial septum and from the distal part of the interosseous membrane. As the fibula is approached, the peroneal artery will be found descending between the flexor hallucis longus and the second fascial septum. Trace the artery downwards. Immediately above the inferior tibiofibular joint it gives off its perforating branch. Now pull the distal part of the flexor hallucis longus medially and follow the peroneal artery to the lateral side of the calcaneus. In order to expose its terminal branches, divide the peroneal retinacula, and, if necessary, displace the peroneal tendons.

TIBIAL NERVE

In the leg this nerve descends under cover of the first fascial septum, and divides into the lateral and medial plantar nerves midway between the calcaneus and the medial malleolus, under cover of the flexor retinaculum. In its upper two-thirds it lies deep to the superficial muscles of the calf, on the fascia of tibialis posterior and on flexor digitorum longus. In the lower third of the leg it is immediately deep to the deep fascia midway between the tendo calcaneus and the medial border of the tibia, and crosses the posterior surfaces of the tibia and ankle joint. The posterior tibial vessels run with it, crossing in front of it from the lateral to the medial side.

Branches

The **muscular** branches arise in the upper part of the leg. They supply the tibialis posterior, flexor hallucis longus, flexor digitorum longus and the deeper part of the soleus.

The **cutaneous** branches spring from the lowest part of the nerve. They are the **medial**

206

calcanean nerves (S. 1) which pierce the flexor retinaculum and supply the skin of the posterior and lower surfaces of the heel.

The **articular** branches are small twigs that arise from the lowest part of the nerve and supply the posterior part of the capsule of the ankle joint.

POPLITEAL ARTERY

This artery ends at the distal border of the popliteus, where it divides into two branches— the anterior and posterior tibial arteries. At the same point the **venae comitantes** of those arteries join together to form the popliteal vein.

Anterior Tibial Artery

Only a small part of this artery is found in this region, for it passes forwards almost at once through the interosseous membrane to the front of the leg. While in the back of the leg it gives off only the small **posterior recurrent** branch which runs upwards under cover of the popliteus muscle to the back of the knee joint.

Posterior Tibial Artery

This is the larger of the two terminal branches of the popliteal trunk, as it carries the main blood supply to the foot. It begins at the distal border of the popliteus muscle, and passes downwards and slightly medially in company with the tibial nerve to end in the hollow between the medial malleolus and the calcaneus, by dividing into the lateral and medial plantar arteries under cover of the flexor retinaculum.

It is closely accompanied by two **venae comitantes,** which are connected with each other by small veins that cross in front of the artery and behind it, and it has the same general relations as the tibial nerve.

Branches. The **circumflex fibular artery,** which may arise from the anterior tibial, runs laterally round the neck of the fibula to supply muscles and skin.

A **nutrient artery** springs from the posterior tibial close to its origin and enters the nutrient foramen of the tibia. It is remarkable on account of its large size.

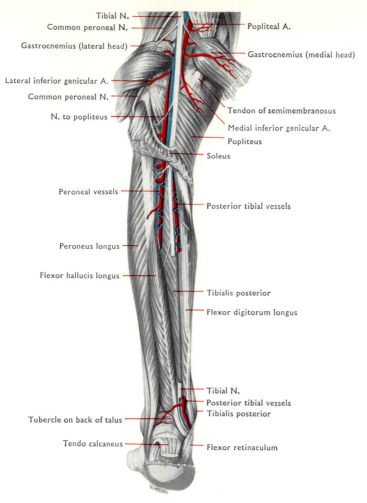

Labels on figure:
Tibial N.
Common peroneal N.
Gastrocnemius (lateral head)
Lateral inferior genicular A.
Common peroneal N.
N. to popliteus
Peroneal vessels
Peroneus longus
Flexor hallucis longus
Tubercle on back of talus
Tendo calcaneus
Popliteal A.
Gastrocnemius (medial head)
Tendon of semimembranosus
Medial inferior genicular A.
Popliteus
Soleus
Posterior tibial vessels
Tibialis posterior
Flexor digitorum longus
Tibial N.
Posterior tibial vessels
Tibialis posterior
Flexor retinaculum

FIG. 139 Deep dissection of back of leg.

The **muscular branches** supply the deep muscles and the soleus, and **cutaneous branches** are given to the skin on the medial side of the leg.

A **communicating branch** arises about 2 cm. above the calcaneus, and passes laterally, either in front of the flexor hallucis longus or behind it, to join the peroneal artery [FIGS. 133, 139].

Medial calcanean branches pierce the flexor retinaculum, and accompany the nerves of the same name.

Peroneal Artery. This is the largest branch of the posterior tibial. It arises about 2 cm. below the commencement of the parent trunk, and running obliquely downwards and laterally, under cover of the soleus, it reaches the fibula, along which it descends deep to the flexor hallucis longus. It passes behind the inferior tibiofibular and ankle joints, medial

207

to the peroneal tendons, and breaks up into a number of **lateral calcanean** branches.

In addition to the terminal branches, it supplies: (1) **muscular** branches; (2) a **nutrient** branch to the fibula; and (3) a **perforating** branch, which pierces the interosseous membrane near the inferior tibiofibular joint, and descends over the lower part of the fibula into the dorsum of the foot.

The peroneal artery is sometimes as large as the continuation of its parent trunk. Its communication with the posterior tibial artery may then be large, or its perforating branch may partially or entirely replace the dorsalis pedis artery.

DEEP MUSCLES

The deep muscles in the back of the leg are the popliteus, the tibialis posterior and the two long flexors of the toes.

Popliteus

The popliteus muscle arises by a stout, round tendon from the anterior part of the popliteal groove of the femur within the capsule of the knee joint. The tendon pierces the posterior part of the capsule of the knee joint, and the fleshy fibres which arise from the tendon are directed medially and downwards. They spread out to obtain insertion into the posterior surface of the tibia above the soleal line, and also into the fascia which covers the muscle.

Nerve supply: the **tibial nerve.** Its nerve can now be seen hooking round the distal margin of the muscle to reach the anterior surface. Action: it flexes the knee and medially rotates the leg at the beginning of the movement of flexion.

The flexors of the toes and the posterior tibial muscle arise from the fascial septa and the interosseous membrane, as well as from the bones of the leg.

Flexor Hallucis Longus

The long flexor of the big toe arises chiefly from the posterior surface of the fibula, below the origin of the soleus. After passing behind

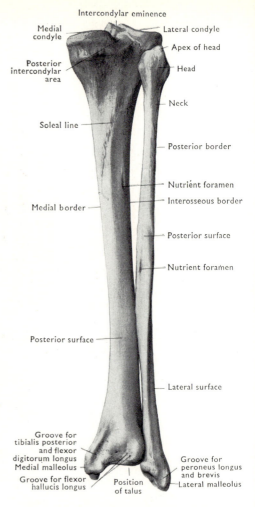

FIG. 140   Right tibia and fibula (posterior aspect).

the ankle joint, its tendon occupies a deep groove on the posterior surface of the talus. It then runs forwards under the flexor retinaculum, grooves the inferior surface of the sustentaculum tali and passes through the sole of the foot, to be inserted into the terminal phalanx of the big toe.

Nerve supply: the **tibial nerves.** Action: it flexes the interphalangeal and metatarso-

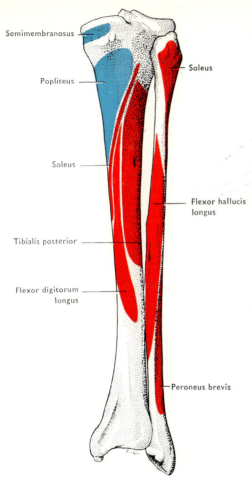

Semimembranosus

Popliteus

Soleus

Soleus

Flexor hallucis longus

Tibialis posterior

Flexor digitorum longus

Peroneus brevis

FIG. 141 Posterior aspect of bones of leg to show attachments of muscles.

phalangeal joints of the big toe, and plantar flexes and may help to invert the foot.

Flexor Digitorum Longus [FIGS. 139, 143]

The long flexor of the toes arises from the posterior surface of the tibia, below the popliteus, and medial to the vertical ridge. After crossing superficial to the distal part of the tibialis posterior, its tendon grooves the lower end of the tibia lateral to that of the

tibialis posterior. It passes into the sole of the foot deep to the flexor retinaculum and divides into four tendons each of which is inserted into the terminal phalanx of one of the lateral four toes.

Nerve supply: the **tibial nerve.** Action: it flexes the interphalangeal and metatarsophalangeal joints of the lateral four toes, and assists in plantar flexion and inversion of the foot.

Tibialis Posterior

The posterior tibial muscle takes origin from the interosseous membrane and the adjoining parts of the posterior surfaces of the tibia and fibula [FIGS. 130, 139, 141]. Its superior end is bifid, the anterior tibial vessels passing forward between the two osseous attachments. Distally the tibialis posterior inclines medially, under the flexor digitorum longus, and its strong, flattened tendon grooves the back of the medial malleolus under cover of the flexor retinaculum. It enters the sole and is inserted chiefly into the tuberosity of the navicular bone and the medial cuneiform bone, and by slips into the other tarsal bones (except the talus) and the middle three metatarsals.

Nerve supply: the **tibial nerve.** Action: it plantar flexes and inverts the foot.

Flexor Retinaculum

This thickened band of the deep fascia bridges across the hollow between the medial malleolus and the medial process of the tubercle of the calcaneus, and is attached to both of them. Its proximal border is continuous with the investing deep fascia of the back of the leg and with the septum which covers the deep muscles [p. 203], the latter forming the greater part of the retinaculum. Its distal or anterior margin is continuous with the deep fascia of the medial part of the sole, and gives attachment to the abductor hallucis muscle which lies deep to it.

Deep to the retinaculum the tendons of tibialis posterior, flexor digitorum longus, and flexor hallucis longus pass into the sole of the foot with the neurovascular bundle between the latter two.

Synovial Sheaths

The tendons are isolated from one another, and from the vessels and nerve, by septa which pass from the deep surface of the retinaculum to ridges on the adjacent bones. To demonstrate the septa, slit open the retinaculum for a

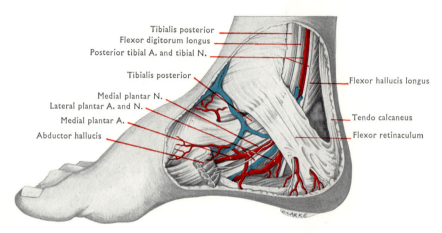

Tibialis posterior
Flexor digitorum longus
Posterior tibial A. and tibial N.
Tibialis posterior
Medial plantar N.
Lateral plantar A. and N.
Medial plantar A.
Abductor hallucis

Flexor hallucis longus
Tendo calcaneus
Flexor retinaculum

Fig. 142 Dissection of medial side of ankle, showing the relations of the flexor retinaculum.

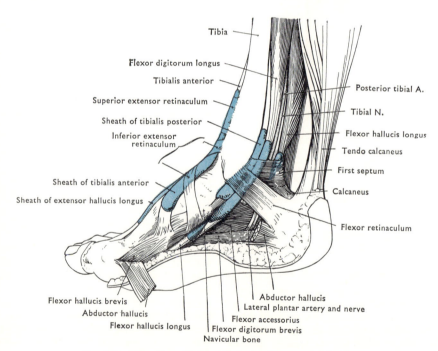

Tibia
Flexor digitorum longus
Tibialis anterior
Superior extensor retinaculum
Sheath of tibialis posterior
Inferior extensor retinaculum
Sheath of tibialis anterior
Sheath of extensor hallucis longus

Posterior tibial A.
Tibial N.
Flexor hallucis longus
Tendo calcaneus
First septum
Calcaneus
Flexor retinaculum

Flexor hallucis brevis
Abductor hallucis
Flexor hallucis longus
Abductor hallucis
Lateral plantar artery and nerve
Flexor accessorius
Flexor digitorum brevis
Navicular bone

Fig. 143 Dissection of leg and foot showing synovial sheaths.

short distance along the line of each tendon. Each of those three compartments will then be seen to be lined with a glistening **synovial sheath.** The dissector should investigate the extent of each sheath as far as possible with the aid of a blunt probe. The sheaths end proximally about 2 cm. above the medial malleolus. Distally, the sheath of the tibialis posterior reaches the insertion of the tendon into the navicular bone. The sheath of the flexor digitorum longus extends to about the middle of the foot. The sheath of the flexor hallucis longus may reach as far as the insertion of the tendon, but sometimes cannot be traced beyond the middle of the first metatarsal bone [FIG. 143].

NERVES AND VESSELS OF THE KNEE JOINT

At different stages of the dissection of the thigh and the leg, articular nerves and vessels that supply the knee joint have been found, and have been partly dissected. Study them now as a whole by following the nerves as far as the fibrous capsule of the joint, and cleaning the vessels around the joint, note their chief anastomoses.

DISSECTION. Find the nerves to the vasti, and trace their articular filaments down through each muscle to the knee. Clean the descending branch of the lateral circumflex artery and the descending genicular artery and their branches as far as possible. Find the branch that the posterior division of the obturator nerve sends into the adductor magnus; trace it into the muscle, and follow its longest filament: it emerges from the muscle and becomes the genicular branch.

Trace the superior genicular nerves and vessels to the capsule of the joint, and note the middle genicular nerve and vessels as they pierce the popliteal ligament of the knee. The proximal part of the inferior lateral genicular nerve has probably been destroyed. Find the inferior internal artery and trace it to the fibular collateral ligament of the joint; the nerve may be found alongside the artery there. Divide the biceps a little above the joint, and pull it downwards to expose the fibular collateral ligament more fully. Clean the ligament from end to end and trace the nerve and artery forwards between it and the fibrous capsule.

Follow the inferior medial genicular nerve and vessels along the upper border of the popliteus to the tibial collateral ligament. Turn the tendons of the sartorius, gracilis and semitendinosus forwards and pick up the nerve and vessels at the anterior border of the ligament and trace them onwards.

Now find the commencement of the anterior tibial artery, and secure its posterior recurrent branch. It passes upwards in front of the popliteus. Therefore, cut the popliteus near its lateral end, turn it medially, trace its nerve to its deep surface, and look for the branch which the nerve sends to the superior tibiofibular joint. Then follow the recurrent artery to its termination. Lastly turn to the front of the limb. Find the anterior recurrent branch of the anterior tibial artery and the recurrent genicular nerve; trace them upwards through the tibialis anterior to the knee.

Nerves of Knee Joint

The knee joint is richly supplied with nerves. No less than ten distinct branches may be traced to it.

The **femoral nerve** supplies three branches, one from each of the nerves to the vasti, to the anterosuperior part of the joint. The largest is from the nerve to vastus medialis and accompanies the descending genicular artery.

The **common peroneal nerve** supplies:

1. The superior lateral genicular nerve descends into the popliteal fossa and supplies the superolateral part of the joint by passing deep to biceps and through the lateral intermuscular septum above the lateral femoral condyle.

2. The inferior lateral genicular nerve is small and sometimes absent. It may arise with the preceding nerve, and curving downwards and forwards over the lateral head of gastrocnemius, reaches the inferior part by passing between the capsule and the fibular collateral ligament.

3. The recurrent genicular nerve consists of a twig or two reaching the antero-inferior part of the joint from the first branch to tibialis anterior.

The **tibial nerve** supplies:

1. The superior medial genicular nerve which runs medially round the femur above the medial condyle, deep to adductor magnus,

211

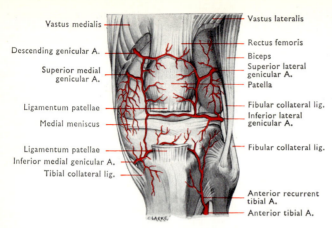

Labels on figure:
Vastus medialis
Descending genicular A.
Superior medial genicular A.
Ligamentum patellae
Medial meniscus
Ligamentum patellae
Inferior medial genicular A.
Tibial collateral lig.

Vastus lateralis
Rectus femoris
Biceps
Superior lateral genicular A.
Patella
Fibular collateral lig.
Inferior lateral genicular A.
Fibular collateral lig.
Anterior recurrent tibial A.
Anterior tibial A.

CLARKE

FIG. 144   Arterial anastomosis on front and sides of left knee joint.

and through vastus medialis to the supero-medial part of the joint.

2. The middle genicular nerve runs forwards through the fibrous capsule to the cruciate ligaments within the capsule.

3. The inferior medial genicular is the largest of the articular nerves. It runs along the upper border of popliteus, and passing forwards between the shaft of the tibia and the tibial collateral ligament, curves superiorly to the inferomedial part of the capsule.

The **obturator nerve** sends a genicular branch through the adductor magnus to join the beginning of the popliteal artery and run with it to the posterior aspect of the knee joint.

Anastomosis around Knee Joint

Eight arteries take part in this anastomosis [FIGS. 119, 144]. They are the five genicular branches of the popliteal artery, the two re-current branches of the anterior tibial, and the descending genicular branches of the femoral and lateral circumflex arteries. Like the articular arteries at other joints, they ramify to form rich networks around the knee; and these plexuses give branches to the soft parts that cover the joint as well as to the bones, ligaments and synovial membranes—the largest branches being those that enter the bone to supply the marrow.

212

The anastomoses are most numerous on the front and sides of the joint. In a well-injected specimen, three distinct arches are seen connecting the vessels of the lateral and medial sides—one amidst the superficial fibres of the quadriceps immediately above the patella, another under cover of the ligamentum patellae immediately below the patella, and the third on the tibia immediately above the insertion of the ligamentum patellae [FIG. 144].

The middle genicular artery takes little share in the network, for it is spent chiefly in the cruciate ligaments and fat in the interior of the joint.

Anastomosis around Ankle Joint

On the **lateral side** of the joint there are communications between branches of the following arteries: (1) lateral malleolar; (2) perforating branch of peroneal; (3) terminal part of peroneal; and (4) lateral tarsal.

On the **medial side** of the joint the medial malleolar branch of the anterior tibial anastomoses with small twigs from the medial calcanean branches of the posterior tibial [FIG. 152].

THE SOLE OF THE FOOT

Before beginning the dissection, revise the surface anatomy [p. 185], and note that the skin is specially thick over the heel, on the ball of the foot, and, to a lesser extent, along the lateral border of the foot; on all those parts the weight of the body presses in the erect posture. Other noticeable features are the shortness of the toes as contrasted with the length of the fingers, and the fact that the longest digit of the foot is either the first or the second, and not the middle digit as in the hand.

DISSECTION. **Reflexion of Skin. Place the** limb on the table with the sole of the foot, toes downwards, facing the dissector and the front of the ankle resting on a block. Two incisions are required—one along the middle line of the sole from the heel to the root of the middle toe; the other across the sole at the roots of the toes. Reflect the skin to the lateral and medial sides. Make also a longitudinal incision along each toe, and reflect the skin from the toes.

SUPERFICIAL FASCIA

Along the lateral border of the foot, at the ball of the foot, and at the heel, it is thick, tough and granular. It is traversed by tough, fibrous bands which connect the skin with the deep fascia, and subdivide the fatty tissue into small, tight lobules, making it firm and resilient.

Under the heel the superficial fascia contains branches of the **medial calcanean vessels** and **nerves.** Further forwards it is supplied by unnamed branches of the medial and lateral plantar nerves. On the sides of the toes it contains the **plantar digital vessels** and **nerves.** Near the webs of the toes, and superficial to the digital vessels and nerves, there is a weak band of fibres called the superficial transverse metatarsal ligament, less conspicuous than the corresponding ligament of the palm [FIG. 145].

DISSECTION. **Trace the** medial calcanean arteries and nerves to their distribution.

The superficial fascia may now be removed. Divide it along the middle line of the sole, and turn it laterally and medially, cleaning the deep fascia at the same time. As you approach the margins of the foot note the longitudinal furrow on each side, and secure the small vessels and nerves that pass from the plantar vessels and nerves through the furrows to reach the skin.

Proceed cautiously as you approach the intervals between the heads of the metatarsal bones, for there the metatarsal arteries and digital nerves are unprotected by the deep fascia. The nerves and vessels which go to the medial side of the big toe and to the lateral side of the little toe are especially liable to injury, for they perforate the deep fascia further proximally than the others. Look for the superficial transverse metatarsal ligament at the roots of the toes.

Trace the digital nerves and arteries forwards along the sides of the toes. Then clean the superficial fascia from the big toe and from one, at least, of the others.

DEEP FASCIA

The deep fascia of the plantar surface of the foot and toes is now brought into view. Study the deep fascia of the toes first.

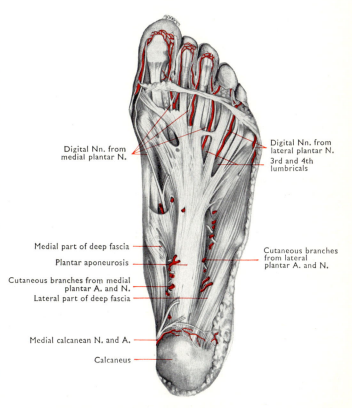

Digital Nn. from medial plantar N.

Digital Nn. from lateral plantar N.
3rd and 4th lumbricals

Medial part of deep fascia

Plantar aponeurosis

Cutaneous branches from medial plantar A. and N.

Lateral part of deep fascia

Cutaneous branches from lateral plantar A. and N.

Medial calcanean N. and A.

Calcaneus

FIG. 145 Superficial dissection of sole of foot to show plantar aponeurosis. The skin and superficial fascia, except the superficial transverse ligament, have been removed, and the fibrous flexor sheaths partially opened.

Fibrous Flexor Sheaths

On each toe the deep fascia is thickened to form a curved plate, the fibrous flexor sheath, which is attached to the margins of the first and second phalanges (only the first in the big toe) and to the margins of the plantar liga-ments of the joints. It forms with them a tunnel which holds the long and short flexor tendons against the phalanges, and is lined with the synovial sheath which envelops the tendons. Distally the fibrous flexor sheath is attached to the base of the terminal phalanx beyond the insertion of the long flexor tendon. Proximally it is continuous with the slips of the plantar aponeurosis, *q.v.* It is thick and strong opposite the phalanges, but thin and weak opposite the joints so that it does not hamper their movements. Slit open one of the fibrous sheaths to see the tendons and the synovial sheath, and then proceed to study the deep fascia.

The deep fascia of the sole is divisible into parts: (1) medial, (2) intermediate and (3) lateral. The division is indicated by a differ-ence in the density of the three parts and by two shallow furrows which traverse the foot in a longitudinal direction. Each of the three portions is in relation to a muscle which takes part of its origin from it.

The **medial part** is the thin fascia that covers the abductor hallucis. The **lateral part** covers the abductor digiti minimi. It is stronger than the medial portion, especially laterally, where it is thickened to form a strong band that stretches from the lateral process of the cal-canean tuber to the base of the fifth metatarsal bone [FIGS. 145, 146].

Plantar Aponeurosis

The **intermediate part** covers the flexor digitorum brevis. It stands out in marked contrast to the lateral and medial parts in point of strength and density, and is called the **plantar aponeurosis.** Its posterior end is narrow, and is attached to the medial process of the calcanean tuber. It expands as it passes forwards and, near the heads of the metatarsal bones, it splits into five processes which proceed towards the toes and are bound together by transverse fibres. In the interval between each two of those digital processes lie a plantar metatarsal artery, a plantar digital nerve, and a lumbrical muscle.

Trace the processes forwards. One goes to the root of each toe; there it sends forwards a few superficial fibres to the skin of the creases of the toes, and then divides into two slips. The two slips diverge from each other and pass towards the dorsum of the foot, embrac-ing the flexor tendons of the toe; their distal edges fuse with the proximal end of the fibrous flexor sheath; their ends are attached to the margins of the plantar ligament of the meta-tarsophalangeal joint and to the deep trans-verse ligaments of the sole.

An **intermuscular septum** [FIG. 145] springs from each margin of the plantar aponeurosis along the lines of the longitudinal furrows, and both pass into the sole. They lie one on each side of the flexor digitorum brevis, and form partitions which separate it from the abductor hallucis and the abductor digiti minimi. They give partial origin to those muscles, and fuse with the layer of fascia that covers their deep surfaces.

DISSECTION. To demonstrate these septa make a transverse incision through the plantar aponeurosis about 2-3 cm. in front of its posterior end and a longitudinal cut through the middle of the aponeurosis, in front of that; raise the divided aponeurosis and turn it laterally and medially. As the margins of the flexor digitorum brevis are approached the septa are brought into view. As the anterior part of the aponeurosis is reflected, avoid injury to the plantar digital arteries and nerves, for they lie close to its deep surface.

MUSCLES AND TENDONS OF THE SOLE

The muscles and tendons of the sole are disposed in four layers separated by fascial partitions in which the plantar vessels and nerves and their branches lie.

DISSECTION. Remove the deep fascia from the abductor muscles, taking care to avoid injury to the digital nerve to the lateral side of the little toe and the digital nerve and artery to the medial side of the big toe. To avoid injuring those structures, pull on each reflected portion of the plantar aponeurosis in turn, and freeing it from the septum at the side of the flexor digitorum brevis, reflect the remaining part of the plantar fascia, dissecting close to its deep surface.

Before proceeding further with the dissection, identify the structures exposed by the removal of the deep fascia [Fig. 146].

The abductor hallucis and the abductor digiti minimi lie along the medial and lateral borders of the sole, with the flexor digitorum brevis between, dividing into tendons to the lateral four toes. Two spaces separate these three muscles, and in the medial of these can be seen: part of the tendon of flexor hallucis longus, the digital artery and nerve to the medial side of the big toe, and the flexor hallucis brevis on a deeper plane. In the lateral space are found: the digital nerves and vessels to the little toe, and the flexor digiti minimi on a deeper plane, with part of an interosseous muscle lying deeper still. Between the tendons of flexor digitorum brevis, and lying medial to that to the second toe, are the digital vessels and nerves and the lumbrical muscles.

DISSECTION. Cut down into the posterior part of the interval between the abductor hallucis and the flexor digitorum brevis, and secure the posterior parts of the medial and lateral plantar nerves and arteries. Follow the medial plantar nerve forwards and secure the muscular branches to flexor digitorum brevis and abductor hallucis that arise from its trunk. Then trace its four digital branches forwards to the toes, securing: (1) a branch to flexor hallucis brevis from the most medial one, (2) a muscular branch to the first lumbrical from the second, and (3) a communicating branch from the fourth to a digital branch of the lateral plantar nerve [Fig. 146]. At the same time clean the medial plantar artery and its branches.

Next cut down into the interval between the flexor digitorum brevis and the abductor digiti minimi, just behind the base of the fifth metatarsal bone, and secure the lateral plantar artery and the trunk of the lateral plantar nerve, before the nerve divides into its superficial and deep divisions. The artery and the deep division of the nerve bend medially and pass out of sight. Follow the superficial division of the nerve forwards, and secure: (1) the branches to the flexor digiti minimi brevis and interossei of the fourth interosseous space; (2) its two digital branches to the fourth and

fifth toes. Clean also the arteries which accompany the nerves.

Now divide the flexor digitorum brevis across its middle; turn the anterior part forwards to the toes, and the posterior part backwards, defining its attachments; at the same time clean the part of the abductor digiti minimi that passes deep to it. Lastly detach the abductor hallucis from the calcaneus (but not from the flexor retinaculum) and turn it medially, thus exposing the greater part of the lateral plantar vessels and nerve, the tendon of the flexor digitorum longus, with its lumbrical muscles, and the flexor digitorum accessorius attached to it, and the tendon of the flexor hallucis longus on the medial side of the flexor digitorum.

Clean the lateral plantar nerve and its branch to the abductor digiti minimi which lies far back, close to the processes of the tuber calcanei, and the branch to the flexor accessorius, a little further forward. Next clean the lateral plantar artery and its branches. Finally clean the muscles and tendons.

FIRST LAYER OF MUSCLES

These are the short flexor of the toes and the abductors of the big toe and little toe.

Flexor Digitorum Brevis

This muscle arises from the medial process of the tuber calcanei and from the fascia and the septa. About the middle of the sole it divides into four fleshy slips which end in slender tendons which enter the fibrous flexor sheaths of the lateral four toes and are inserted into the middle phalanges.

Nerve supply: the **medial plantar nerve.** Action: it flexes the first interphalangeal and the metatarsophalangeal joints of the lateral four toes.

Abductor Hallucis

The abductor of the big toe arises from the flexor retinaculum, and from the medial process of the tuber calcanei. Its strong tendon is joined by fibres of the medial belly of the flexor hallucis brevis, and it is inserted into the medial side of the base of the proximal phalanx of the big toe.

Nerve supply: the **medial plantar nerve.** Action: it abducts the big toe from the second toe.

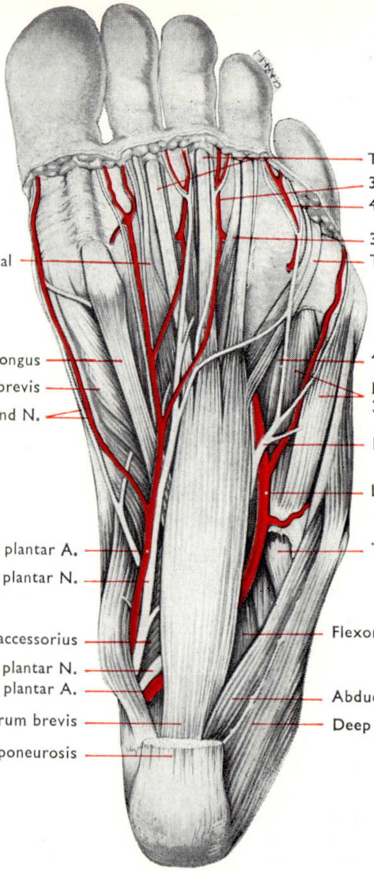

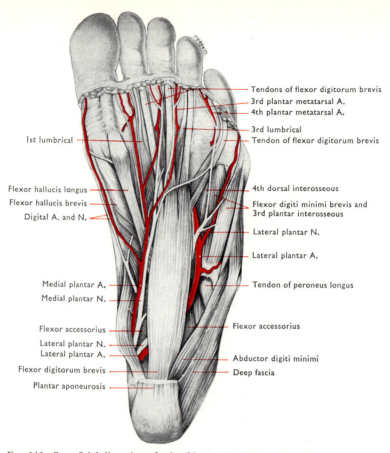

Tendons of flexor digitorum brevis
3rd plantar metatarsal A.
4th plantar metatarsal A.
3rd lumbrical
Tendon of flexor digitorum brevis
Ist lumbrical
Flexor hallucis longus
Flexor hallucis brevis
Digital A. and N.
4th dorsal interosseous
Flexor digiti minimi brevis and
3rd plantar interosseous
Lateral plantar N.
Lateral plantar A.
Tendon of peroneus longus
Medial plantar A.
Medial plantar N.
Flexor accessorius
Flexor accessorius
Lateral plantar N.
Lateral plantar A.
Abductor digiti minimi
Flexor digitorum brevis
Deep fascia
Plantar aponeurosis

FIG. 146 Superficial dissection of sole of foot. The plantar aponeurosis has been removed. The abductor digiti minimi and the abductor hallucis have been pulled aside.

Abductor Digiti Minimi

The abductor of the little toe arises from both processes of the tuber calcanei, partly therefore under cover of the flexor digitorum brevis. Its tendon is inserted into the lateral side of the base of the proximal phalanx of the little toe. The lateral portion of the muscle is often inserted into the base of the fifth metatarsal bone and is called the **abductor of the fifth metatarsal bone.**

Nerve supply: the **lateral plantar nerve.** Action: it abducts the little toe from the fourth toe.

DISSECTION. Separate the abductor hallucis from the flexor retinaculum, and turn it medially; then divide the retinaculum until the origins of the plantar arteries and nerves are exposed.

Medial Plantar Nerve (L. 4, 5; S. 1)

This is the larger of the two terminal branches of the tibial nerve. It arises, deep to the flexor retinaculum, midway between the calcaneus and the medial malleolus, and passes under cover of the abductor hallucis, to appear with the medial plantar vessels in the interval between that muscle and the flexor

digitorum brevis, under cover of the deep fascia [FIGS. 146, 151].

Branches. The **cutaneous twigs** spring from the trunk of the nerve; they pierce the deep fascia in the line of the medial intermuscular septum and supply the skin of the medial part of the sole.

The **first digital nerve** arises far back and runs a comparatively long course to reach the medial side of the big toe. The **other three** diverge as they run forwards, superficial to the flexor tendons and the lumbricals, towards the clefts between the medial four toes. Each divides into two branches which run along the adjacent sides of two toes, and the most lateral digital nerve sends a communicating branch to the superficial part of the lateral plantar nerve. They supply the skin on the plantar surfaces of the medial three and a half toes, the skin on the dorsal surfaces of their terminal phalanges, and their joints and ligaments.

The digital distribution of the medial plantar nerve closely resembles that of the median nerve in the hand.

The **muscular branches** go to four muscles of the sole:

Abductor hallucis.
Flexor digitorum brevis.
Flexor hallucis brevis.
First lumbrical.

Lateral Plantar Nerve (S. 1, 2)

The lateral plantar nerve is the smaller terminal branch of the tibial nerve, and corresponds to the ulnar nerve in the palm of the hand. It begins, deep to the flexor retinaculum, midway between the medial malleolus and the calcaneus, and runs anterolaterally with the lateral plantar vessels, between the first and second layers of muscles, towards the base of the fifth metatarsal bone. Here it ends by dividing into superficial and deep branches [FIG. 147]. At its termination it is either deep to the flexor digitorum brevis, or to the deep fascia in the interval between that muscle and the abductor digiti minimi.

Branches. The trunk of the nerve gives off **muscular** branches to the **abductor digiti minimi** and the **flexor**

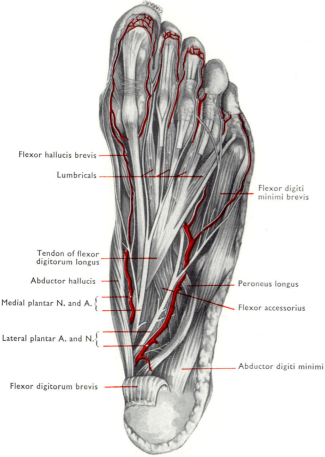

Flexor hallucis brevis

Lumbricals

Flexor digiti minimi brevis

Tendon of flexor digitorum longus

Abductor hallucis

Medial plantar N. and A.

Peroneus longus

Flexor accessorius

Lateral plantar A. and N.

Abductor digiti minimi

Flexor digitorum brevis

FIG. 147   Dissection of sole of foot.   Most of the flexor digitorum brevis has been removed.

digitorum accessorius, and **cutaneous** branches which pass between the flexor digitorum brevis and the abductor digiti minimi, and supply the skin of the lateral part of the sole.

The **superficial branch** [FIGS. 146, 147] divides into:

The **lateral digital branch** runs forwards along the lateral side of the little toe. The **medial digital branch** crosses the flexor tendons of the little toe and divides into two branches which run along the contiguous sides of the fifth and fourth toes. It communicates with the fourth digital branch of the medial plantar nerve. These digital branches are distributed to the little toe and the lateral half of the fourth toe in the same way as the digital branches of the medial plantar nerve to the other toes.

Muscular twigs from the stem, or lateral digital branch, supply the flexor digiti minimi brevis and the third plantar and fourth dorsal interosseous muscles.

The **deep branch** is really the continuation of the lateral plantar nerve. It curves medially and forwards, between the third and fourth layers of muscles, towards the first metatarsal bone, and it will be dissected later. Its branches supply the adductor of the big toe, the lateral three lumbricals, most of the interossei, and the intertarsal and tarsometatarsal joints.

Medial Plantar Artery

The medial plantar artery arises, as a terminal branch of the posterior tibial, under cover of the flexor retinaculum. Usually small, it is accompanied by venae comitantes and the medial plantar nerve, and it ends by joining the digital branch which the first metatarsal artery sends to the medial side of the big toe [FIG. 152].

It supplies adjacent muscles and the skin of the medial part of the foot, and, according to its size, it may give off one or more **digital** branches to accompany the digital branches of the medial plantar nerve [FIG. 151].

Lateral Plantar Artery

The lateral plantar artery is the larger of the two terminal branches of the posterior tibial artery. It is accompanied by venae comitantes and the lateral plantar nerve, and runs across the sole to the fifth metatarsal bone near its base. It then runs medially with the deep branch of the nerve, and crossing the sole for the second time forms the **plantar arch.** The arch lies deep in the sole, and terminates at the proximal extremity of the first intermetatarsal space by joining the end of the dorsalis pedis artery [FIG. 152]. The arch will be dissected later.

The part of the artery now exposed supplies the adjacent muscles and the skin of the lateral and posterior parts of the sole.

DISSECTION. Detach the abductor digiti minimi from its origin, and turn it forwards in order that a good display may be obtained of the second stratum of the sole.

SECOND LAYER OF MUSCLES AND TENDONS

This layer is made up of the tendons of the two long flexors of the toes, with the flexor accessorius, and the four lumbrical muscles.

As the tendon of the **flexor hallucis longus** enters the sole it grooves the plantar surface of the sustentaculum tali [FIG. 171] and inclines medially, passing deep to the tendon of the flexor digitorum longus, which inclines laterally, to reach the middle of the foot. Here the latter receives the insertion of the **flexor digitorum accessorius** and divides into the four tendons which give origin to the **lumbrical muscles,** and passes to the four lateral toes. Where the long tendons cross each other, the tendon of the flexor hallucis longus gives a slip to the deep surface of the tendon of flexor digitorum longus. Variable in size, this slip may pass into the medial one, two, or three branches of the latter tendon.

DISSECTION. Turn over the tendons of the flexor digitorum and trace the fibres of the slip of the flexor hallucis into them. Then follow the tendons of the long and short flexors to the toes, and open one of the fibrous flexor sheaths.

Flexor Digitorum Accessorius

This muscle arises by two heads which embrace the calcaneus and the long plantar

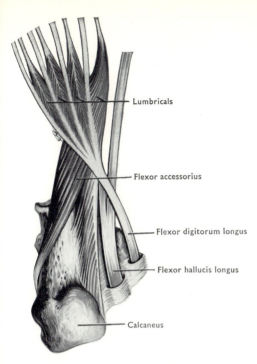

Lumbricals

Flexor accessorius

Flexor digitorum longus

Flexor hallucis longus

Calcaneus

FIG. 148   Second layer of muscles and tendons in sole of foot.

ligament. The **medial head,** wide and fleshy, springs from the medial surface of the calcaneus ; the **lateral head,** narrow, pointed and tendinous, takes origin from the lateral margin of the plantar surface of the calcaneus. The muscle is inserted into the tendon of the flexor digitorum longus in the middle of the sole.

Nerve supply : the **lateral plantar nerve.** Action : it is a direct flexor of the toes, and pulls the tendons of the long flexor muscle into line with the toes upon which they operate.

Lumbrical Muscles

The lumbrical muscles of the foot are more slender than those of the hand and arise from the tendons of the flexor digitorum longus in the manner shown in FIGURE 148. Their tendons cross the medial sides of the metatarsophalangeal joints of the lateral four toes, and each is inserted into the base of the proximal phalanx and slightly into the extensor expansion [see p. 191].   Nerve supply : the **first lumbrical** is supplied by the **medial plantar nerve,** the others by the **lateral plantar nerve.**

Flexor Tendons in the Toes

In the digits, the tendons lie enclosed in synovial sheaths in the osteofibrous canals formed by the fibrous flexor sheaths, the phalanges, and plantar ligaments of the joints.

The **tendon of the flexor hallucis longus,** after giving its slip to the tendon of the flexor digitorum longus is inserted into the base of the terminal phalanx of the big toe.

The four smaller toes each receive a tendon of the **flexor digitorum longus** and a tendon of the **flexor digitorum brevis.** Opposite the proximal part of the first phalanx the short flexor is superficial ; but, at the middle of the phalanx, it is perforated by the tendon of the long flexor, which passes forwards to be inserted into the base of the terminal phalanx, whilst the two parts of the tendon of the short flexor are attached to the margins of the second phalanx.

Synovial Sheaths of the Digits

Each sheath begins in the sole near the middle of the metatarsal bone, and extends to the insertion of the long flexor tendon, *i.e.,* to the **base** of the terminal phalanx. The sheath of the little toe is usually continuous with the sheath that envelops the main tendon of the flexor digitorum longus.

The sheath has two layers : one lines the canal, the other clothes the tendons, enveloping them separately ; the two layers are continuous with each other at the ends of the sheath.   The sheath facilitates the play of the tendons when the muscles are in action, for the opposed surfaces of the layers are smooth and glistening, and are separated by a film of synovia.

The sheath forms folds called **vincula** which pass between the tendons and the bones, and carry small arteries to the tendons. In each sheath there are two **vincula brevia,** short triangular folds at the insertions of the tendons, exactly similar to those found in the

219

fingers [FIG. 74, p. 108]. The **vincula longa** are slender bands, irregular in number and position, that pass between the two tendons and between the tendons and the first phalanx.

The deep division of the lateral plantar nerve and the plantar arterial arch are partially exposed, but they will be more fully displayed at a later stage.

THIRD LAYER OF MUSCLES

The muscles of this layer are the adductor and short flexor of the big toe and the short flexor of the little toe [FIG. 149].

Flexor Hallucis Brevis

The short flexor of the big toe arises from the cuboid bone and from adjoining slips of the tendon of the tibialis posterior. It is narrow and tendinous at its origin, but it soon widens to form two partly separated fleshy bellies which ultimately divide to be inserted by tendons—one on each side of the base of the proximal phalanx of the big toe, fusing with the plantar ligament of the metatarsophalangeal joint. The medial tendon is inserted in common with the abductor hallucis, and the lateral tendon with the adductor; there is a sesamoid bone in each tendon of insertion [FIG. 173].

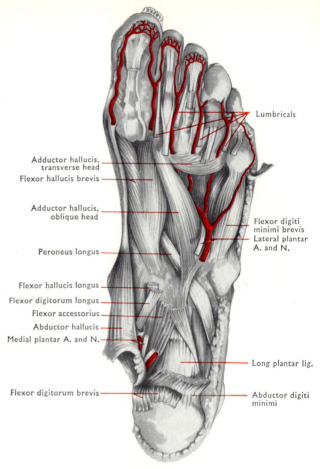

FIG. 149   Deep dissection of sole of foot.

Nerve supply: the **medial plantar nerve.** Action: it flexes the metatarsophalangeal joint of the big toe.

Adductor Hallucis

The adductor of the big toe has two separate heads [FIG. 149].

The **oblique head** arises from the fibrous sheath of the peroneus longus tendon and from the bases of the second, third and fourth metatarsal bones. The **transverse head** springs from the plantar ligaments of the lateral four

220

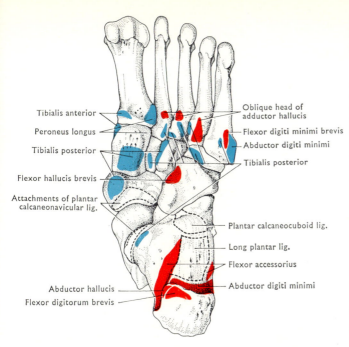

Tibialis anterior

Peroneus longus

Tibialis posterior

Flexor hallucis brevis

Attachments of plantar calcaneonavicular lig.

Abductor hallucis

Flexor digitorum brevis

Oblique head of adductor hallucis

Flexor digiti minimi brevis

Abductor digiti minimi

Tibialis posterior

Plantar calcaneocuboid lig.

Long plantar lig.

Flexor accessorius

Abductor digiti minimi

Fig. 150 Muscle attachments to left tarsus and metatarsus (plantar aspect). See Fig. 171.

nerve. Action : it flexes the little toe at the metatarso-phalangeal joint.

DISSECTION. Clean all those muscles from end to end, but avoid injury to the branches of the deep division of the lateral plantar nerve—especially its branches to the lumbrical muscles. Clean also the exposed part of the plantar arterial arch. Divide the common tendon of insertion of the abductor and flexor hallucis brevis; turn the two muscles aside and find the sesamoid bones in the tendons of the flexor brevis.

Sesamoid Bones in the Foot

Two small sesamoid bones—each about 1.5×0.8 cm.—are found in the tendons of the flexor hallucis brevis as they fuse with the plantar ligament of the metatarsophalangeal joint. These bones replace that ligament almost entirely, and their upper surfaces are smooth for articulation with the lower surface of the head of the metatarsal bone, which is grooved for their reception. The medial part of the ball of the foot owes its size and firmness largely to them.

Radiographs sometimes disclose minute nodules of bone in one or more of the other metatarsophalangeal joints ; it will be seen later that a sesamoid bone or a sesamoid cartilage is developed in the tendons of both the peroneus longus and the tibialis posterior as they enter the sole.

DISSECTION. Detach the flexor hallucis brevis and the oblique head of the adductor from their origins and turn them towards their insertion in order to display the entire length of the plantar arterial arch, the deep branch of the lateral plantar nerve, and the termination of the dorsalis pedis artery. As you raise the oblique head of the adductor, secure its nerve and retain it. Then clean the deep branch of the lateral plantar nerve and trace its branches; the branch to the

metatarsophalangeal joints. The two heads converge as they approach the root of the hallux and blend to be inserted, with the lateral tendon of the short flexor, into the lateral side of the base of the proximal phalanx.

Nerve supply : the **deep branch** of the **lateral plantar nerve.** Action : the oblique head adducts and flexes the big toe ; the transverse head draws the roots of the toes closer together and accentuates the curvature of the transverse arch made by the metatarsal bones.

Flexor Digiti Minimi Brevis

The short flexor of the little toe is a single fleshy slip which springs from the base of the fifth metatarsal bone and the fibrous sheath of the peroneus longus tendon. It is inserted into the lateral side of the base of the proximal phalanx of the little toe. Nerve supply : the **superficial branch** of the lateral plantar second lumbrical needs especial care. Lastly clean the plantar arch and its branches.

Deep Branch of Lateral Plantar Nerve

This branch arises from the parent trunk near the base of the fifth metatarsal bone. It curves medially and forwards towards the medial side of the foot, and it ends in the deep surface of the oblique head of the adductor hallucis.

It is deeply placed in the sole, immediately proximal to the plantar arterial arch. It rests against the interosseous muscles and the proximal parts of the metatarsal bones, under cover of the flexor tendons, the lumbrical muscles and the oblique head of the adductor hallucis.

Branches. The **muscular branches** supply the two heads of the adductor hallucis, the lateral three lumbrical muscles, the medial three dorsal interossei and the medial two plantar interossei. The branches to the transverse head and to the lumbricals emerge from under cover of the oblique head and run distally to these muscles; the branch to the second lumbrical passes across the upper surface of the transverse head.

The articular branches are fine filaments that arise from the stem of the nerve and from its muscular branches; they supply the intertarsal and tarsometatarsal joints.

Plantar Arch

The plantar arterial arch is the continuation of the lateral plantar artery across the sole of the foot. It runs from the level of the base of the fifth metatarsal bone to the base of the first interosseous space, where it is joined by the terminal portion of the dorsalis pedis artery. It is concave proximally [FIGS. 151, 152], is accompanied by two venae comitantes, and lies immediately in front of the deep branch of the lateral plantar nerve; its relations are therefore the same as those of the nerve.

Branches. Articular branches arise from the concavity of the arch, and run backwards to supply the intertarsal and tarsometatarsal joints.

Three posterior perforating branches pass upwards through the lateral three intermetatarsal spaces and join the corresponding dorsal metatarsal arteries.

Three **plantar metatarsal arteries** run forwards opposite the lateral three spaces. Each gives off an anterior perforating artery and bifurcates into **plantar digital arteries** that supply the contiguous sides of the lateral four toes. The lateral plantar digital artery of the little

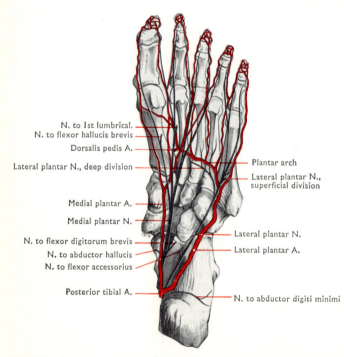

N. to 1st lumbrical.
N. to flexor hallucis brevis
Dorsalis pedis A.
Lateral plantar N., deep division
Medial plantar A.
Medial plantar N.
N. to flexor digitorum brevis
N. to abductor hallucis
N. to flexor accessorius
Posterior tibial A.
Plantar arch
Lateral plantar N., superficial division
Lateral plantar N.
Lateral plantar A.
N. to abductor digiti minimi

FIG. 151 Arteries and nerves of sole of foot. The plantar nerves and their branches are black.

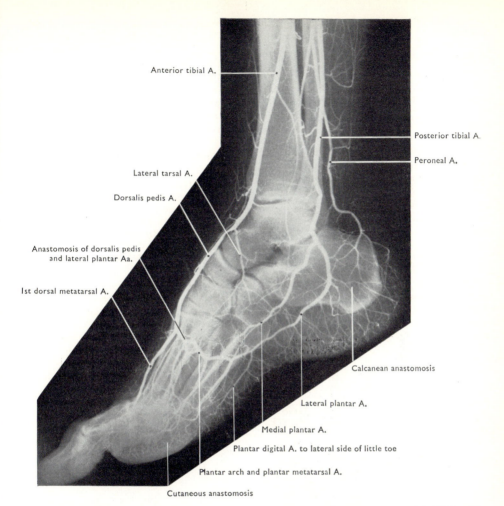

Anterior tibial A.

Posterior tibial A.

Peroneal A.

Lateral tarsal A.

Dorsalis pedis A.

Anastomosis of dorsalis pedis
and lateral plantar Aa.

1st dorsal metatarsal A.

Calcanean anastomosis

Lateral plantar A.

Medial plantar A.

Plantar digital A. to lateral side of little toe

Plantar arch and plantar metatarsal A.

Cutaneous anastomosis

Fig. 152   Lateral radiograph of foot after injection of the arteries with X-ray-opaque material. Cf. Fig. 151.

toe springs independently from the lateral extremity of the arch.

As in the hand, the digital arteries unite, opposite the terminal phalanx, to form an arch from which fine branches are sent to the pad of the toe and the bed of the nail.

First Plantar Metatarsal Artery. This artery arises from the plantar end of the dorsalis pedis, at the point where the dorsalis pedis joins the plantar arch. It runs forwards to the

cleft between the big toe and the second toe, where it divides into two plantar digital arteries for the supply of the adjacent sides of the first and second toes. Before it divides, it gives off the plantar digital artery to the medial side of the big toe. This joins the terminal part of the medial plantar artery.

DISSECTION. Detach the transverse head of the adductor hallucis from its origin and turn it towards

223

the hallux to display the deep transverse ligaments of the sole.

Deep Transverse Metatarsal Ligaments

This name is given to the strong, flat bands that lie between the heads of the metatarsal bones. They are attached to the margins of the plantar ligaments of the metatarsophalangeal joints, and through them to the bases of the proximal phalanges, so that the transverse ligaments prevent the roots of the toes from spreading apart. The lumbrical muscles and the plantar digital vessels and nerves pass forwards across the plantar surfaces of the transverse ligaments; the interosseous muscles cross their dorsal surfaces.

FOURTH LAYER OF MUSCLES
AND TENDONS

The muscles are the interossei, and the tendons are those of the peroneus longus and tibialis posterior.

Owing to the arched arrangement of the skeleton of the foot, the more medial **inter-** osseous muscles are very deeply placed as seen from the plantar aspect though all are close to the dorsal surface. The **tendon of the peroneus longus** crosses the sole obliquely from the lateral to the medial side; the slips of the **tendon of the tibialis posterior** pass laterally and forwards from the medial side. These tendons, crossing the sole obliquely from opposite directions, brace up the foot, and help to maintain both the longitudinal and the transverse arches.

DISSECTION. Clean the interosseous muscles. To follow their tendons, divide the deep transverse ligaments and pull the toes apart. Detach the flexor digiti minimi brevis from its origin and turn it towards its insertion, thus exposing the most lateral interossei more fully. The dorsal interossei should be cleaned on both plantar and dorsal aspects of the foot.

Interossei [Fig. 153]

There are three plantar and four dorsal interossei which lie between the metatarsal bones and arise from them.

The general principle of origin, insertion and

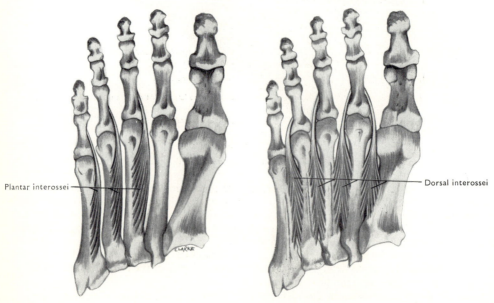

Plantar interossei

Dorsal interossei

Fig. 153   Interosseous muscles of right foot.

action is the same as in the hand [p. 115]. Each **plantar interosseous** arises from the metatarsal bone of the toe upon which it acts, the **dorsal interossei** from the sides of the metatarsals between which they lie. The insertions are mainly into the bases of the proximal phalanges and also, though less effectively, into the extensor expansions [p. 191].

Nerve supply: the **lateral plantar nerve**. Action: the **plantar interossei** adduct the lateral three toes towards the second toe; the **dorsal interossei** abduct the second, third and fourth toes from the middle line of the second

toe (cf. hand). In addition, they flex the metatarsophalangeal joints and help, feebly, to extend the interphalangeal joints.

DISSECTION. Put tension upon the tendon of the tibialis posterior. Clean its principal insertion and the various slips which it sends forwards and laterally. Then pull upon the tendon of the peroneus longus; cut through the fibrous bridge that holds it in place in the groove on the cuboid bone, and follow the tendon to its insertion.

Tendon of Tibialis Posterior

This tendon enters the sole and divides into two parts. The larger medial part is inserted

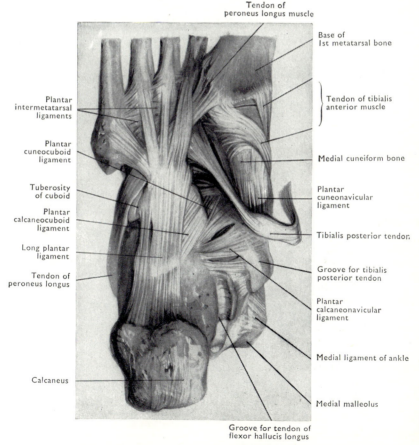

Tendon of peroneus longus muscle

Base of 1st metatarsal bone

Plantar intermetatarsal ligaments

Plantar cuneocuboid ligament

Tuberosity of cuboid

Plantar calcaneocuboid ligament

Long plantar ligament

Tendon of peroneus longus

Calcaneus

Tendon of tibialis anterior muscle

Medial cuneiform bone

Plantar cuneonavicular ligament

Tibialis posterior tendon

Groove for tibialis posterior tendon

Plantar calcaneonavicular ligament

Medial ligament of ankle

Medial malleolus

Groove for tendon of flexor hallucis longus

FIG. 154   Plantar aspect of tarsal and tarsometatarsal joints.

into the tuberosity of the navicular bone and the adjoining part of the lower surface of the medial cuneiform bone. The lateral part lies in a groove on the plantar surface of the navicular bone and divides into slips which spread out from it to every bone of the tarsus except the talus, and also to the bases of the second, third and fourth metatarsal bones.

The tendon of the tibialis posterior enters the sole on the plantar surface of the **plantar calcaneonavicular ligament** or 'spring ligament'. This strong ligament stretches from the sustentaculum tali of the calcaneus to the navicular bone, and supports the head of the talus. Thus the tendon also supports the talus and, at this point, contains a sesamoid nodule of fibrocartilage which may be ossified to become a sesamoid bone. The tendon is separated from the ligament by the distal part of its synovial sheath.

Tendon of Peroneus Longus

This tendon turns round the lateral margin of the cuboid and runs medially across the sole, in the groove on its plantar surface which is bridged over and converted into a synovial-lined tunnel by fibrous tissue derived from the long plantar ligament. The tendon, free to slide in its synovial sheath within the tunnel, is inserted into the base of the first metatarsal bone and the adjacent part of the medial cuneiform bone.

Just before the tendon enters the tunnel, it is thickened and contains a nodule of fibrocartilage or a sesamoid bone which plays upon a facet situated on the posterior margin of the lateral end of the groove on the cuboid. It helps to maintain the transverse arch of the foot.

DISSECTION. Bring the dissection of the sole of the foot to an end by disarticulating the proximal end of the first metatarsal bone. A good view is thus obtained of the continuity between the dorsalis pedis artery and the plantar arch.

THE JOINTS OF THE LOWER LIMB

The **hip joint** was dissected before the limb was removed from the body.

THE KNEE JOINT

The distal end of the femur, the patella and the proximal end of the tibia take part in the formation of the knee joint, which is the largest and most complicated joint in the body.

In all positions of the joint, the patella is in contact with the femur and the femur with the tibia. The bones do not interlock with one another, but the areas of contact are large and the ligaments and surrounding muscles are strong; dislocation of the joint is therefore rare, in spite of the many strains to which it is subjected.

The femoral condyles are partly separated from the tibial condyles by two sharply curved pieces of fibrocartilage called the **menisci**; they lie on the marginal parts of the tibial condyles [FIG. 163], and, being wedge-shaped in section, they slightly deepen the surfaces for articulation with the femoral condyles. In the interior of the joint there are two very strong ligaments which pass from the top of the tibia to the two femoral condyles; they cross each other, and are called therefore the **cruciate ligaments** of the knee; and they take the chief part in holding the femur and tibia together.

The three bones of the joint are united also by: (1) an imperfect **fibrous capsule,** which envelops the joint incompletely, and (2) by supplementary bands which have been partly examined already—namely, the **fibular collateral** and **tibial collateral ligaments** of the knee, the **oblique popliteal ligament,** and the **ligamentum patellae** which serves as an anterior ligament.

DISSECTION. Remove the popliteal vessels and nerves and the muscles that surround the knee joint. Leave portions of the tendons of the biceps femoris, semimembranosus, sartorius, semitendinosus, gracilis and popliteus, and also small pieces of the heads of the

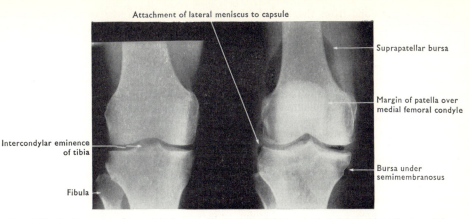

Attachment of lateral meniscus to capsule

Suprapatellar bursa

Margin of patella over medial femoral condyle

Intercondylar eminence of tibia

Bursa under semimembranosus

Fibula

FIG. 155 Radiographs of two right knees. That on the right has had air injected into the knee joint. Air being translucent to X-rays, appears dark and therefore outlines the joint cavity, and makes the margins of some soft tissues visible.

gastrocnemius, in order that their connexions with the ligaments of the joint may be studied. Define the margins of the ligamentum patellae.

ARTICULAR CAPSULE

The fibrous capsule is thin, wide and membranous at the back, thicker and shorter at the sides, and is replaced anteriorly by the patella, the ligamentum patellae, and the tendon of the quadriceps—an arrangement which allows the full range of flexion.

Attachments

Laterally and posteriorly it is attached to the condyles of the tibia and femur close to their articular margins, and to the intercondylar line of the femur. Anteriorly it is attached to the oblique lines on the front of the tibia which run from the articular margins to the sides of the tuberosity, and superior to this, blends with the edges of the ligamentum patellae, the patella, and the quadriceps tendon.

The capsule gives origin to some of the muscle fibres of the lateral head of gastrocnemius, plantaris and popliteus. It is perforated opposite the back of the lateral tibial condyle by the tendon of popliteus, and at the back of the medial femoral condyle where the synovial membrane of the joint

becomes continuous with the bursa under the medial head of gastrocnemius.

Accessory Structures

The fibrous capsule is supplemented and strengthened by accessory ligaments, by

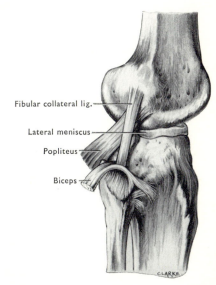

Fibular collateral lig.

Lateral meniscus

Popliteus

Biceps

C. CLARKE

FIG. 156 Fibular collateral ligament of right knee joint.

227

tendons or expansions from them, and by deep fascia. The ligamentum patellae, the patella, and the tendon of the quadriceps replace it in front. At the back it is strengthened by the oblique popliteal ligament. The tibial collateral ligament of the joint overlies it on the medial side, and the fibular collateral ligament on the lateral side. In the intervals that separate those two ligaments from the ligamentum patellae, the capsule is subcutaneous and is strengthened by the fascia lata and expansions from the lateral and medial vasti which fuse with it; these expansions from the vasti are called the **patellar retinacula.**

Ligamentum Patellae. The patellar ligament is a strong, thick band, about 5 cm. long and 2·5 cm. wide. It extends from the apex and the lower part of the deep surface of the patella to the smooth, upper part of the tuberosity of the tibia. Its superficial fibres are directly continuous, anterior to the patella, with the central part of the tendon of the quadriceps femoris. The upper part of its deep surface is separated from the synovial membrane by a mass of loose fatty tissue—the **infrapatellar pad of fat;** the lower part is separated from the anterior surface of the upper end of the tibia by the deep infrapatellar bursa [Fig. 158].

Fibular Collateral Ligament. This is a cord, nearly 5 cm. long, which extends from the lateral epicondyle of the femur to the head of the fibula. Superiorly it fuses with the underlying capsule, but elsewhere they are separ-

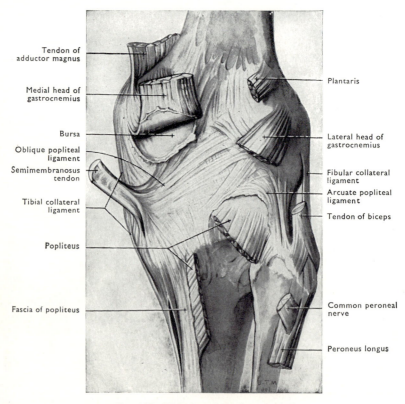

Tendon of adductor magnus

Medial head of gastrocnemius

Bursa

Oblique popliteal ligament

Semimembranosus tendon

Tibial collateral ligament

Popliteus

Fascia of popliteus

Plantaris

Lateral head of gastrocnemius

Fibular collateral ligament

Arcuate popliteal ligament

Tendon of biceps

Common peroneal nerve

Peroneus longus

FIG. 157   Right knee joint from behind.

ated by fatty tissue which transmits the inferior lateral genicular vessels [FIG. 144]. Inferiorly it pierces the tendon of biceps just superior to its insertion into the fibula. The tendon of popliteus passes deep to the ligament, but is separated from it by the articular capsule, and both these structures intervene between the ligament and the lateral meniscus [FIG. 156].

Tibial Collateral Ligament. This is a broad flat band lying in the plane of the capsule. It arises from the medial femoral epicondyle and receives some fibres of the adductor magnus attached immediately above. Passing downwards and slightly forwards, the deepest fibres are attached to the medial meniscus and the margin of the medial tibial condyle, while the remaining fibres cross the anterior part of the insertion of semimembranosus, and extend on to the upper fourth of the tibial shaft close to its medial border, and posterior to the insertions of sartorius, gracilis and semitendinosus. In this part it is separated from the tibia by the inferior medial genicular vessels and nerve.

Oblique Popliteal Ligament of Knee. The oblique popliteal ligament is readily demonstrated if the tendon of the semimembranosus is pulled upon. It is a broad slip that springs from that tendon at the back of the medial condyle of the tibia; it spreads upwards and laterally towards the lateral femoral condyle, fusing with the fibrous capsule.

DISSECTION. Cut across the quadriceps femoris immediately above the patella, prolong each end of the incision downwards, about 3–4 cm. behind the patella, to the condyles of the tibia, and turn the patella downwards.

Next split the lower part of the quadriceps, and turn the two parts aside to expose the suprapatellar bursa. Open the bursa, if that was not done when the quadriceps was split. Explore the interior of the bursa and note the size of the opening by which it communicates with the knee joint.

INTERIOR OF THE KNEE JOINT

When the joint is laid open in this way, the semilunar cartilages, the cruciate ligaments and the synovial membrane, including its infrapatellar fold are visible. The **infrapatellar synovial fold** is the first structure to be noticed. It is a triangular ridge of synovial membrane that covers the mass of fat behind the patellar ligament and extends upwards and backwards to be attached to the anterior margin of the intercondylar notch of the

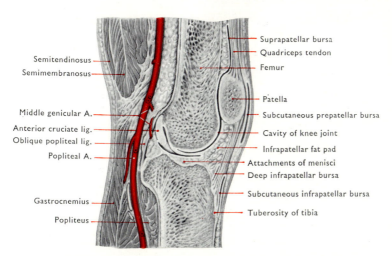

FIG. 158 Sagittal section of right knee joint to show extension of cavity into suprapatellar bursa. The popliteal vein is not shown.

femur [Figs. 158, 160]. Its lateral edges fade out on to the upper surface of the tibia as the alar folds. The **infrapatellar pad of fat** fills up the interval between the patella, femur and tibia, and adapts itself to the varied forms which that recess assumes in the different movements of the joint.

Synovial Membrane

The synovial membrane of the knee joint is more extensive than that of any other joint. It lines the fibrous capsule and covers the intracapsular parts of the tibia and femur up to the margins of the articular cartilage, which it overlaps.

At the sides it is reflected also on to the upper and lower capsular margins of the menisci. In the middle part of the back of the joint the synovial membrane leaves the capsule and passes anteriorly to cover the sides and the front of the cruciate ligaments, leaving the posterior one connected with the fibrous capsule by areolar tissue [Fig. 160].

At the front of the joint the synovial membrane covers the posterior surface of the infrapatellar pad of fat, which separates it from the ligamentum patellae, but not the patella. Superiorly it forms the **suprapatellar bursa**, a large, saccular extension of the joint cavity between the femur and the tendon of quadriceps. The synovial membrane lines the deep surface of the tendon of quadriceps, and a hand-breadth above the patella it is reflected posteriorly on to the front of the femur, extending inferiorly on it to overlap the margin of its patellar articular surface. This bursa allows free movement of the tendon of quadriceps on the lower end of the femur and facilitates the full range of flexion and extension. The articularis genus muscle [p. 153] is attached to the upper limit of the synovial membrane.

The tendon of popliteus is separated from the joint cavity by the synovial membrane which partially surrounds it on the medial side, separating it from the lateral condyle of the femur and the lateral meniscus. This part of the synovial lining extends out through the capsule deep to popliteus and between it and the superior tibiofibular

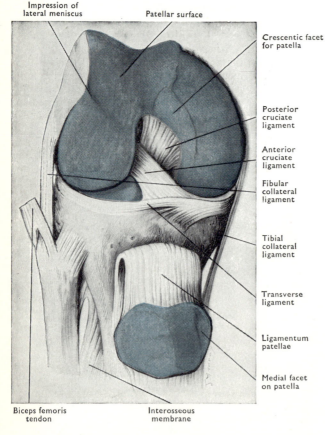

Impression of lateral meniscus Patellar surface

Crescentic facet for patella

Posterior cruciate ligament

Anterior cruciate ligament

Fibular collateral ligament

Tibial collateral ligament

Transverse ligament

Ligamentum patellae

Medial facet on patella

Biceps femoris tendon Interosseous membrane

Fig. 159 Dissection of right knee from the front: patella and patellar ligament turned down.

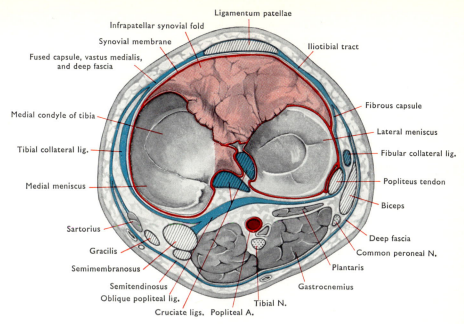

Infrapatellar synovial fold

Ligamentum patellae

Synovial membrane

Fused capsule, vastus medialis, and deep fascia

Iliotibial tract

Medial condyle of tibia

Fibrous capsule

Tibial collateral lig.

Lateral meniscus

Medial meniscus

Fibular collateral lig.

Sartorius

Popliteus tendon

Gracilis

Biceps

Semimembranosus

Deep fascia

Semitendinosus

Common peroneal N.

Oblique popliteal lig.

Plantaris

Cruciate ligs. Popliteal A.

Gastrocnemius

Tibial N.

Fig. 160 Transverse section through right knee joint and its surroundings showing relations of synovial membrane.

joint, and is sometimes continuous with the synovial membrane of that joint.

DISSECTION. Divide the infrapatellar synovial fold and remove the infrapatellar pad of fat. Open and examine the bursa between the ligamentum patellae and the tibia. Then turn the limb round, dissect away the intermediate part of the posterior portion of the capsule, and trace the middle genicular artery (which pierces it) forwards to the cruciate ligaments.

Remove the areolar tissue from the back of the cruciate ligaments, and the synovial membrane from their front and sides, and define their attachments to the femur and tibia. Lastly define the connexions of the menisci.

Movements at the Knee Joint

The chief movements at the knee joint are flexion and extension. The leg can be bent backwards until the calf comes into contact with the back of the thigh; but in extension the movement is stopped when the leg comes into line with the thigh. In that position the joint is firmly locked; the anterior cruciate,

the tibial and fibular collateral ligaments, and the posterior part of the capsule, with the oblique popliteal ligament, are taut; and the leg and thigh are converted into a rigid column of support. In flexion, however, the ligaments mentioned are relaxed, and a considerable amount of rotation is allowed, which is most free when the leg is at right angles to the thigh.

The muscles acting on it are: *Extensors:* the four parts of the quadriceps femoris. *Flexors:* biceps femoris, sartorius, gracilis, semitendinosus, semimembranosus and popliteus. Of these, only biceps is inserted on the lateral side of the leg. *Medial rotators of the leg:* Popliteus, gracilis, sartorius, semitendinosus and semimembranosus. *Lateral rotator of the leg:* biceps femoris.

The articular surfaces of the femur show a number of separate areas:

1. The patellar surface of the femur is a well marked groove, the lateral lip of which

is more prominent and longer than the medial, and helps to prevent lateral displacement of the patella [Fig. 159].

2. Postero-inferiorly the patellar surface is continuous with the two condyles, and is separated from each by a faint oblique line running towards the intercondylar notch. Each of these lines is the anterior edge of a groove which lodges the corresponding meniscus in full extension of the knee.

3. The anterior part of the medial condyle shows a faint anteroposterior line which separates off a crescentic facet adjacent to the intercondylar notch.

The articular surface on the patella is divided into larger lateral, and smaller medial, parts by a vertical ridge, and each part is divided into three facets, one above the other.

A faint vertical line cuts off a narrow strip along the medial border, the perpendicular facet.

In full flexion of the knee the posterior surfaces of the condyles articulate with the tibia, while the patella is in contact with the lateral and crescentic facets, through its upper lateral and perpendicular facets respectively. As the knee is extended, the patella slides upwards on the femur, passing first on to its middle and then its lower facets as full extension is reached. The femoral condyles roll backwards on the tibia and its attached menisci, the points of contact with the tibia moving steadily forwards on the femoral condyles. The lateral condyle, having a shorter anteroposterior extent than the medial, reaches full extension earlier, the lateral meniscus fit-

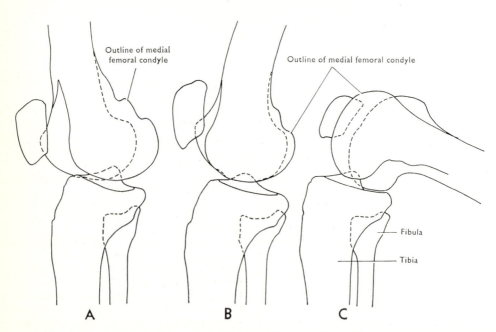

Fig. 161   Tracings of three positions of the right knee joint taken from radiographs of three phases of flexion of the knee with the foot firmly fixed on the ground.   In this way there is no movement of the tibia and fibula and the full effects of rotation are visible in the femur. The tracings are viewed from the medial side, the parts that are hidden by the more medial structures are shown as broken lines.   A. Position of full extension with the femur fully rotated medially and the knee joint locked.   B. Slight flexion.   Note that there has been considerable lateral rotation of the femur, so that the outlines of the condyles are nearly superimposed. This movement occurs at the very outset of flexion.   C. Considerable flexion of the knee with further lateral rotation of the femur on the tibia.

ting into the groove between the condyle and the patellar surface. The medial condyle continues to slide backwards, producing a medial rotation of the femur which screws it home on to the tibia and the medial meniscus, and finally tightens the anterior cruciate, the tibial and fibular collateral, and the posterior capsular ligaments of the knee, thus turning the limb into a rigid pillar [FIG. 161].

Flexion begins with lateral rotation of the femur (medial rotation of the tibia) produced by popliteus. This 'unlocks' the joint and allows the remainder of the movement to take place.

An account of the part played by the menisci and a fuller account of the relations of the bones to one another are given in the large textbooks of anatomy. In reading a full account, the student must not lose sight of the fact that the knee joint is essentially a hinge. The bolt of the hinge passes through the femoral attachments of the fibular collateral, tibial collateral, and cruciate ligaments; subject to the control of muscles, the ligaments suspend the leg after the manner of the ropes of a swing, and some rotation is therefore possible as soon as they are relaxed.

DISSECTION. In order to obtain a proper view of the attachments of the cruciate ligaments, saw the femur across immediately above the joint, and divide the distal part of the bone by a sagittal saw-cut that ends in the intercondylar notch between the two cruciate ligaments.

Note that the fibular collateral ligament of the joint and the anterior cruciate ligament are fixed to opposite sides of the lateral condyle. The tibial collateral ligament and the posterior cruciate ligament are attached to the opposite sides of the medial condyle. Divide the tibial collateral

ligament of the joint in order to free the medial condyle and to give greater space for the study of the cruciate ligaments.

Cruciate Ligaments of Knee

The cruciate ligaments are so named because they cross each other like the limbs of the letter X.

The **anterior cruciate ligament** springs from the anterior part of the tibial intercondylar area on the upper surface of the tibia, and proceeds upwards, backwards and laterally, to gain attachment to the posterior part of the medial surface of the lateral condyle of the femur [FIGS. 159, 162].

The **posterior cruciate ligament** springs from the posterior part of the tibial intercondylar area. It passes upwards, forwards and a little medially, and is attached to the anterior

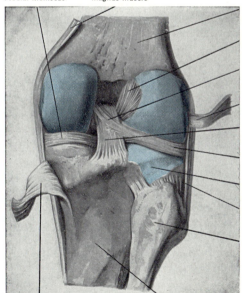

Medial meniscus — Tendon of insertion of adductor magnus muscle — Popliteal surface of femur — Anterior cruciate ligament — Posterior meniscofemoral ligament — Tendon of popliteus muscle — Posterior cruciate ligament — Lateral meniscus — Groove on tibia for tendon of popliteus muscle — Fibular collateral ligament — Head of fibula — Tendon of semimembranosus muscle (turned down) — Popliteal surface of tibia

FIG. 162 Right knee joint opened from behind by the removal of posterior part of the articular capsule.

portion of the lateral surface of the medial condyle [FIG. 159]. It receives one or sometimes two strong slips from the posterior horn of the lateral semilunar meniscus [FIG. 163].

These ligaments hold the femur to the tibia and prevent it from sliding backwards (anterior cruciate) or forwards (posterior cruciate) on the flat, upper tibial surface, except as part of the movement of flexion and extension. The latter movements are permitted because the femoral attachments of these ligaments lie on the axis of these movements. The anterior cruciate ligament tends to tighten in extension of the knee joint, the posterior in flexion, but they do not restrict these movements.

Menisci

The menisci are two crescentic plates of fibrocartilage which are placed on the condylar surfaces of the tibia. They deepen the surfaces upon which the condyles of the femur roll, and, being movable, fill up the gaps which would otherwise arise during the movements of the joint. They are thick towards the circumference of the joint but thin away to a fine, free concave edge internally. Both surfaces are smooth and articular.

The convex external margins of the menisci are attached to the capsule of the joint, and through it to the edges of the tibial condyles, except where the tendon of popliteus and its synovial pouch intervene between the capsule and the lateral meniscus. Anteriorly and posteriorly they are attached to the tibial intercondylar area by fibrous extremities or **horns**. The **lateral meniscus** being nearly circular, in keeping with the more spherical lateral femoral condyle, its horns are attached close together, the posterior to the intercondylar eminence, the anterior immediately in front of this. In addition it gives a strong slip to the posterior cruciate ligament, and is attached anteriorly to the medial meniscus by the tra nsverse ligament of the keen [FIG. 163].

The **medial meniscus** is more oval in shape (its long axis being anteroposterior in keeping with the elongated medial femoral condyle) and its horns are attached further apart ; the anterior, to the most anterior part of the intercondylar area ; the posterior, between the intercondylar eminence and the posterior cruciate ligament.

In sudden turning movements with the foot on the ground and the knee semiflexed, the femur may be forcibly rotated medially on the tibia. In such a movement the medial femoral condyle pivots around the spherical lateral condyle, and sliding violently backwards

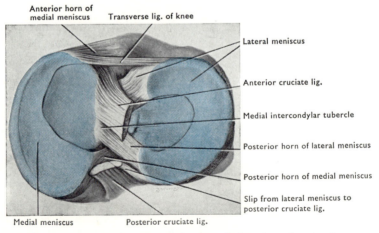

Anterior horn of medial meniscus — Transverse lig. of knee — Lateral meniscus — Anterior cruciate lig. — Medial intercondylar tubercle — Posterior horn of lateral meniscus — Posterior horn of medial meniscus — Slip from lateral meniscus to posterior cruciate lig. — Medial meniscus — Posterior cruciate lig.

FIG. 163   Upper end of tibia with menisci and attached portions of cruciate ligaments.

while under pressure, may catch the margin of the medial meniscus between it and the tibia and tear or avulse the cartilage. This injury is most likely to involve the medial meniscus, partly because it is held rigid by adherence to the tibial collateral ligament, and partly because of the range of sliding movement which the medial femoral condyle can undertake in rotation without flexion or extension. If the torn piece of cartilage becomes wedged between the articular surfaces, the joint becomes 'locked'.

DISSECTION. Carefully define the attachments of the fibrous horns of the menisci.

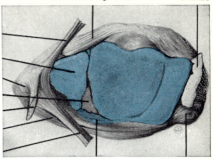

FIG. 164 Surfaces of tibia and fibula which articulate with the talus at the ankle joint.

Transverse Ligament of the Knee. This is a fibrous band which stretches across from the anterior part of one semilunar cartilage to the corresponding part of the other, and by means of it the one cartilage is partly controlled and partly accompanied by the other in its displacement during the movements of the femur on the tibia.

DISSECTION. Divide the fibular collateral ligament, the cruciate ligaments, and the remains of the fibrous capsule close to their femoral attachments, and examine the tibial attachments of the cruciate ligaments and menisci.

THE ANKLE JOINT

The ankle joint is a synovial joint of the hinge variety. It is a joint of great strength; its stability is ensured not only by its powerful ligaments and the tendons around it, but also by the close interlocking of the articulating surfaces.

The trochlea of the talus is inserted into the deep socket between the lateral and medial malleoli, and bears on them and the distal end of the tibia. The socket is deepened posteriorly by the inferior part of the posterior tibiofibular ligament, and some tension and spring is given to the socket by the strong tibiofibular

ligaments and the flexibility of the fibula. Thus, if the talus is forced against the lateral malleolus, it can move slightly outwards and, acting on the tibiofibular ligaments as a fulcrum, spring the shaft of the fibula medially; in extreme cases this may lead to fracture of the fibula in the leg.

DISSECTION. Remove the remains of the flexor and extensor retinacula, and cut through and displace the tendons which are in relation with the joint, but do not remove them. Review the anastomoses between the arteries around the joint [p. 212], and, if possible, secure the twigs from the deep peroneal and tibial nerves which supply the joint. Then clean carefully the anterior and posterior ligaments of the joint, both of which are extremely thin and easily injured.

Ligaments of Ankle Joint

In conformity with the movements of a hinge joint, the main ligaments are lateral and medial, the anterior and posterior parts of the capsule being thin and consisting mainly of transversely placed fibres. Thus the weak **anterior** part of the capsule extends from the anterior margin of the distal end of the tibia to the superior surface of the neck of the talus, and the very delicate **posterior** part passes from the posterior margin of the distal end of the tibia and the posterior tibiofibular ligament to the posterior surface of the body of the talus.

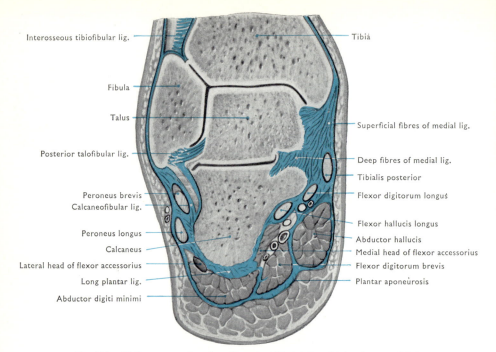

Interosseous tibiofibular lig.

Fibula

Talus

Posterior talofibular lig.

Peroneus brevis

Calcaneofibular lig.

Peroneus longus

Calcaneus

Lateral head of flexor accessorius

Long plantar lig.

Abductor digiti minimi

Tibia

Superficial fibres of medial lig.

Deep fibres of medial lig.

Tibialis posterior

Flexor digitorum longus

Flexor hallucis longus

Abductor hallucis

Medial head of flexor accessorius

Flexor digitorum brevis

Plantar aponeurosis

FIG. 165   Oblique coronal section through ankle joint and talocalcanean joint.

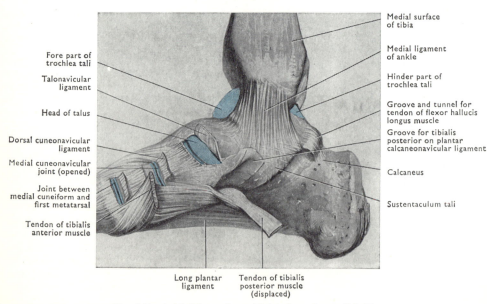

Fore part of
trochlea tali

Talonavicular
ligament

Head of talus

Dorsal cuneonavicular
ligament

Medial cuneonavicular
joint (opened)

Joint between
medial cuneiform and
first metatarsal

Tendon of tibialis
anterior muscle

Medial surface
of tibia

Medial ligament
of ankle

Hinder part of
trochlea tali

Groove and tunnel for
tendon of flexor hallucis
longus muscle

Groove for tibialis
posterior on plantar
calcaneonavicular ligament

Calcaneus

Sustentaculum tali

Long plantar
ligament

Tendon of tibialis
posterior muscle
(displaced)

FIG. 166   Ankle joint and tarsal joints from the medial side.

Medial (deltoid) Ligament. This is extremely strong, and radiates from the lower border of the medial malleolus to a long distal attachment extending from the body of the talus posteriorly, along the sustentaculum tali, the neck of the talus, the medial edge of the plantar calcaneonavicular (spring) ligament, to the tuberosity of the navicular bone. Thus the medial ligament not only strengthens the ankle joint, but also holds the calcaneus and navicular bones against the talus, and by supporting the plantar calcaneonavicular ligament, on which the head of the talus rests, it supports the medial side of the foot and helps to maintain the medial longitudinal arch.

DISSECTION. Remove the anterior and posterior ligaments in order to bring the ligaments on the sides of the joint more fully into relief. Clean these ligaments and define their attachments.

Lateral Ligament. The lateral ligament consists of three bands, of which the anterior and posterior talofibular ligaments **are** thickenings of the capsule, while the calcaneofibular ligament is a separate band with fatty tissue between it and the capsule.

The **anterior talofibular ligament** is a flattened band which passes medially from the anterior border of the lateral malleolus to the neck of the talus immediately in front of the fibular facet [FIGS. 164, 167].

The **posterior talofibular ligament** is much stronger. It runs almost horizontally, medially and backwards, from the fossa of the lateral malleolus to the posterior process of the talus [FIGS. 164, 165, 167].

The posterior tubercle of the talus is usually ossified from a separate centre, and appears in radiographs as a separate bone until fusion with the rest of the talus occurs. Its presence should be kept in mind in studying radiographs of injured ankles, especially in children. Rarely it fails to fuse with the body of the talus and remains in the adult as the os trigonum.

The **calcaneofibular ligament** is a round cord which passes postero-inferiorly from the distal

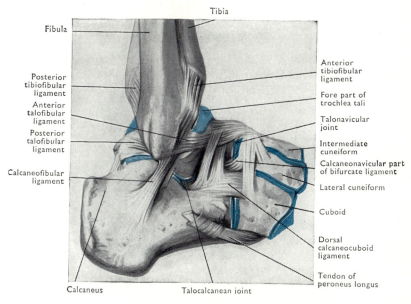

Fig. 167 Ligaments of lateral side of ankle joint and dorsum of tarsus.

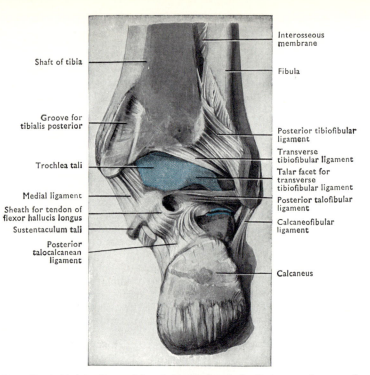

Shaft of tibia

Groove for
tibialis posterior

Trochlea tali

Medial ligament

Sheath for tendon of
flexor hallucis longus

Sustentaculum tali

Posterior
talocalcanean
ligament

Interosseous
membrane

Fibula

Posterior tibiofibular
ligament

Transverse
tibiofibular ligament

Talar facet for
transverse
tibiofibular ligament

Posterior talofibular
ligament

Calcaneofibular
ligament

Calcaneus

Fig. 168   Ankle joint dissected from behind and part of articular capsule removed.

end of the lateral malleolus to the lateral surface of the calcaneus [Figs. 165, 167, 168]. It functions also as an accessory ligament of the talocalcanean joint.

Synovial Membrane

The synovial membrane lines the fibrous capsule, and sends a short process upwards into the narrow interval between the tibia and the fibula below the interosseous ligament. In front and behind it covers fatty pads in relation to the anterior and posterior ligaments.

Relations

Anteriorly the ankle joint is close to the surface, and is covered by the tendons, vessels and nerve passing into the foot from the anterior compartment of the leg [Fig. 131. p. 194.]

Posteriorly it is some distance from the surface because of the presence of the tendo calcaneus and the pad of fat between them. The tendons of flexor hallucis and flexor digitorum, and the posterior tibial vessels and tibial nerve sweep medially across its posterior surface to enter the medial side of the foot. The tibialis posterior on the medial side, and the peronei on the lateral side, turn round the corresponding malleolus and come into relation with the sides of the ankle joint.

DISSECTION. Cut through the anterior talo-fibular ligament, the calcaneofibular ligament, and the anterior part of the medial ligament ; separate the articular surfaces and examine them.

Movements

If the trochlea tali and its socket are examined, it will be seen that the surfaces for

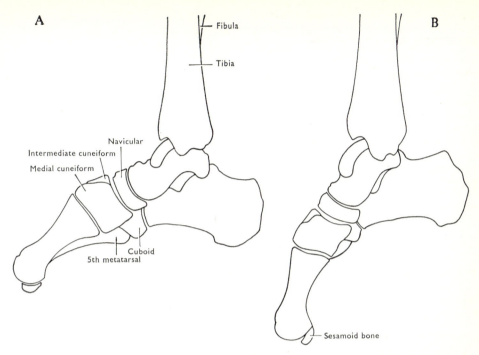

A

- Fibula
- Tibia

Navicular
Intermediate cuneiform
Medial cuneiform

Cuboid
5th metatarsal

B

Sesamoid bone

FIG. 169   Outline drawings of two radiographs of the same foot. In B the foot has been plantar flexed without any other movement. Note that virtually all of this movement takes place at the ankle joint, but that there is also slight flexion of the bones forming the medial longitudinal arch on each other; the distance between the medial process of the tuber calcanei and the head of the first metatarsal being 7 mm. less in B than in A. Note also how the latter movement, produced by the plantar flexors, has increased the height of the longitudinal arch.

articulation with the malleoli are wider apart anteriorly, and that the socket is also broader in front. It follows that when the muscles of the anterior compartment contract and the foot is dorsiflexed, the talus fits snugly into the socket and lateral movements are resisted. On the other hand when the muscles of the posterior compartments of the leg contract and the foot is plantar flexed, the talus is slightly loose and some lateral movement is possible. In standing, therefore, the maximum stability of the ankle is obtained.

In *dorsiflexion*, the calcaneofibular and posterior talofibular bands, the greater part of the medial ligament, and the posterior part of the capsule are put on the stretch. In *plantar-flexion*, the anterior talofibular ligament, the anterior fibres of the medial ligament, and the anterior part of the capsule are tense.

THE TIBIOFIBULAR JOINTS

The fibula articulates with the tibia by both of its ends. The **proximal tibiofibular joint** is a synovial joint. The **distal joint** is held together by ligaments that do not enclose a cavity, and the only movements possible are those allowed by slight stretching and twisting of the ligaments. The **interosseous membrane** is common to both joints.

DISSECTION. Preparatory to the examination of the tibiofibular joints, remove the foot by dividing the remains of the ligaments of the ankle joint. Clean and define the ligaments that connect the ends of the

239

fibula with the tibia. Detach the muscles from the bones of the leg and from both surfaces of the interosseous membrane, and clean the membrane.

Interosseous Membrane of Leg

This strong membrane stretches across the interval between the tibia and the fibula, and greatly extends the surface for the origin of muscles. It is attached to the interosseous borders of the two bones and is composed of strong, oblique fibres which run downwards and laterally from the tibia to the fibula. In the upper part of the membrane, immediately below the lateral condyle of the tibia, there is an oval opening for the passage of the anterior tibial vessels, and a small aperture, a short distance above the ankle joint, transmits the perforating branch of the peroneal artery. The tibialis posterior and flexor hallucis longus take partial origin from the back of it; the tibialis anterior, long extensors of the toes and peroneus tertius from the front. The membrane is supplied by a branch from the nerve to the popliteus.

PROXIMAL TIBIOFIBULAR JOINT

This joint is between the head of the fibula and the lateral condyle of the tibia. The bones are united by a fibrous capsule attached near the margins of the articular facets. This capsule is strengthened, in front and behind (especially in front), by oblique fibres that run downwards and laterally from the tibia to the head of the fibula. The tendon of the popliteus and its synovial pouch cross the upper part of the back of the joint, and the pouch is sometimes continuous with the synovial membrane of the joint through a hole in the capsule; in this way the joint may be indirectly in communication with the knee joint. The lateral ligament of the knee and the tendon of the biceps cross the upper surface of the joint.

The joint is supplied by twigs from the nerve to the popliteus and the recurrent genicular nerve.

DISTAL TIBIOFIBULAR JOINT
[Figs. 164–8]

This joint is constructed upon a stronger plan, because the strength of the

ankle joint very largely depends upon its integrity.

The joint is formed between the rough surface on the medial side of the lower end of the fibula and the fibular notch of the tibia. The bones, however, are not in contact with each other, but separated by the interosseous ligament which binds them together. Sometimes the interosseous ligament does not quite reach the distal end of the tibia. In such cases there is a narrow strip coated with cartilage for articulation with the uppermost part of the articular facet of the lateral malleolus.

In addition to the interosseous ligament, there are ligamentous bands in front of and behind the joint.

The **interosseous ligament** is the chief bond at this joint. It is thick and very strong, and is composed of short fibres that pass between the opposing bony surfaces.

The **anterior** and **posterior tibiofibular ligaments** are strong, flat bands that pass upwards and medially from the front and the back of the uppermost part of the lateral malleolus to the distal end of the tibia. They conceal the interosseous ligament. The posterior ligament is continuous inferiorly with a strong, narrow band of yellowish fibres attached to the whole length of the posterior border of the distal surface of the tibia and to the malleolar fossa of the fibula. It projects downwards as a lip from the posterior border of the socket of the ankle joint [Figs. 164, 168] and articulates with a special facet on the posterolateral part of the body of the talus.

DISSECTION. To see the interosseous ligament and appreciate its shortness and thickness, saw across the bones of the leg about 5 cm. from the distal end of the tibia, and then split them by a coronal saw cut. The interosseous ligament will then be seen, and also the narrow articular interval between the distal portions of the bones, when it exists.

THE JOINTS OF THE FOOT

The joints of the foot are very numerous. All the bones of the foot—tarsal and metatarsal bones and phalanges—enter into their formation; and they are classified therefore as:

1. Intertarsal joints.
2. Tarsometatarsal joints.
3. Intermetatarsal joints.

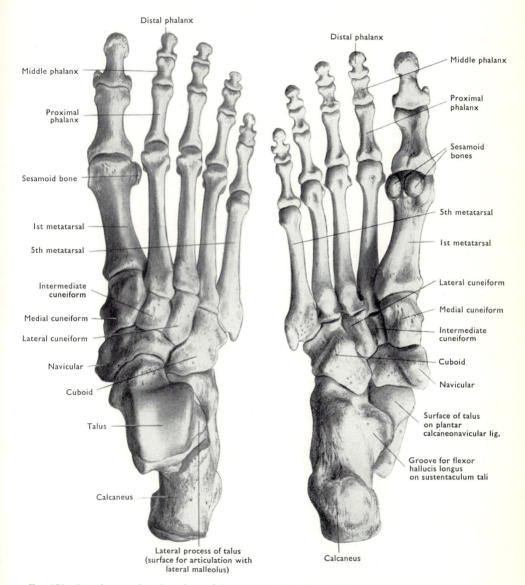

Distal phalanx

Middle phalanx

Proximal phalanx

Sesamoid bone

Ist metatarsal

5th metatarsal

Intermediate cuneiform

Medial cuneiform

Lateral cuneiform

Navicular

Cuboid

Talus

Calcaneus

Lateral process of talus (surface for articulation with lateral malleolus)

Distal phalanx

Middle phalanx

Proximal phalanx

Sesamoid bones

5th metatarsal

Ist metatarsal

Lateral cuneiform

Medial cuneiform

Intermediate cuneiform

Cuboid

Navicular

Surface of talus on plantar calcaneonavicular lig.

Groove for flexor hallucis longus on sustentaculum tali

Calcaneus

FIG. 170 Superior or dorsal surface of bones of right foot.

FIG. 171 Inferior or plantar surface of bones of right foot.

241

4. Metatarsophalangeal joints.
5. Interphalangeal joints.

ARCHES OF THE FOOT

The tarsal and metatarsal bones are bound together by ligaments, and are disposed in the form of two arches, viz., a longitudinal and a transverse, the foot having the general shape of a half-dome. The integrity of these arches is maintained : (1) by the shape of the bones ; (2) by the tension of the ligaments and the plantar aponeurosis ; and (3) by muscular action in which both the short muscles of the sole and the long muscles, through the bracing action of their tendons, take a share.

Longitudinal Arch

This arch presents a greater height and a wider span along the medial side of the foot than along the lateral side. The talus lies at the summit of this arch and, in a sense, is its 'keystone' [FIG. 172]. The **posterior pillar** is short and solid, being formed by the calcaneus alone. The **anterior pillar,** much longer, comprises the rest of the tarsal bones, and the metatarsus. Further, the anterior pillar is divided into a medial column composed of the

navicular, the three cuneiforms, and the medial three metatarsal bones, and a lateral column composed of the cuboid and the lateral two metatarsals.

The talus, lying at the summit of the arch, receives the weight of the body and transmits it : (1) Posteriorly towards the heel through its subtalar joint with the calcaneus. (2) Anteriorly, through its head, to the medial longitudinal arch by its articulation with the navicular. (3) To the lateral side of the foot through both of its articulations with the calcaneus.

The head of the talus fits into a deep socket between the anterior end of the calcaneus and the navicular, and appears between them on the plantar surface. It is prevented from driving them apart and flattening the arch, by the presence of the plantar calcaneonavicular (spring) ligament which fills the gap, binds the navicular to the sustentaculum tali (on which the head of the talus also rests) and completes the socket for the head [FIG. 174]. All the other ligaments on the plantar surfaces of the bones of the foot play a part in maintaining the arches of the foot, and they are assisted by the extensive insertion of tibialis posterior

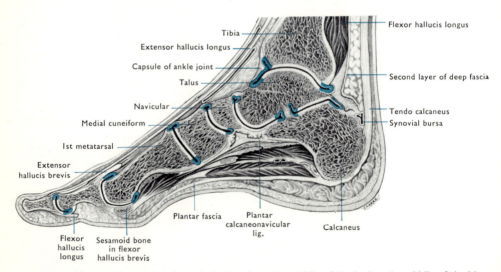

Tibia
Extensor hallucis longus
Capsule of ankle joint
Talus
Navicular
Medial cuneiform
1st metatarsal
Extensor hallucis brevis
Flexor hallucis longus
Sesamoid bone in flexor hallucis brevis
Plantar fascia
Plantar calcaneonavicular lig.
Flexor hallucis longus
Second layer of deep fascia
Tendo calcaneus
Synovial bursa
Calcaneus

FIG. 172   Oblique sagittal section through the foot from the middle of the heel to the middle of the big toe.   Synovial membrane, blue.

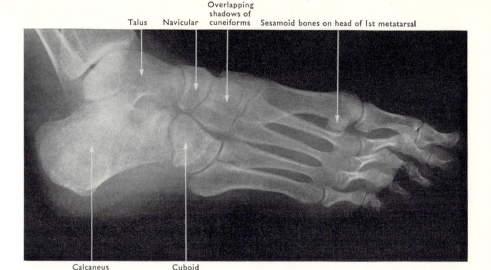

Talus   Navicular   Overlapping shadows of cuneiforms   Sesamoid bones on head of 1st metatarsal

Calcaneus   Cuboid

FIG. 173   Oblique radiograph of the left foot. It is only in this view that most of the foot bones are visible separately.

and by the tendon of peroneus longus, but more especially by the plantar aponeurosis which joins the two ends of the arch and acts as a 'tie beam'.

Transverse Arch of the Foot

This is seen to best advantage across the line of the tarsometatarsal articulations. The inferior surfaces of the cuneiforms and the metatarsal bases are narrow transversely, and are held tightly together by plantar and interosseus ligaments, and by the tendon of peroneus longus. This arrangement gives the plantar surface in this region a much smaller transverse radius of curvature than the dorsal surface, thus forming a well-defined transverse arch.

DISSECTION. **Remove all the muscles and tendons from the tarsus and metatarsus. Clean and define the ligaments on the various surfaces.**

SUBTALAR JOINT

This is a simple, gliding synovial joint between the large, slightly concave, cylindrical facet on the lower surface of the body of the talus and the corresponding facet on the middle of the upper surface of the calcaneus. It is surrounded by a **fibrous capsule,** which is attached to the bones near the margins of the articular facets. The medial and calcaneofibular ligaments of the ankle joint, and the ligament of the neck of the talus, which extends inferolaterally from it to the calcaneus, act as accessory ligaments to this joint.

TALOCALCANEONAVICULAR JOINT

This joint consists of the articulation of the head of the talus with the navicular bone and the upper surface of the plantar calcaneonavicular ligament, and the inferior surface of the neck and adjacent part of the body of the talus with the anteromedial part of the calcaneus, including the sustentaculum tali. These articular surfaces, approximating to a ball-and-socket joint, are contained within a single articular capsule composed of a number of ligaments: medially, the medial ligament of the ankle joint; posteriorly, part of the interosseus talocalcancan ligament; laterally,

243

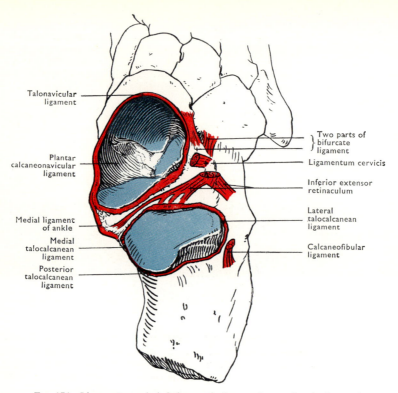

Labels on figure:
Talonavicular ligament
Plantar calcaneonavicular ligament
Medial ligament of ankle
Medial talocalcanean ligament
Posterior talocalcanean ligament
Two parts of bifurcate ligament
Ligamentum cervicis
Inferior extensor retinaculum
Lateral talocalcanean ligament
Calcaneofibular ligament

FIG. 174 Ligaments and inferior articular surfaces of subtalar and talocalcaneonavicular joints seen from above after removal of the talus.

the calcaneonavicular ligament; superiorly, the talonavicular ligament.

The **interosseous talocalcanean ligament** [FIG. 174] consists of the adjacent parts of the capsules of the subtalar and the talocalcaneonavicular joints. These are thickened and lie in the tunnel between the talus and calcaneus (sinus tarsi) and have the stem of the inferior extensor retinaculum attached between them at the lateral end of the floor of the sinus tarsi [p. 195]. The interosseous talocalcanean ligament is an important element in the movements of inversion and eversion, *q.v.*, allowing the calcaneus, carrying the rest of the foot with it, to pivot on the talus around the ligament. The **ligament of the neck of the talus,** lying at the lateral end of the sinus tarsi, limits the movement of inversion.

DISSECTION. Divide the various ligaments which hold the talus in place, and remove the bone. Clean the divided interosseous ligament, and examine its attachment on both the talus and the calcaneus. Clean the lateral calcaneonavicular ligament on the lateral margin of the socket.

Examine the **talus,** and note: (1) The large facet on the lower surface for articulation at the subtalar joint. (2) The convex surface in front for articulation with the navicular. (3) An elongated facet on the lower surface of the head, neck, and body for articulation with the upper surface of the anterior part of the calcaneus and of the sustentaculum tali; it may be divided into two parts by a ridge or by a groove. (4) A triangular facet, between (2) and (3), for articulation with the spring ligament.

Examine also the corresponding parts of the **calcaneus** and of the socket for the head of the talus; the facet on the sustentaculum tali is frequently cut off from the rest of the anterior articular surface of the calcaneus.

Calcaneonavicular Ligaments

Although the calcaneus does not articulate with the navicular bone, it is connected with it by the powerful calcaneonavicular ligaments.

The **plantar calcaneonavicular ligament,** or 'spring' ligament, is a triangular sheet, thick and dense—almost fibrocartilaginous in texture—that plays an important part in maintaining the longitudinal arch of the foot. It stretches from the anterior margin of the sustentaculum tali to the plantar surface of the navicular bone, and fills up the angular interval between the two bones.

The head of the talus rests on it. The deltoid ligament is attached to its medial margin and braces it up. The tendon of the tibialis posterior is in close contact with it and supports it inferiorly; and, lateral to that, it is separated only by a little fat from the tendons

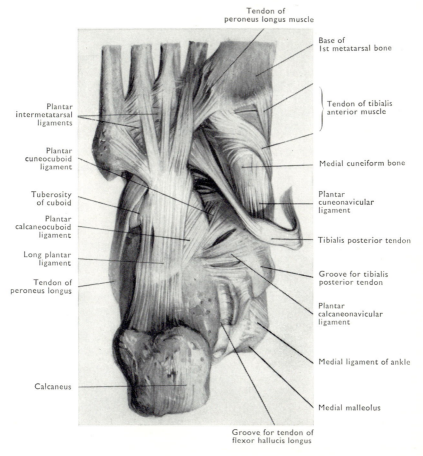

Tendon of peroneus longus muscle

Base of 1st metatarsal bone

Tendon of tibialis anterior muscle

Plantar intermetatarsal ligaments

Plantar cuneocuboid ligament

Medial cuneiform bone

Tuberosity of cuboid

Plantar cuneonavicular ligament

Plantar calcaneocuboid ligament

Tibialis posterior tendon

Long plantar ligament

Groove for tibialis posterior tendon

Tendon of peroneus longus

Plantar calcaneonavicular ligament

Calcaneus

Medial ligament of ankle

Medial malleolus

Groove for tendon of flexor hallucis longus

FIG. 175   Plantar aspect of tarsal and tarsometatarsal joints.

of the long flexors at their point of crossing each other.

The **calcaneonavicular ligament** is placed deeply in the anterior part of the depression between the calcaneus and the lateral aspect of the head of the talus; it is the medial part of a V-shaped band, called the **bifurcate ligament,** which springs from the calcaneus and immediately divides into the calcaneonavicular ligament and the calcaneocuboid ligament. The calcaneonavicular ligament stretches from the anterior part of the upper surface of the calcaneus to the lateral surface of the navicular bone; it forms a part of the socket for the head of the talus.

CALCANEOCUBOID JOINT

The calcaneocuboid joint does not communicate with the cavities of neighbouring joints. The **fibrous capsule** surrounds the joint, and is strengthened by the calcaneocuboid, and plantar calcaneocuboid ligaments. The capsule is supplemented, on its plantar aspect, by the long plantar ligament.

The **calcaneocuboid ligament** is the lateral part of the 'bifurcate ligament'. It springs from the anterior part of the upper surface of the calcaneus and passes to the medial surface of the cuboid bone.

The **long plantar ligament** is a long, strong band whose importance in maintaining the arch of the foot is surpassed only by that of the spring ligament. It has a wide attachment on the plantar surface of the calcaneus, in front of the medial and lateral processes. It extends forwards to be attached to both lips of the groove on the cuboid bone, and its superficial fibres are prolonged into slips that are fixed to the bases of the second, third, and fourth metatarsal bones. The part of it that bridges across the groove of the cuboid forms a fibrous sheath for the tendon of the peroneus longus and holds it in place.

DISSECTION. Define the margins of the long plantar ligament. Slip the knife between the ligament and the anterior part of the calcaneus, and carry it backwards, detaching the ligament from the bone. Turn the ligament forwards to expose the plantar calcaneocuboid ligament, and clean that ligament.

The **plantar calcaneocuboid ligament** is placed under cover of the long plantar ligament—all except its medial edge. It is a wide band composed of strong fibres, nearly 2·5 cm. in length. They spring from the anterior part of the plantar surface of the calcaneus, and extend to the plantar surface of the cuboid behind its ridge. The ligament is broader than the long plantar ligament and can be seen at the medial border of the latter before it is reflected.

TRANSVERSE TARSAL JOINT

The talonavicular and calcaneocuboid joints are quite separate from each other; but they lie very nearly in the same transverse plane [FIG. 170] and together are often called the 'transverse tarsal joint'. Owing to the slope of the foot, the talonavicular joint is above the calcaneocuboid joint, as well as medial to it; and it is noteworthy, in relation to the part that these joints play in the movements of **inversion** and **eversion** of the foot, that the ligaments that cross the transverse tarsal joint are, with the exception of the talonavicular, all attached behind to the calcaneus, thus tending to link the anterior part of the foot with the calcaneus in these movements.

SMALLER JOINTS OF TARSUS

The remaining joints of the tarsus are of relatively small size compared with those described already, and they are of less importance, for the bones are so tightly bound together that the movement between them is very slight; the bones are all united by **dorsal** and **plantar ligaments,** and the rough parts of their contiguous surfaces give attachment to **interosseous ligaments.** The joints are named after the bones which form them—cuneonavicular, intercuneiform, cuneocuboid and cubonavicular.

DISSECTION. Divide the dorsal ligaments and draw the bones apart in order to see the interosseous ligaments.

The **navicular** bone articulates with the three **cuneiform** bones and is united to them by dorsal and plantar ligaments.

The **cuneiform** bones lie in front of the navicular. They articulate side by side, and are closely bound by dorsal, plantar and interosseous ligaments.

The **cuboid** bone lies inferolateral to the navicular and cuneiform bones. It articulates with the lateral cuneiform bone and, occasionally, with the navicular; and it is united to both of them by dorsal, plantar and interosseous ligaments.

Movements of Joints of Tarsus

At most of the intertarsal joints only slight gliding of one bone on another takes place, *e.g.*, when the arches of the foot are depressed by the weight of the body; but at the **subtalar** and **talocalcaneonavicular joints** the bones not only glide but can also rotate to a moderate degree on each other, giving rise to the movements of the foot called eversion and inversion. In **inversion,** the sole is turned medially and the medial border of the foot is raised. **Eversion** is the opposite movement, in which the sole is turned laterally and the lateral border of the foot raised: it is more restricted than inversion. Movements of gliding and slight rotation at the **calcaneo-cuboid joint** are associated with inversion and eversion, but the principal factor is the movement of the rest of the foot on the talus, as can be shown by fixing the calcaneus, and thereby greatly reducing the range of these movements. Inversion and eversion can occur with the weight of the body on the foot, as in adjusting the foot to rough ground, but all movements are most easily studied on one's own foot off the ground. The possible extent of the movements of individual bones should be tested, and the line of pull of the tendons that pass from the leg into the foot should be observed. The muscles that evert the foot are the three peronei; the chief invertors are the tibialis anterior and posterior.

The arches of the foot are maintained mainly by the ligaments of the plantar surface, especially the plantar calcaneonavicular, the long plantar, and the plantar aponeurosis; but muscles acting on the foot also assist. Thus tibialis anterior raises the medial longitudinal arch, and tibialis posterior has a similar action by drawing the navicular against the head of the talus, and tightening up the plantar surface of the foot through its widespread insertion into the tarsal and metatarsal bones. The long and short flexors draw the ends of the arch together and assist the plantar aponeurosis. Peroneus longus, passing across the sole of the foot, not only helps to raise the transverse arch, but can evert the anterior part of the foot, while tibialis posterior produces an inverting effect on the posterior part. Thus a twisting force is applied to the foot, and this effectively raises the medial longitudinal arch.

TARSOMETATARSAL JOINTS

The bases of the first three **metatarsal bones** articulate with the three **cuneiform bones,** and the bases of the fourth and fifth articulate with the **cuboid bone.** The metatarsal bones are very firmly attached to the cuneiform and cuboid bones by dorsal, plantar and interosseous ligaments.

There are only two constant interosseous ligaments. The most medial one—thick and strong—passes from the medial cuneiform to the base of the second metatarsal; the lateral one connects the lateral cuneiform to the base of the fourth (and sometimes of the third) metatarsal, and shuts off the lateral from the middle part of the tarsometatarsal articulation. A weaker interosseous band may pass from the lateral cuneiform to the base of the second metatarsal.

DISSECTION. To bring the interosseous ligaments into view, divide the dorsal ligaments and bend the metatarsus forcibly towards the sole.

Note that the line of articulation is irregularly indented; the base of the second metatarsal bone being wedged in a kind of socket between the medial and lateral cuneiform bones [FIG. 170].

Articular Surfaces and Movements

The **first metatarsal bone** rests against the medial cuneiform bone; and this joint has a separate synovial cavity. It has a slightly greater range of movement than the rest of the series.

The **second metatarsal** articulates with the intermediate cuneiform; but its base is grasped by the anterior parts of the medial and lateral cuneiform bones, with both of which it articulates, and with both of which it may be connected by interosseous ligaments. This metatarsal, therefore, possesses extremely little power of independent movement, a feature which makes it particularly liable to fracture when sudden stresses are applied to the distal part of the foot.

The **third metatarsal** articulates with the lateral cuneiform, against which the medial margin of the base of the fourth metatarsal also rests. The synovial membrane of the second and third joints is continuous with that of the joint between the medial two cuneiform bones, and through that with the synovial membrane of the cuneonavicular joint.

The bases of the **fourth** and **fifth metatarsal bones** articulate with the cuboid. The cavity of the joint is separate from the other tarso-metatarsal joints, and more movement is permitted than in the case of the third.

INTERMETATARSAL JOINTS

The bases of the lateral four metatarsal bones articulate with one another, and are very firmly bound together by dorsal, plantar and interosseous ligaments.

DISSECTION. To bring the interosseous ligaments into view, divide the dorsal ligaments and forcibly separate the bases of the bones from one another.

Joint Cavities of the Foot

There are six separate joint cavities included in the intertarsal, tarsometatarsal, and inter-metatarsal articulations as a whole :

1. Talocalcanean.
2. Talocalcaneonavicular.
3. Calcaneocuboid.
4. Cuneonavicular, with extensions.
5. Medial cuneometatarsal.
6. Cubometatarsal, with extension.

Note that the cuneonavicular joint is prolonged forwards between the cuneiforms,

and also between the cuboid and the lateral cuneiform; moreover, it extends beyond the tarsus and is continuous with the cavities that separate the bases of the second, third, and fourth metatarsal bones from the cuneiform bones and from one another.

The interosseous ligament which passes from the lateral cuneiform (frequently from the cuboid) to the fourth metatarsal bone separates this complex tarsal cavity from the cavity between the cuboid and the fourth and fifth metatarsals. That cavity is itself prolonged forwards between the bases of those two metatarsals.

DISSECTION. Remove the abductor, adductor, and flexor brevis of the big toe, detaching them from the first phalanx and separating them carefully from the sesamoid bones. Next divide the deep transverse metatarsal ligaments on each side of the second toe if that has not been done) and trace the tendons of the interosseous muscles of the first two spaces to their insertion into the extensor expansion. Raise the extensor tendons from the joints of the first and second (toes, separating them carefully from the synovial membranes. Then clean the ligaments on the sides and plantar surfaces of those joints.

METATARSOPHALANGEAL JOINTS

These joints are between the heads of the metatarsal bones and the bases of the proxi-mal phalanges. In extension the base of the phalanx articulates with the distal surface of the head of the metatarsal, and in flexion with its plantar surface.

The **fibrous capsule** surrounds the joint, and is attached to the bones near the margins of the articular surfaces. It is thickened at the sides to form the collateral ligaments; its plantar part is greatly thickened to form the plantar ligament; its dorsal part is formed by the extensor tendon, which is lined with the synovial membrane.

Each **collateral ligament** is a thick, triangular band whose apex is attached to the pit and tubercle on the side of the head of the meta-tarsal bone. From that attachment its fibres radiate to the side of the base of the phalanx and to the margin of the plantar ligament.

The **plantar ligament** is a thick, dense, fibrous

248

plate. It forms part of the socket for the head of the metatarsal bone and articulates with the plantar surface of the head when the toes are straight. It is attached firmly to the base of the phalanx, and loosely to the neck of the metatarsal bone, and moves with the phalanx. Its margins give attachment to the fibrous flexor sheath, to the slips of the plantar aponeurosis, and to the deep transverse metatarsal ligaments. As part of the tunnel for the flexor tendons its plantar surface is concave from side to side, and is lined with the synovial flexor sheath.

The plantar ligament of the first metatarsophalangeal joint is almost all replaced by the **sesamoid bones** in the two tendons of the flexor hallucis brevis, which groove the plantar surface of the head of the metatarsal bone. Minute sesamoid nodules are developed occasionally in the plantar ligaments of some of the other joints. The first metatarsophalangeal joint is much the largest, owing to the size of the bones and the presence of the sesamoids.

DISSECTION. Pull the extensor tendons out of the way; divide the synovial membrane on the dorsum of the joint and the collateral ligaments at the sides. Flex the toe; examine the attachments of the plantar ligament, and note the sesamoid bones that replace it in the joint of the big toe.

Movements

The metatarsophalangeal joints are condyloid joints and therefore permit flexion, extension, abduction, adduction, and circumduction, but not rotation. Flexion and extension are brought about by the long and the short flexors and extensors, the flexors being aided by the interossei and the lumbricals. Abduction and adduction take place from and to the middle line of the second toe and are carried out by the interossei [p. 224], the abductor of the little toe and the special abductor and adductor of the big toe.

INTERPHALANGEAL JOINTS

These are constructed on the same plan as the metatarsophalangeal joints; but the movements are more restricted.

Movements

An interphalangeal joint is a simple hinge joint, permitting only flexion and extension; lateral movements are prevented by the pulley-shaped head of the proximal bone and the tightness of the collateral ligaments. In the lesser toes, at rest, the joints are, to a varying degree, in a state of partial flexion. The interphalangeal joint of the hallux is operated on by the long extensor and long flexor. The interossei and the lumbrical muscles aid the extensors in extending the joints of the other toes, and the interossei are the chief agents in extending the distal joints; the distal joint is flexed by the long flexor, and the proximal joint by the short flexor aided by the long flexor.

HALLUX VALGUS AND HAMMER TOE

The first metatarsophalangeal joint is often enlarged and deformed, with permanent lateral displacement of the big toe. This condition, known as hallux valgus, is more common in women than in men; dissectors should take any opportunity that presents itself in the dissecting-room to examine the relations of the parts in such cases.

Lateral displacement of the toe having begun, and the medial aspect of the capsule of the metatarsophalangeal joint having stretched, the extensors of the great toe lie at an angle to the phalanges and tend progressively to swing the toe further laterally. As a result the head of the first metatarsal becomes obvious on the medial side of the foot, and being subject to pressure, an adventitious bursa tends to form over it. This can become inflamed and produce a painful swelling or bunion.

The flexor tendons and the sesamoid bones are displaced laterally, and the head of the metatarsal and the sesamoids are often enlarged and irregular from osteo-arthritis.

In **hammer toe,** the toe (usually the second) is permanently dorsiflexed at the metatarsophalangeal joint, and the normal flexion at the interphalangeal joints is accentuated. Such a deformity may be due to weakness of the lumbrical muscles which flex the metatarsophalangeal and extend the interphalangeal joints.

INDEX

This index contains references to figures illustrating the bones of the limbs. These have been introduced so that the student may rapidly identify any bony structure mentioned in the text even when he does not have the dried bones to hand. The entries in the index refer to the page on which the illustration appears and they are marked with an asterisk thus : Olecranon, 43, 89*, 111*. Bold figures indicate main references or descriptions, *e.g.*, Ankle, joint, **235**.